KU-556-705

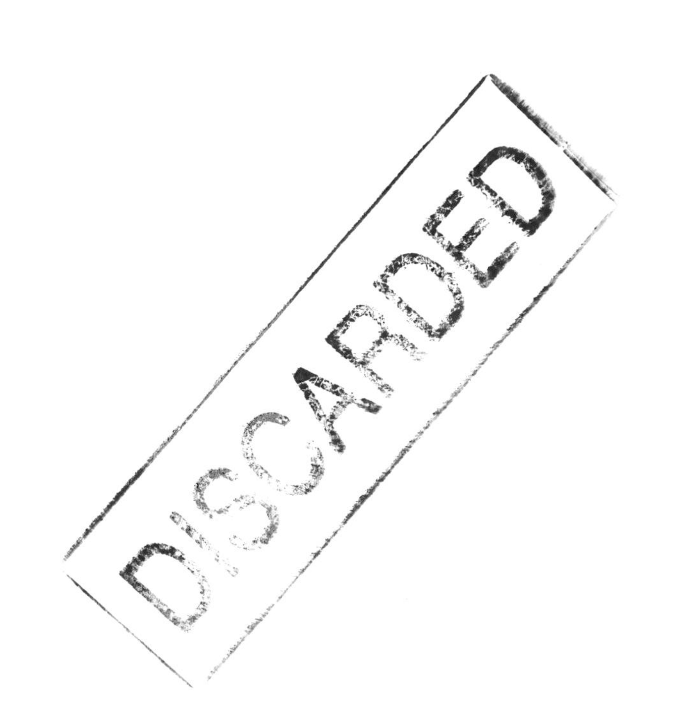
DISCARDED

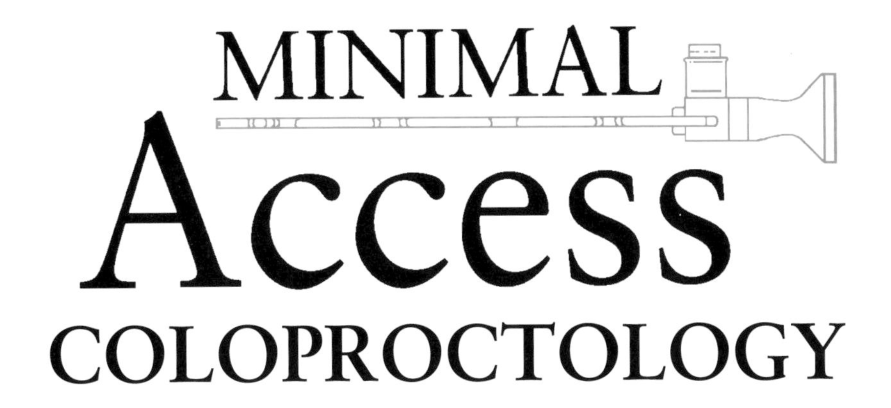

Edited by

Maurice E Arregui

Director of Fellowship in Laparoscopy, Endoscopy and Ultrasound, St Vincent Hospital and Health Care Center, Indianapolis, Indiana, USA

and

Jonathan M Sackier

Associate Professor of Surgery, University of California, San Diego, California, USA

Foreword by Marvin L Corman, MD

Sansum Medical Clinic, Santa Barbara, California, USA

Series Editor: R David Rosin, Consultant Surgeon, St Mary's Hospital, London

RADCLIFFE MEDICAL PRESS, OXFORD AND NEW YORK

Radcliffe Medical Press Ltd
18 Marcham Road, Abingdon, Oxon, OX14 1AA, UK

Radcliffe Medical Press, Inc
141 Fifth Avenue, New York, NY 10010, USA

British Library Cataloguing in Publication Data

A catalogue record for this book is available from the British Library.

ISBN 1 870905 68 7

Library of Congress Cataloguing-in-Publication Data is available

Typeset by AMA Graphics Ltd, Preston
Printed and bound in Spain

Contents

List of Contributors

Mark B Anderson, University of California San Diego, San Diego, California, USA

Robert W Beart Jr, University of Southern California Healthcare Consultation Center, Los Angeles, California, USA

Michael Bouvet, UCSD Medical Center, San Diego, California, USA

Armin Brueggemann, Staedtische Kliniken Kassel, Kassel, Germany

Douglas A Dorsay, University of South Carolina School of Medicine, Columbia, South Carolina, USA

L Peter Fielding, St Mary's Hospital, Waterbury, Connecticut, USA

Kenneth A Forde, College of Physicians and Surgeons of Columbia University, New York, New York, USA

Morris E Franklin, Texas Endosurgery Institute, San Antonio, Texas, USA

Ricardo Goes, University of Southern California Healthcare Consultation Center, Los Angeles, California, USA

Philip H Gordon, McGill University Teaching Hospital, Montreal, Quebec, Canada

Frederick L Greene, University of South Carolina School of Medicine, Columbia, South Carolina, USA

John G Hunter, Emory University School of Medicine, Atlanta, Georgia, USA

Joseph C Iraci, Park City Hospital, Bridgeport, Connecticut, USA

Moises Jacobs, University of Miami School of Medicine, Miami, Florida, USA

Jean-Michel Loubeau, Lenox Hill Hospital, New York, USA

Robert F Nagan, St Vincent Hospital and Health Care Center, Indianapolis, Indiana, USA

Santhat Nivatvongs, Mayo Medical School, Rochester, Minnesota, USA

Margret Oddsdottir, Emory University School of Medicine, Atlanta, Georgia, USA

Gustavo Plasencia, University of Miami School of Medicine, Miami, Florida, USA

Jonathan M Sackier, UCSD Medical Center, San Diego, California, USA

Lee Smith, George Washington University Medical Center, Washington DC, USA

Felicien M Steichen, Institute for Minimally Invasive Surgery, St Agnes Hospital, White Plains, New York, USA

Roger Welter, Princess Marie-Astrid Hospital, Differdange, Luxembourg

Foreword

It is always a special privilege to be asked to write a commentary for a colleague's book. *Minimal Access Coloproctology* is a new concept of a text which is directed not only to that of minimal access surgery (ie laparoscopy), but also to that of minimal access procedures for anorectal problems that do not involve the use of the laparoscope. Dr Gordon comments in his chapter that procedures such as hemorrhoidectomy and operations for anal fistula and incontinence, among others, do indeed fall into the category of being minimally invasive. Therefore, the ambulatory management of anorectal problems is included within these pages.

The most exciting advances in the field of general surgery and, specifically, colon and rectal surgery, have been realized with the advent of laparoscopically-assisted colon surgery. It seems that with every issue of surgical journals, there are different, innovative approaches to the management of what hitherto had been traditional, standard surgical techniques. Arregui and Sackier have gathered a group of luminaries and pioneers to advise us. Have laparoscopic procedures facilitated or hindered us in the management of appendicitis, rectal prolapse, volvulus and colorectal malignancies? Are laparoscopic partial colectomy, abdominoperineal resection, total colectomy and the complex and sophisticated stapling and suture techniques abominations or beneficences? The various contributors attempt to answer the question 'Is laparoscopic-assisted colectomy a major advance in technology or is it technology in search of an application?'

A unique value to this monograph is the often introduced philosophical commentary concerning the appropriateness of this new technology to the field of colon and rectal surgery.

Dr Fielding addresses existential considerations, including ethical issues, training and credentialing and the importance of standards, such as the establishment of a laparoscopy registry. Along these lines, the American College of Surgeons is developing guidelines for evaluating individuals for the purpose of awarding surgical privileges in new technologies. Obviously, the final step in the process will be to establish the value of the new technology in an individual's practice.

At this time of controversy, concern and excitement in the field of general and colon and rectal surgery, Arregui and Sackier's book is a welcome addition, especially so, since it presents such a critical objective review of many of these issues.

Marvin L Corman, MD
Sansum Medical Clinic
January 1995

Preface

This volume is one in a series of books on minimal access surgery. It is testimony to the philosophy that a few short years ago, there were no books to be found on this subject, and now a series is warranted. The academic activity surrounding these less invasive procedures has been an impressive sight to behold! National societies have grown, such as the Society of American Gastrointestinal Endoscopic Surgeons (SAGES); or have been formed, such as the European Association of Endoscopic Surgery (EAES), Endoscopic and Laparoscopic Surgeons of Asia (ELSA) and, indeed, an International Federation of Surgical Endoscopic Societies (IFSES). Meetings are held, world congresses are organized, journals circulated, and the Mayo stand in the operating room is forever replete with new and enticing tools of our trade.

Whilst it is easy to be swept away with enthusiasm for minimal access surgery, the surgeon is well advised to use a degree of objective cynicism when evaluating the benefit of new techniques and an equal measure of self-deprecation and humility before incorporating them into his or her armamentarium. Not all diseases are best treated by the minimally invasive route and not all surgeons are meant to be endoscopic surgeons. Only with the use of such restraint will we avoid damaging the good name of our profession and injuring our patients.

It is salutatory to remember that although laparoscopy was introduced at the turn of the century and had a number of proponents in the early 1900s, it was not until the widespread acceptance of laparoscopic cholecystectomy in the 1980s that the way opened for the innovative surgeon, armed with trocar and laparoscope, to attempt new feats. Disorders of the colon, anus and rectum are the grist to the mill for today's surgeons, and it was inevitable that the lure of the laparoscope would be too compelling for the colorectal or interested general surgeon.

In this book we have gathered some of the leading experts in the world on these subjects, who are renowned not only for their depth of knowledge, but for their honesty, integrity and the critical lights with which they illuminate their subject. Prior to the fervor of laparoscopic approaches, many of these surgeons were practicing minimally invasive approaches, including endoscopic polypectomies, sclerotherapy, rubber band ligation of hemorrhoids, transanal endoscopic microsurgery, etc.

This textbook begins with the history of colorectal surgery, which reminds us that any changes in the generally accepted norm of practice are often met with resistance and controversy. In the subsequent chapters colonoscopy, less invasive rectal surgery, transanal endoscopic surgery and laparoscopic appendectomy are described, followed by the new, developing techniques in minimally invasive approaches to the staging of colorectal cancer, including intraoperative radioimmuno-localization with monoclonal antibodies to colorectal tumor antigens, and laparoscopic ultrasound. The techniques of laparoscopic staging of colorectal malignancies will most likely be a requisite for laparoscopic approaches to these cancers. Several chapters present the exciting new laparoscopic approaches to colectomy as well as an in-depth discussion of the necessary tools. The final chapter probes critically the philosophical considerations for laparoscopic coloproctology.

We hope the reader will enjoy *Minimal Access Coloproctology*. We, as editors, have been stimulated by the task of preparing this tome and truly believe that the adage of the laparoscopic surgeon is the byword for the future of medicine – less is more!

Maurice E Arregui, MD, FACS
Jonathan M Sackier, MD, FRCS
January 1995

Acknowledgements

I dedicate this book to my parents, Alvina and Efrain, who set the stage for my academic development.

MEA

I would like to dedicate this book to my family for all their support and encouragement.

JMS

1

History and Principles of Colonic and Rectal Surgery

ROBERT F NAGAN

Written surgical history dates back to at least 4000 BC. Records dating back to the ancient civilizations of Babylon, Assyia and Egypt list surgical techniques not only for wound care and injuries but also for dislocations, fractures and tumors. Trephinations seems to have been done as early as the New Stone Age; they were also done in the Neolithic period in many parts of Europe, and by primitive tribes in both North and South America. Amputations were represented in cave paintings in prehistoric times in Europe. Circumcision probably originated in Ancient Egypt, and carvings from the Stone Age suggest that this operation was also done then. If so, this represents the earliest record of any operation. However, real advances in surgery were prevented by the lack of knowledge about anatomy and body function, along with the complete lack of understanding of infection, the limiting influence of supernatural ideas about disease, and of course the inability to achieve more than minimal pain relief.

More knowledge of disease, anatomy, blood circulation, sepsis and anesthesia had to develop before surgery could really advance. Even then, surgical procedures for colonic problems did not really start until well into the 18th century.

The only exception to this was in the treatment of rectal fistulas. In about 420 BC, Hippocrates recognized and treated rectal fistulas in largely the same way as often employed today. He twisted a folded strand, perhaps of linen and horse hair, and inserted it into the fistula while his left index finger was in the rectum. This hand-made ligature was then tied and tightened each day until it cut completely through. He even recognized the importance of not letting it heal too quickly! The first to recommend the introduction of a sound into the fistula and then pulling it out of the anus and cutting down on the tract was Paul of Agena (Greco-Roman School) a thousand years later in AD 600. He also described complicated fistulas.

John of Arderne's writings in the early 14th century are considered landmarks in the history of rectal surgery. His treatment by ligation and knife was similar to that of Hippocrates and Paul of Aegina. He also devised special instruments and advised against the use of corrosive agents.

Heister of Helmstedt, in his published *General System of Surgery*, advised injecting the tract(s) with milk in order to open and drain them completely.

Hippocrates accurately described hemorrhoids. His treatment included the application of hot irons and dilation. Four hundred years later Celsus was the first to use needle and thread in the treatment of hemorrhoids.

No additional advances in rectal surgery were really made until the advent of anesthesia and sepsis. Alligham's textbook in 1895[1] listed 13 different methods of the treatment of hemorrhoids including the Whitehead operation which has now been abandoned.

Historical records show that primitive tribesmen found (probably by accident) that stabbing the distended abdomen of an animal frequently relieved its pain. There is also an ancient text that reports that Praxagorus in 400 BC actually opened the abdomen and incised the bowel to treat distension, but the patient probably did not survive. There are many other records of fecal drainage following traumatic wounds with only a few survivors.

The first planned cecostomy was probably done by Alexis Littre in France in 1710. He proposed and succeeded in bringing a part of the colon to the abdominal wall where it could act as an anus. In 1776, Pillore[2] found a hard tumor in the rectum, made a transverse incision and created a colostomy. The patient died 20 days later, but the obstruction had partially cleared. This may have been the first use of a transverse incision.

In 1783 DuBoise performed a colostotomy in a child with imperforate anus. The patient died 10 days later. Duret[3] performed a left iliac colostomy some 15 years later. This is the first report of a modern-type colostomy, and was also done for a case of imperforate anus.

Colostomy for cancer of the rectum was first performed by Amussat[4] in France in 1839. He advocated colostomy as a routine measure for obstruction due to cancer. He was a great anatomist and contributed a great deal to the advancement of both right and left-sided colostomies for obstruction. He said that an 'artificial anus is a grave infirmity but it is not insupportable'. Of the 29 cases reviewed by Amussat, only four survived. A pupil of Amussat, John Erickson, introduced his operation in England around 1841.

In 1865 the Englishman Nathanial Ward urged physicians perform lumbar colostomy in all cases as soon as rectal cancer was recognized, not just in those who were obstructed.

J F Reybard in 1844 reported a successful case of resection of a part of the sigmoid colon for ca. Bilroth also performed a colon resection in 1879 and added a colostomy. There were only 10 cases of colon resection reported by 1880.

Ether (introduced in 1846) and chloroform (in 1847) made it possible to undertake more abdominal surgery, but the mortality rate made the risks of the procedure prohibitively high. In the words of Sir James Simpson: 'A man laid on an operating table in one of our hospitals is exposed to more chances of death than was the English soldier on the field of Waterloo.' Even the first ovariotomies had a mortality rate of over 30%.

Even after Lister had published his first results in 1867, using his antiseptic system, his principles were accepted only slowly and sporadically.

In 1884, W H Heineke[5] described a multiple-stage operation in which the loop containing the tumor was exteriorized before removal. Later a spur crushing clamp was used to create a single opening which could be closed later.

Maydl[6] advocated delayed opening of the bowel to allow adhesions to develop, and D Colley further suggested even leaving the tumor loop intact for several days.

In 1885 Weir[7] reported resection of the colon for ca and bringing just the proximal end out as a colostomy. Mikulicz-Radecki's obstructive resection technique was not reported until 1902[8], 12 years after Block of Copenhagen had performed a similar operation.

A few immediate reconstructions were also being reported, but the mortality rate was often over 50%. Mickulicz-Radecki[8] reported 16 cases with only 12.5% mortality using his technique.

The Murphy button for anastomosis was introduced in 1892[9]. Mayo reported 14 cases using the Murphy button with the loss of only two patients[10]. Durham's report on the button in the *Annals of Surgery* in 1894 showed less success, but the Murphy button and a vegetable plate version were used quite extensively until 1911.

During World War II exteriorizations and colostomies were frequently the procedures considered most advisable for intestinal wounds. In the postwar years, the use of intestinal and systemic sulfonamids, streptomycin, tetracycline and neomycin made it possible to perform more and more extensive colonic resections with immediate anastomosis. Developments in anesthesia, our greater understanding of nutrition, fluid and electrolytes, and the improvements in transfusions, all helped to make the advances possible.

Foget, Lisfranc, Verneuil and others had performed quite limited, extraperitoneal excisions of the rectum. The more adequate excision known as the abdominal–perineal operation was probably at least partially described by Von Volkman in 1887, but Czerny actually performed this type of removal in 1883. He had attempted to do just local removal of the rectum, but the lesion was higher than he thought so he opened the abdomen and removed the rectosigmoid area. His patient did not survive.

Lockhart-Mummery succeeded in developing a technique in which he did a preliminary loop colostomy and then later did a perineal resection of the rectum. His operation was not satisfactory for high rectal or low sigmoid lesions, and it did not remove the regional nodes. The collective experience at St Mark's Hospital using his technique from 1910 to 1931 on 370 cases showed a morality rate of 11.6% and five-year survival of 40%.

In 1908 Ernest Miles published his method which included a wide and total excision of the sigmoid colon, mesentery and nodes, the entire rectum including the anal canal, sphincter and parts of the levators. The Miles operation or slight modifications of it is the most commonly accepted operation for rectal cancer in USA and Europe.

Kraske's operation, which preserves the anus and sphincter, had too much morbidity and never became very popular. Another version, the Bacon–Babrock–Block operation too often resulted in incontinence. It did not become popular. Other modifications such as the Turnbull–Cutail and Maunsell–Weir operation were also tried.

Hartman's (1923) method was developed because of the high morbidity and mortality associated with low anastomosis. He simply closed the rectal stump and established a colostomy. This method could be used entirely intraperitoneally and the rectum could be excised almost down to the anal ring.

Improvements in anesthesia, antibiotics and techniques began to make primary anastomosis possible. Wangeneteen (1943), Mayo[10], Dixon and others reported success with both high anterior resections (just above the peritoneal reflexion) and low anterior resections (below the peritoneal reflexion), but pointed out that it should not be done for large tumors and that it required meticulous dissection and anastomosis. The risk of anastomotic leakage and abscess remains greater than for other colon resections even in the best hands, and the overall long-term cure rate may be lower.

At the present time, the combined operation for rectal cancer remains the standard which other procedures must achieve. Decreased morbidity and mortality, and increased survival rates, can now only be improved by earlier diagnosis, and possibly by improvements in radiation and chemotherapy.

Today, as in the past, surgeons are trying to make an intelligent, honest choice about the best approach to colon surgery. Improvements in instruments and increasing experience with laparoscopic techniques have made it possible to do colonic resections. Valid statistics to demonstrate that this type of resection equals or is better than the open methods of treatment will not be available at least until the turn of the century.

References

1 Allingham H (1985) Cancer of colon removed in colotomy. *Br Med J*, **2**:963–6.

2 Pillore H (1776) *Brit For Med Chir Rev*, **18**:452.

3 Duret C (1798) *Récueil Pér Soc Méd Paris*, **4**:45.

4 Amussat JZ (1983) *Mémoire sur la Possibilité d'Etablir un Anus Artificiel dans le Région Lombaire sans Pénétrer le Peritoine*. Paris, Baillière.

5 Heineke WH (1884) *Compendium der chirurgischen Operations und Verbandlehre*, 3rd edn., Erlangen, E Besold.

6 Maydl K (1886) Zur Technik der Kolotomie. *Zbl Chir*, **15**:433–9.

7 Weir R (1885) Resection of the large intestine for carcinoma. *Ann Surg*, **3**:469–89.

8 Mikulicz-Radecki J von (1902) Chirurgischen Erfahrunger über das Darmacarzinom. *Arch Klin Chir*, **69**:28.

9 Murphy JB (1892) Cholecysto-intestinal, gastrointestinal, entero-intestinal Anastomosis and Approximation without Sutures. *Chicago Med Rec*, **3**:803–40.

10 Mayo CH (1895) Gastroenterostomy by means of the Murphy button with table of late cases of anastomosis by this method. *Ann Surg*, **21**:41–4.

2

Colonoscopy for the Management of Benign Colorectal Conditions

KENNETH A FORDE

Introduction

The colonoscopic management of benign and malignant neoplastic polyps is addressed in Chapter x, and the management of colonic volvulus is dealt with in Chapter 8. This chapter will be devoted to the other benign conditions.

Non-neoplastic polyps

Hyperplastic polyps

Hyperplastic polyps are the most common colonic polyps encountered endoscopically, especially in the rectum. Usually pale pink in color and sessile in shape, they tend to be small and to have no demonstrable malignant potential. Unless biopsied, however, it may not be possible to differentiate them from tiny adenomas. In fact, some tiny polyps contain both adenomatous and hyperplastic epithelium[1]. Since these would be expected to have the same propensity for malignant change as adenomas, it is important to recognize and remove them. On the other hand, not every tiny mucosal excrescence needs to be removed at the time of colonoscopy, especially if the patient is going to be followed up regularly. When we encounter these tiny polyps, especially above the rectum, in a young patient or one who would not ordinarily be followed, it is our practice to sample them in case adenomatous tissue is demonstrable. It is still debatable whether patients with hyperplastic polyps should ungergo total colonoscopy. There is some evidence to suggest that individuals with hyperplastic polyps above the rectosigmoid colon are more likely to have adenomatous polyps, but this has been challenged[2–4].

Inflammatory polyps

Lymphoid hyperplasia

Lymphoid hyperplasia appears as tiny nodular mucosal elevations which are biopsied only to exclude minute adenomas from which they are not always grossly distinguishable.

Fibrous polyps

These are encountered in the anal canal and represent old internal haemorrhoids. They need only symptomatic treatment.

Juvenile polyps

Juvenile polyps occur most commonly in children. Grossly they may mimic adenomas and are commonly multiple. In a small percentage of patients they are associated with adenomas and carcinoma. Polyps of mixed juvenile and adenomatous histology are occasionally encountered and are treated like adenomatous polyps. Solitary juvenile polyps are usually removed if associated with bleeding, prolapse (per anum) or intussusception or, in the older child, to rule out adenomatous histology. In younger children they have been known to disappear, presumably through auto-amputation.

Inflammatory pseudopolyps

These represent islands of exuberant granulation tissue and are usually encountered in patients with inflammatory bowel disease. They have no malignant potential. They may persist even when the disease is in remission, and they occur singly or in clusters. They tend to be friable, often capped with ulceration and exudate. Rarely, they may be of mixed histology, usually adenomatous and inflammatory. 'Giant pseudopolyposis' refers to large masses of pseudopolyp formation which may mimic villous adenoma or carcinoma and which has occasionally been demonstrably the cause of colonic obstruction[5].

Inflammatory bowel disease

Most patients with inflammatory bowel disease can be managed without colonoscopy. However, flexible endoscopy has a role in specific aspects of their diagnosis and therapy.

Differential diagnosis

Especially in the absence of rectosigmoid involvement, it may be difficult to distinguish between ulcerative colitis and Crohn's disease. Other inflammatory conditions (infectious, ischemic, antibiotic-related) may have endoscopic appearances similar to these two conditions. The endoscopic appearance, even with biopsy, may often not be pathognomonic.

	Ulcerative colitis	Crohn's colitis
Early	Edema Erythema Vascular pattern lost	Aphthous ulcers Normal vascular pattern
Moderate	Granularity Friability	Linear ulcers Cobblestoning
Late	Discrete ulcers Pus	Confluent linear ulcers Friability
General	Rectum usually involved In-continuity involvement	+– rectal involvement Skip areas

Table 2.1: Endoscopic features of ulcerative colitis and Crohn's colitis.

However, there are differential features which help in endoscopic diagnosis (Table 2.1). Radiologic abnormalities in patients with long-standing inflammatory bowel disease may raise the possibility of malignancy either through protrusion into the lumen or through stricture. For the former, endoscopic visualization with or without biopsy may settle the issue (Figure 2.1). Strictures are more difficult to evaluate in that it may not be possible to visualize mucosa in or above the stricture (Figure 2.2). However, if no mucosal lesion is seen and biopsy does not retrieve neoplastic tissue, endoscopic cytology of the strictured area, if positive, may indicate the need for resection of a malignancy. In strictures that are demonstrably benign but symptomatic, there is only limited reported experience with endoscopic dilatation for those secondary to inflammatory bowel disease.

Postoperative radiography following resection for Crohn's disease may not be determinate when recurrent disease is suspected, for example, at a colocolic or ileocolic anastomosis. Endoscopic visualization and biopsy may establish the diagnosis. Stomas may also be conveniently examined with flexible endoscopes for evaluation of recurrent disease.

Colon cancer surveillance

Colon cancer surveillance for premalignancy in patients with long-standing universal ulcerative colitis (over 10–12 years) is now regularly undertaken. In Crohn's colitis and left-sided ulcerative colitis, although there is also increased susceptibility to colon cancer, surveillance guidelines are not well established. In surveillance programs, blind biopsies are taken at different levels in the colon and examined microscopically for evidence of dysplasia. Persistent dysplasia is usually accepted as a reason to advise colectomy. There are no firm guidelines on when this surveillance should be initiated and how often it should be undertaken[6].

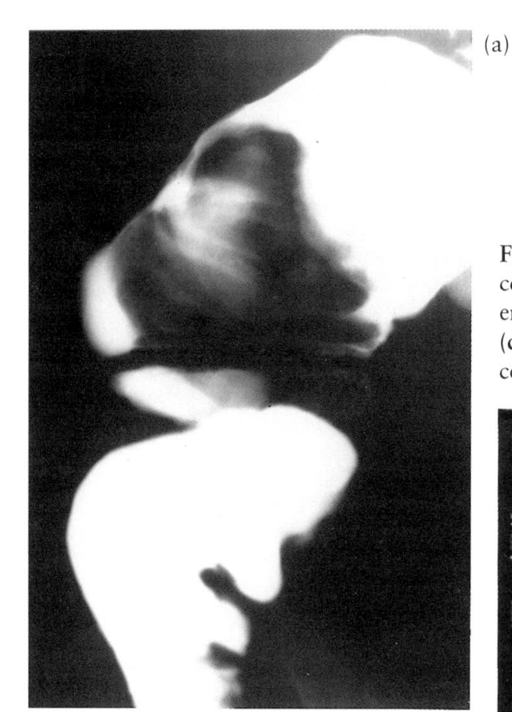

(a)

Figure 2.1: Patient with long-standing ulcerative colitis; (**a**) Ascending colon filling defect on barium enema; (**b**) Friable polypoid lesion at colonoscopy; (**c**) Resected specimen—carcinoma and ulcerative colitis.

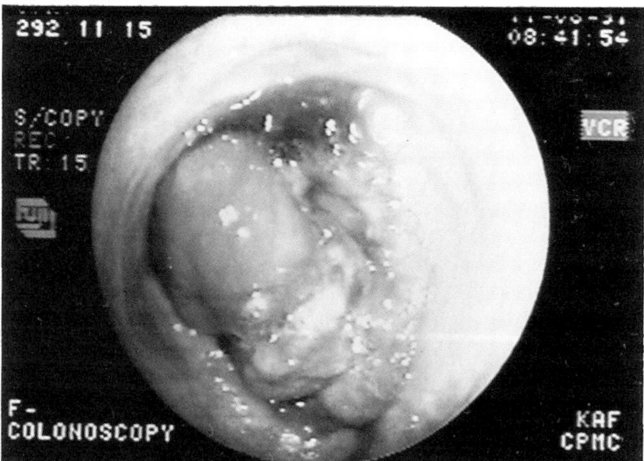

(b)

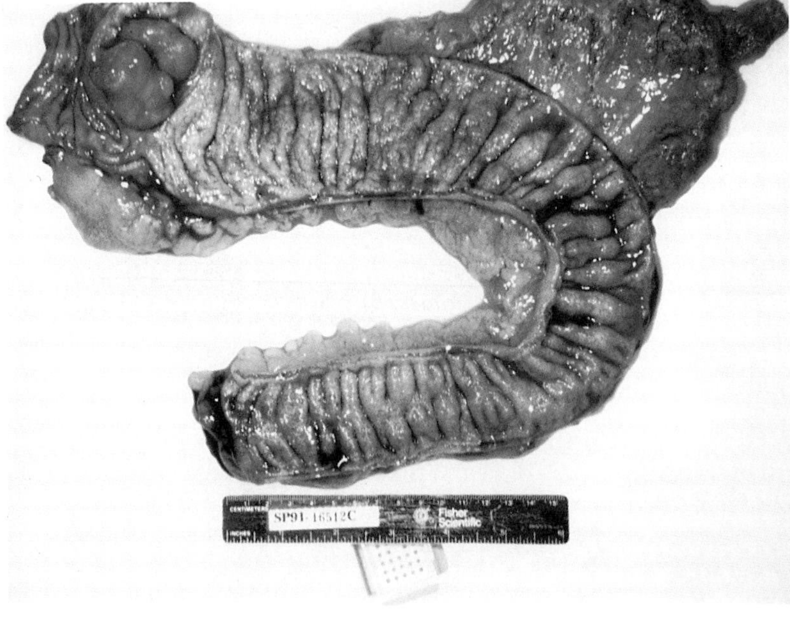

(c)

(a)

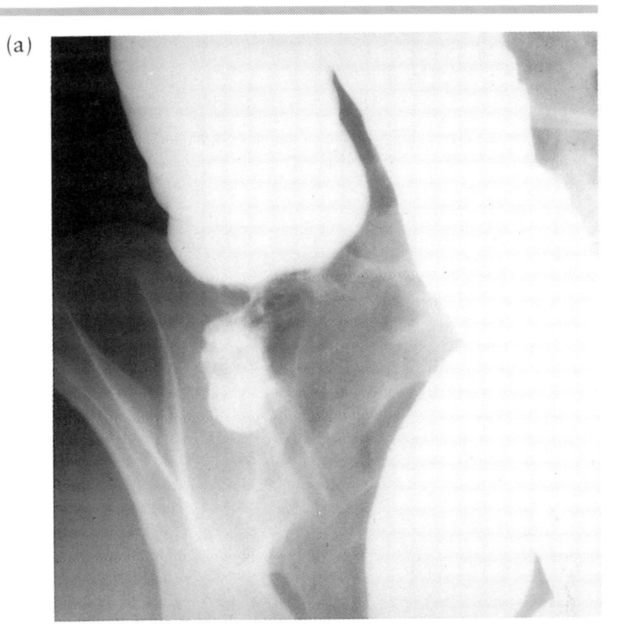

(b)

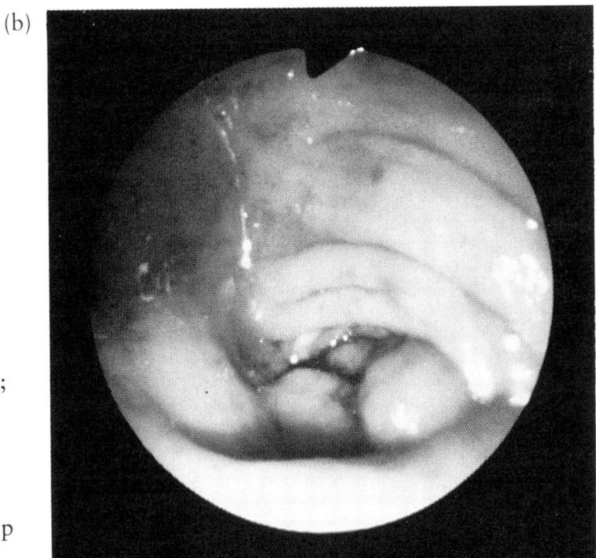

Figure 2.2: Patient with long-standing Crohn's disease; (**a**) Ascending colon stricture on barium enema; (**b**) Colonoscopy: inactive inflammatory bowel disease with stricture and pseudopolyp formation.

Diverticular disease

The evaluation of lower gastrointestinal symptoms (bleeding, change in bowel habits and lower abdominal pain), especially in patients over 40 years of age, frequently necessitates barium enema examination. It is often difficult for radiologists to exclude coexisting polyps or cancer (Figure 2.3) because of problems related to inadequate bowel cleansing, redundant bowel and spasticity in segments involved with extensive diverticulosis. Flexible colonoscopy has been of great value in resolving many of these problems[7]. Like the radiologist,

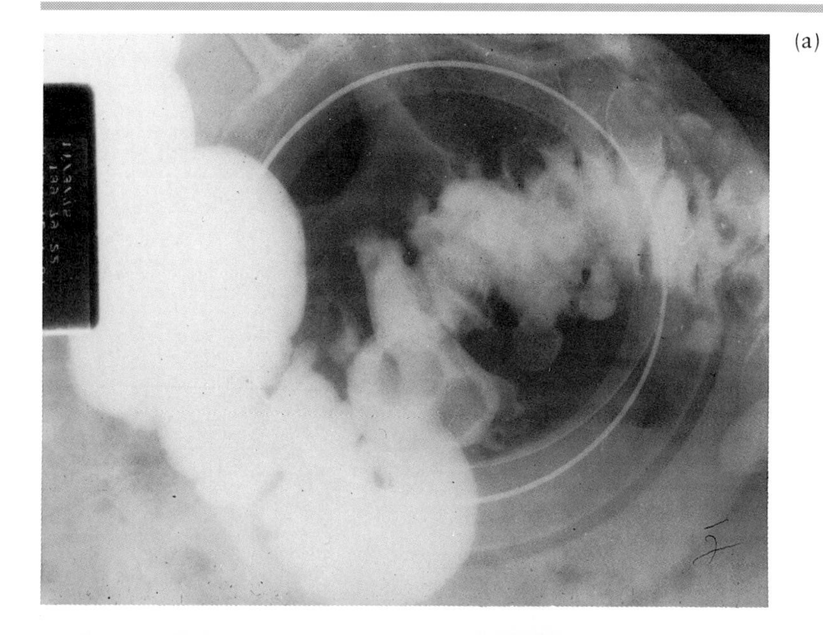

(a)

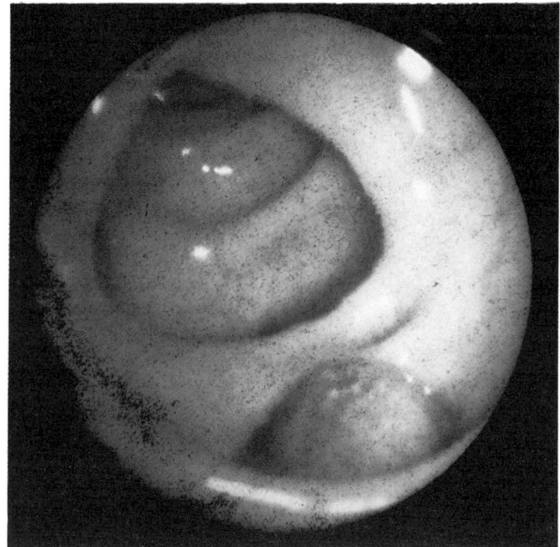

(b)

Figure 2.3: (**a**) Barium enema: diverticulosis with/without carcinoma/polyps; (**b**) Colonoscopy: diverticulosis with inspissated stool.

the endoscopist often finds it more exacting to examine patients with extensive diverticulosis than those with other disease states. The extent of diverticulosis on radiological study does not predict how easy or difficult the endoscopic examination will be.

Patients with acute diverticulitis that is recognized are usually not examined endoscopically for fear of damaging the inflamed bowel. While most patients with acute diverticulitis who require operation usually undergo resection of the diseased bowel, even if anastomosis is not thought advisable, there are still a few patients who require proximal colostomy and left lower quadrant drainage leaving the process in situ. At celiotomy and even on subsequent barium study it may be difficult to tell whether such a process is inflammatory, neoplastic or both. While carcinoma would demand earlier surgical intervention, in diverticulitis it is preferable to allow resolution of the inflammatory reaction before undertaking further surgical intervention. Interim colonoscopy in this situation is frequently helpful in establishing whether or not neoplasm is present, even when barium enema and rigid sigmoidoscopy are inconclusive.

Chronic diverticulitis

A bout of acute diverticulitis may result in marked narrowing of the colonic lumen as the episode resolves. Barium enema may be inconclusive and endoscopic inspection may be definitive in ruling out co-existent neoplasm. Direct brush cytology obtained from a strictured segment is helpful, if positive, even when the colonoscope cannot be passed through the narrowed area (Figure 2.4).

Chronic bleeding

Chronic bleeding from diverticulosis has traditionally been a diagnosis of exclusion. It has been well recorded in the literature that in the patient with chronic lower gastrointestinal bleeding in whom sigmoidoscopy has been negative and barium enema has revealed diverticulosis only, the addition of colonoscopy has been valuable in demonstrating other and important causes of gastrointestinal bleeding[8].

Acute bleeding

Acute bleeding from diverticulosis, usually self-limited, may on occasion be severe enough to be life-threatening (Figure 2.5). Much of the early literature assumed that significant lower gastrointestinal bleeding was caused by diverticulosis because the radiologic demonstration of diverticulosis was the only modality then available. It is now established that there are many causes of massive lower gastro-intestinal bleeding[9,10]. It is important to establish the specific etiology, if possible, in order to achieve optimal management. As will be discussed later in the section on colonic bleeding, emergency colonoscopy, while more difficult, has been performed successfully in patients who are bleeding acutely from diverticulosis.

Colonoscopy, therefore, can be a valuable part of the evaluation of patients with diverticular disease, and it is complimentary to the barium enema. Among its many advantages, it can:

- confirm or deny radiologic suspicion
- avert operative intervention
- discover other unsuspected but significant lesions
- localize sites of acute bleeding.

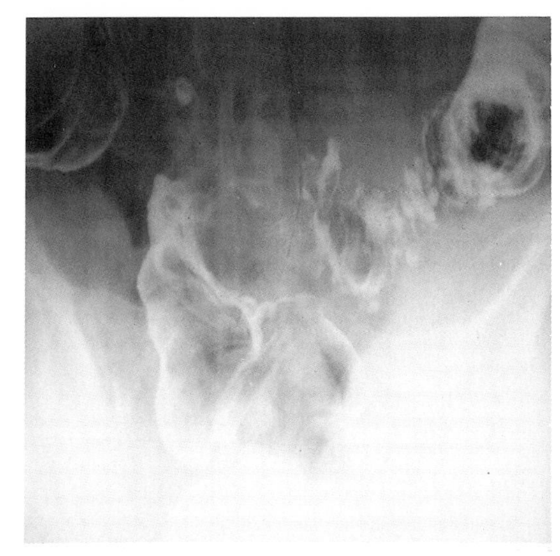

(a)

(b)

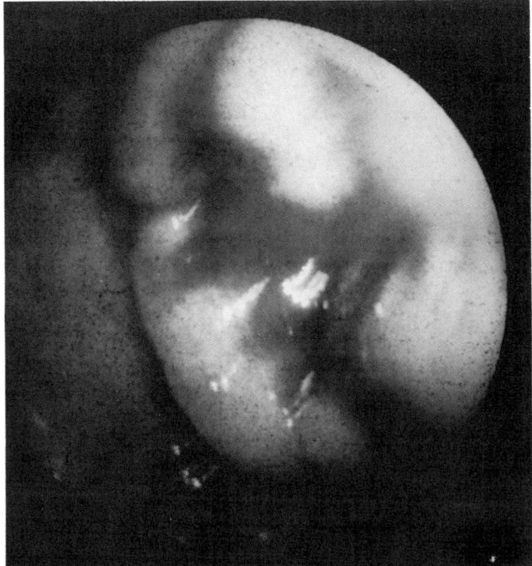

(c)

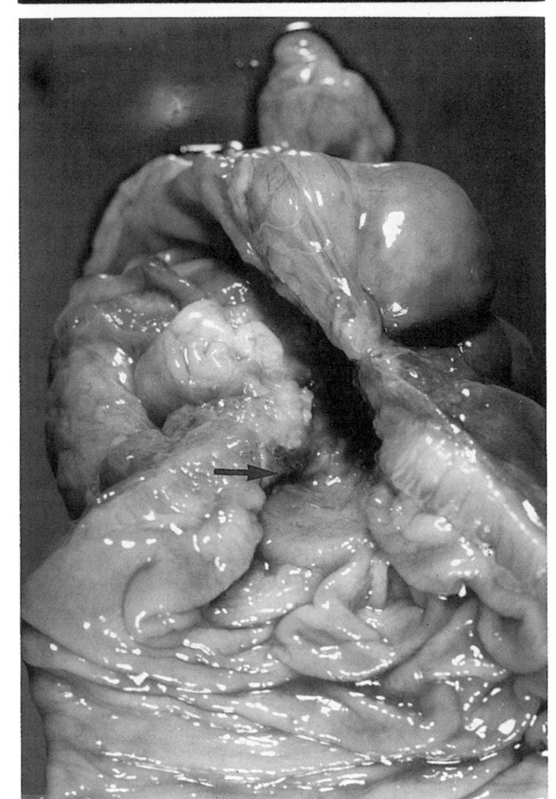

Figure 2.4: (**a**) Barium enema: diverticulosis and stricture; (**b**) Colonoscopy: stricture, biopsy negative cytology positive; (**c**) Resected specimen—carcinoma. Arrow indicates biopsy site.

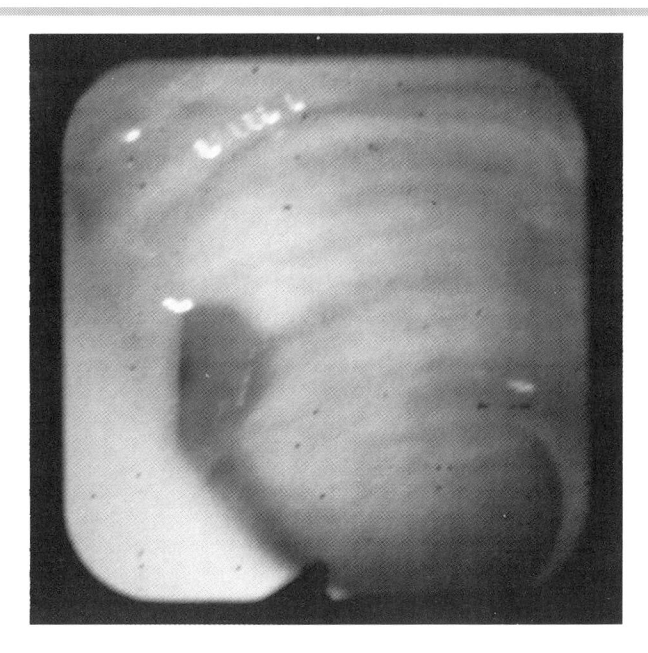

Figure 2.5: Endoscopic view of actively bleeding right colon diverticulum.

Ischemia

Ischemia of the colon may be evaluated colonoscopically under certain conditions. For example, loss of left colon blood supply as in aorto-iliac disease or with sacrifice of the inferior mesenteric artery during vascular reconstruction or at the time of aneurysmectomy, although uncommon, may pose a problem in diagnosis. Poor perfusion of the colon during periods of prolonged hypotension, as might occur during other procedures (for example in open heart surgery), may also result in clinically significant ischemia. Many of these patients are too ill or not sufficiently advanced in their postoperative course to permit radiologic study. Endoscopic examination is nevertheless possible in the recovery room or the intensive care unit to confirm or exclude the suspicion of ischemia. Serial examinations may be necessary in order to follow the evolution of the ischemic insult, as patterns consistent with the various phases of the ischemic process are recognizable endoscopically, ranging from mucosal pallor to submucosal hemorrhage or frank ulceration and necrosis. If the process is recognized as resolving, resection may be averted[11]

Radiation proctitis

Approximately 5–15% of patients who undergo irradiation with gastrointestinal tract in the radiation field will develop some form of enteritis or colitis, which may present as rectal bleeding. Men who have undergone radiation for prostatic or bladder cancer, and women who have undergone similar treatment for pelvic visceral malignancy, not infrequently experience rectal bleeding.

Although it is usually self-limiting and often temporally related to the radiation therapy, it may occur at distant periods, separated sometimes by intervals of several years. In this patient population the specific etiology of the rectal bleeding is important since the differential diagnosis includes recurrent tumor or other primary malignancy. Occasionally such bleeding is severe enough to produce symptomatic anemia and require transfusion. Endoscopic therapy using laser modalities (argon, KTP/532 or Nd:YAG) has been of value in at least the temporary control of bleeding in some of these patients (Figure 2.6)[12–14].

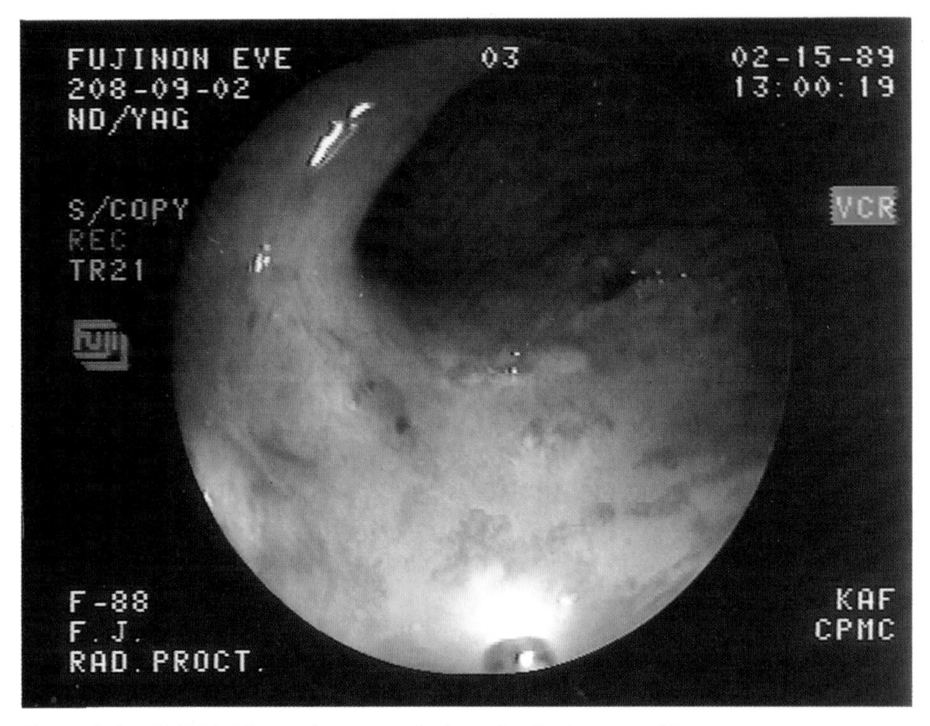

Figure 2.6: Nd:YAG laser photocoagulation of radiation proctitis.

Colonic bleeding

The role of colonoscopy in the diagnosis of lower gastrointestinal bleeding forms has now been well established and some of the problems encountered are increasingly amenable to endoscopic therapy as well. In the management of patients with suspected colonic bleeding there are three clinical situations in which colonoscopy may be of value.

Chronic or minor bleeding

If a lesion has been discovered at sigmoidoscopy and barium enema in a patient with non-active bleeding and this is deemed to require surgical intervention, there must still be concern about the co-existence of other potential sites of hemorrhage. Lesions such as angiodysplasia and some forms of ischemia cannot be identified on barium contrast study, and angiography may not be clinically indicated nor feasible. The additional diagnostic yield of colonoscopy has been well documented in the literature[15].

Recent major hemorrhage

When a patient has bled massively per anum (as judged by symptoms and low hematocrit) but is stable at the time of presentation, early colonoscopy is indicated after the patient has been stabilized and can tolerate the necessary mechanical preparation for the examination. Colonoscopy under such circumstances has been helpful in some patients through the early discovery of neoplasms which require endoscopic or open surgical management. However, in a patient who is no longer bleeding at the time of the examination, any lesion which is found is not necessarily the cause of the recent bleeding. Therefore its removal may not guarantee resolution of the problem.

In the patient who is actively bleeding, and in whom sigmoidoscopy, technetium scanning and selective angiography have not localized a source, colonoscopy may be helpful. In these actively bleeding patients, preparation is usually not feasible (because they are often in shock) nor necessary (since blood is such an excellent cathartic). However, in order to initiate the examination, it is often necessary to evacuate clots from the rectum with the use of irrigation. Many reports in the literature describing emergency colonoscopy for acute lower gastrointestinal bleeding[9], by indicating the type of mechanical preparation used, suggest that these examinations were performed urgently but not in emergency. We would place such examinations in the category of 'recent major hemorrhage'.

A variety of situations may be encountered when colonoscoping patients who are thought to be actively bleeding:

- an actively bleeding lesion
- a significant lesion such as a carcinoma which is not actively bleeding
- bright red blood covering a lesion without evidence of blood elsewhere
- fresh blood in one region with non-bloody contents proximally (indicating a proximal bleeding site)
- fresh blood throughout and a recognizable condition (for example, uremic colitis) for which there is no appropriate surgical therapy
- the cessation of active bleeding, leaving no clue as to the site of origin
- bowel or even more proximal site is suspected when fresh blood issuing from the ileocecal valve, raising suspicions of a small bowel or even more proximal site.

It is possible in over 75% of these patients to identify the specific site, or at least the region, of colonic bleeding[16]. If indicated, therefore, the surgeon may be correctly directed to either limited or extensive colonic resection or to avoiding colonic extirpation altogether. Perhaps the greatest benefit of emergency colonoscopy for bleeding is the clinical evaluation of the rate of hemorrhage. However, it is more difficult and carries a greater potential risk than elective diagnostic colonoscopy. It should therefore be undertaken only by individuals with significant experience and skill in routine colonoscopy.

Endoscopic therapy

Endoscopic therapy for benign lesions identified as the source of recent colonic bleeding is sometimes possible in the absence of active hemorrhage. Polyps may be removed by snare and cautery and areas of angiodysplasia ablated by one of several endoscopic modalities, ranging from monopolar cautery to bipolar and multipolar cautery, heater probe and laser[17]. KTP/532 and argon lasers are particularly suited to the ablation of angiodysplastic lesions (arteriovenous malformations and vascular ectasias) since the laser energy of these modalities is specifically absorbed by hemoglobin pigment (Figure 2.7). The delivery of hemostatic agents to an actively bleeding site has been reported but is not commonly available. In fact, except for immediately regrasping a bleeding polypectomy stalk or irrigating the site through the endoscope with ice saline or dilute epinephrine solution, colonoscopic therapy for acute bleeding is not yet commonly feasible.

Strictures

Colonic strictures, especially in asymptomatic patients, are most frequently diagnosed initially on barium study. Whether or not surgical intervention is indicated depends on the diagnosis and, in this regard, endoscopic evaluation

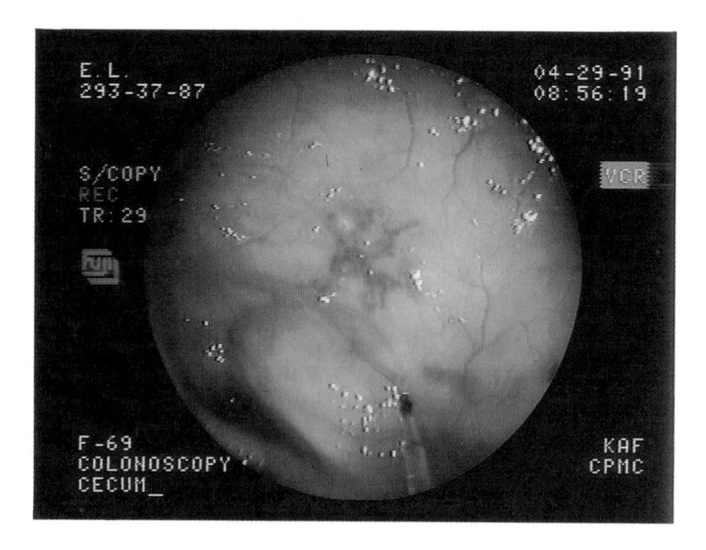

Figure 2.7: KTP/532 laser photocoagulation of cecal vascular ectasia.

is frequently helpful[18]. Strictures occur in a variety of benign conditions, including inflammatory bowel disease and diverticulitis which, in the absence of symptoms of obstruction, may not require operative intervention. The endoscopic examination of patients with strictures is often more challenging and potentially of greater risk unless the examiner takes certain precautions. For example, over-insufflation of the proximal bowel with resultant perforation is a hazard, as is bowel disruption at the point of narrowing from excessively forceful attempts to manipulate the involved segment which may also be fixed. If a stricture cannot be traversed with the colonoscope but one can see the bowel lumen beyond, endoscopy is still useful if a cytology brush (passed beyond the instrument tip through the area of stricture) can harvest malignant cells or tissue. 'Negative' cytology or biopsy does not rule out malignancy.

Selected forms of benign colonic stenosis may now be treated endoscopically, at times obviating the alternative of open surgical intervention. Anastomotic strictures which are symptomatic or which prevent total colonoscopy are in this category but, as in all strictures, it is important to rule out malignancy at the point of stricture. Several methods of endoscopic dilatation are available, and some authors have recommended different instruments (all passed endoscopically) for differing pathology. In our experience[19], dilatation with bougies or through-the-scope balloons are more useful for strictures secondary to inflammatory processes or from external compression (Figure 2.8, 2.9). Electrocautery and laser modalities, as cutting and ablating tools, are recommended for strictures resulting from neoplastic tissue and anastomotic webs.

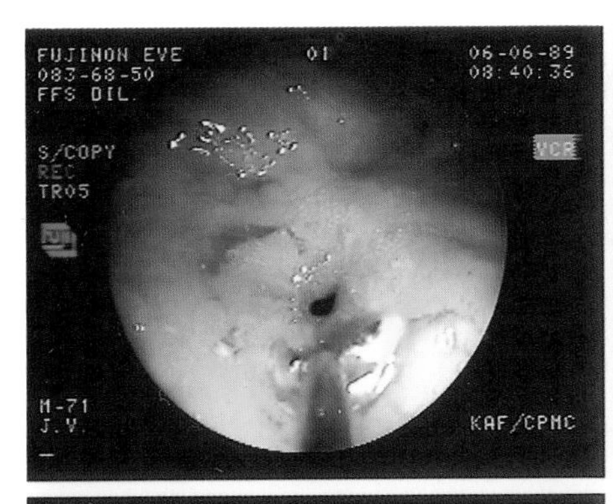

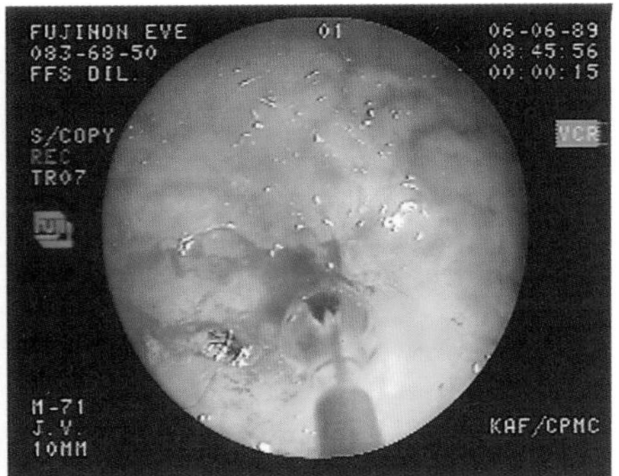

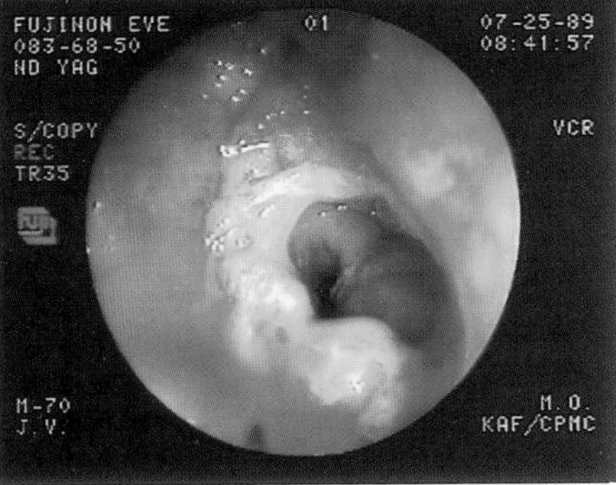

Figure 2.8: Endoscopic balloon dilatation of anastomotic top left stricture: strictured lumen, smaller than adjacent open (7 mm) biopsy forceps. Top right: through-the-scope balloon. Bottom left: dilatation—stricture dilated, proximal bowel now visible.

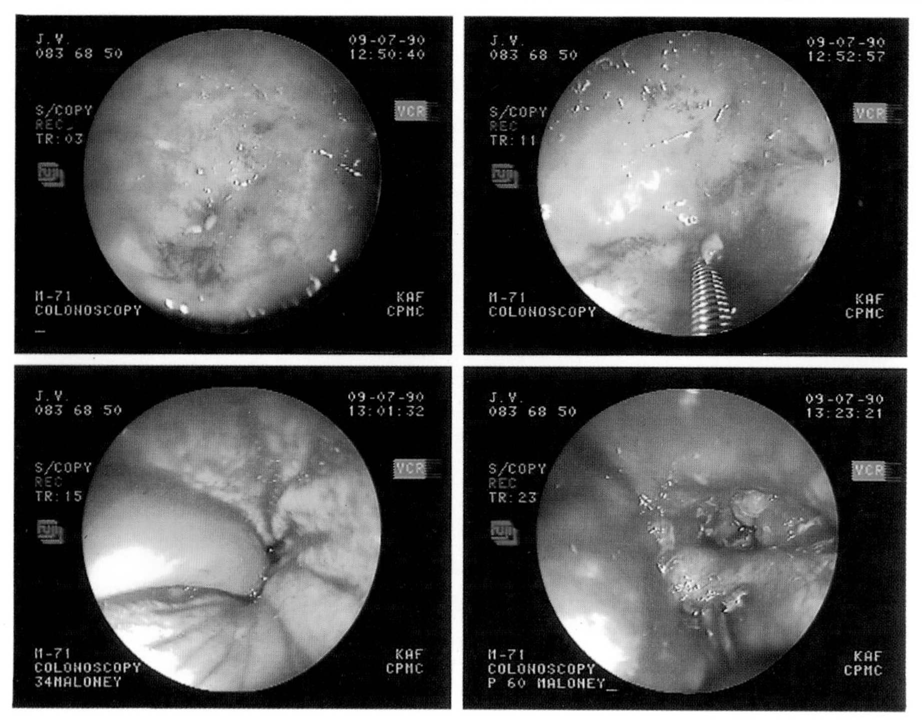

Figure 2.9: Bougie dilatation of anastomotic stricture with endoscopic guidance; Top left: lumen barely discernible in centre. Top right: closed biopsy forceps inserted into tiny lumen. Bottom left: Maloney dilator in stricture. Bottom right: partially dilated stricture, now approximately size of open biopsy forceps (7 mm).

Nonobstructive colonic ileus (Oglivie syndrome)

Colonoscopic decompression has emerged as the most effective means of managing this unusual disorder, and this has decreased the need for tube cecostomy[20]. The procedure may be performed at the bedside, if necessary. However, it is ideally conducted in the endoscopy suite or in an area with fluoroscopic capability so that, if feasible, a large bore catheter may be passed through the endoscope, placed in the proximal colon and left there for continuing decompression, since many of these patients require repeated sessions of decompression.

Foreign body extraction

Most foreign bodies in the colon lodge in the rectosigmoid, within reach of manual or rigid sigmoidoscopic retrieval instruments. Anesthesia, if used at all, may be local. However, foreign bodies may be encountered above this level, and their extraction is often possible using a variety of ingenious endoscopic techniques[21]. The polypectomy snare is the single most useful accessory, and it is advisable to use an overtube when sharp objects are to be extracted. If foreign bodies in the colon appear impacted, then manipulation should be discontinued for fear of causing perforation.

Conclusion

We have attempted to review the most common benign colorectal conditions currently amenable to endoscopic management. The list continues to expand as the technology improves, as public acceptance of minimal access surgery grows, and as more and more practitioners of 'endosurgery' become familiar with the techniques and exploit it with the limitless capacity of human imagination.

References

1 Forde KA (1989) Colonoscopic management of polypoid lesions. *Surg Clin Am.* **69**:1287–1308.

2 Church JM, Fazio VW and Jones IT (1988) Small colorectal polyps-are they worth treating? *Dis Colon Rectum*, **31**:50–3.

3 Provenzale D, Martin ZZ, Holland K L *et al.* (1988) Colon adenomas in patients with hyperplastic polyps. *J Clin Gastro.* **10**:46–9.

4 Cappell MS and Forde KA (1989) Spatial clustering of multiple hyperplastic, adenomatous and malignant colon polyps in individual patients. *Dis Colon Rectum*, **32**:641–52.

5 Forde KA, Gold RP and Weber C (1980) Giant pseudopolyposis and antegrade colonic obstruction: report of a case. *Dis Colon Rectum.* **23**:583–6.

6 Guidelines for Clinical application (1981) *The role of colonoscopy in patients with inflammatory bowel disease.* American Society for Gastrointestinal Endoscopy, PO Box 1565, Manchester, Mass.

7 Forde KA (1977) Colonoscopy in complicated diverticular disease. *Gastrointest Endosc*, **23**:192–3.

8 Guillem JG, Forde KA, Treat MR *et al.* (1987) The impact of colonoscopy on the early detection of colonic neoplasms in patients with rectal bleeding. *Ann Surg.* **206**:601–11.

9 Jensen DM and Machicado GA (1988) Diagnosis and treatment of severe hematochezia: the role of urgent colonoscopy after purge. *Gastroenterol.* **95**:1569–74.

10 Forde KA (1992) Lower gastrointestinal bleeding: the magnitude of the problem. In: Sugawa C, Schuman BM and Lucas C E (Eds) *Gastrointestinal bleeding.* Igaku-Shoin, New York. pp. 13–25.

11 Forde KA, Lebwohl O, Wolff M *et al.* (1979) Reversible ischemic colitis correlation of colonoscopic and pathologic changes. *Am J Gastroenterol.* **72**:182–5.

12 Berken CA (1985) Nd:YAG laser therapy for gastrointestinal bleeding due to radiation colitis. *Am J Gastroenterol.* **80**: 730.

13 Alexander TJ and Dwyer RM (1988) Endoscopic Nd:YAG laser treatment of severe radiation injury of the lower gastrointestinal tract: long-term follow-up. *Gastrointest Endosc.* **34**:407–11.

14 O'Connor JJ (1989) Argon laser treatment of radiation proctitis. *Arch Surg.* **124**:749.

15 Todd GJ and Forde KA (1979) Lower gastrointestinal bleeding with negative or inconclusive radiographic studies: the role of colonoscopy. *Am J Surg.* **138**:627–8.

16 Forde KA and Treat MR (1985) Colonoscopy for lower gastrointestinal bleeding. In: Dent TL, Strodel WE, Turcotte JG *et al.* (Eds) *Surgical endoscopy.* Year Book Medical Publishers, Chicago. p. 261.

17 Jensen DM and Machicado GA (1989) Endoscopic diagnosis and treatment of bleeding colonic angiomas and radiation telangiectasia. *Persp Colon Rectal Surg.* **2**:99.

18 Forde KA and Treat MR (1985) Colonoscopy in the evaluation of strictures. *Dis Colon Rectum.* **28**:699–701.

19 Oz MC and Forde KA (1990) Endoscopic alternatives in the management of colonic strictures. *Surgery.* **108**:513–19.

20 Strodel WE and Brothers T (1989) Colonoscopic decompression of pseudo-obstruction and volvulus. *Surg Clin N Am.* **69**:1327–35.

21 Viceconte G, Viceconte GW, Bogliolo G *et al.* (1982) Endoscopic removal of foreign bodies in the large bowel. *Endoscopy.* **14**:176.

3

Colonoscopy for the Management of Malignant Colorectal Conditions

MICHAEL BOUVET AND JONATHAN M SACKIER

Introduction

Each year there are approximately 156 000 new cases of colorectal cancer diagnosed in the USA[1]. There were an estimated 51 000 deaths from colon cancer and 7 300 from rectal cancer in 1992. Cancer of the colon and rectum is the third most common cause of cancer death in the USA.

Colorectal carcinoma is unique among cancer models because there is a well documented progression from a premalignant to malignant state, the polyp–to–cancer sequence, which occurs on the epithelial surface and is readily accessible to the endoscopist. Since its advent in 1969, colonoscopy has contributed to the better understanding of the pathogenesis, diagnosis and treatment of this disease.

The American College of Surgeons has taken the position that endoscopic training should be an integral part of the education of general surgeons. The American Board of Surgery requires that residents in general surgery training programs have performed a minimum number of endoscopic procedures by the end of their chief year. All gastroenterology fellows are trained in this technique. With the advent of minimal access surgery, endoscopy is becoming more important in the care of patients, especially those afflicted with malignant conditions of the colon and rectum. This chapter discusses the role of colonoscopy in the management of malignant colorectal conditions.

Historical aspects

In June 1969, the first flexible colonoscopic examination was performed by two surgeons, Wolff and Shinya[2], at the Beth Israel Medical Center in New York. Three months later, the first colonoscopic polypectomy was performed by these same surgeons. Before the advent of colonoscopy, surgeons had to rely on rigid sigmoidoscopy and barium enema to make diagnoses. Save for lesions that could be biopsied up to 20 cm with the rigid sigmoidoscope, patients had to undergo celiotomy with open polypectomy for pathologic confirmation, at considerable expense and risk to the patient.

The development and perfection of colonoscopy were at first fraught with technical and procedural difficulties. Opponents claimed that the same information could be obtained from a good barium enema, and argued that colonoscopy was expensive and even dangerous. Through trial and error, however, the technical difficulties were overcome, and improved methods of bowel preparation and fiberoptics made colonoscopy a safer and more reliable means of assessing the large bowel. Eventually the technique was embraced by the surgical community. In 1973, at the meeting of the American College of Surgeons, J Englebert Dunphy labeled the method 'a major contribution to colonic surgery', and Frances Moore called it 'a quantum advance in abdominal surgery'[3].

In 1983 a new feature for viewing the gastrointestinal tract was introduced, the videoendoscope. The endoscopic images are transmitted by a small electronic chip and then displayed on a video monitor. This technological advancement made colonoscopy easier to teach and also provided a hard copy of the endoscopic image available for the patient's chart. Around the same time, the application of lasers to colonoscopy led to the palliative treatment of obstructing lesions of the colon and rectum.

New indications and applications for colonoscopy continue to be evident. The use of intraoperative colonoscopy as an aid to laparoscopic colectomy is one example.

Technique

Equipment

Instruments are of various working lengths, from approximately 115 cm to almost 180 cm (Figure 3.1). They are forward-viewing, with angles of up to

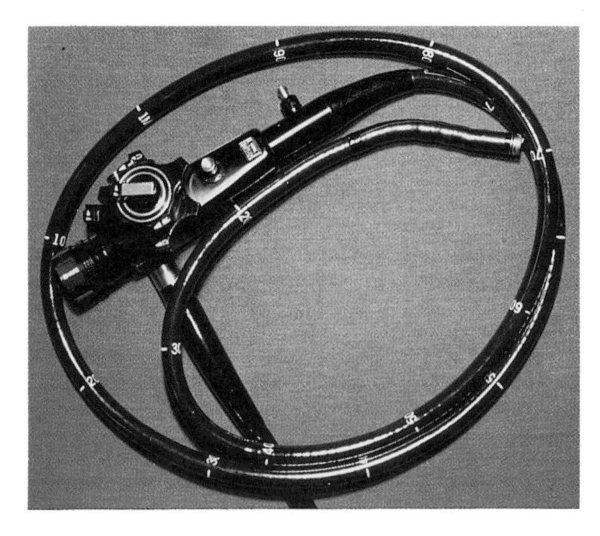

Figure 3.1: A standard colonoscope.

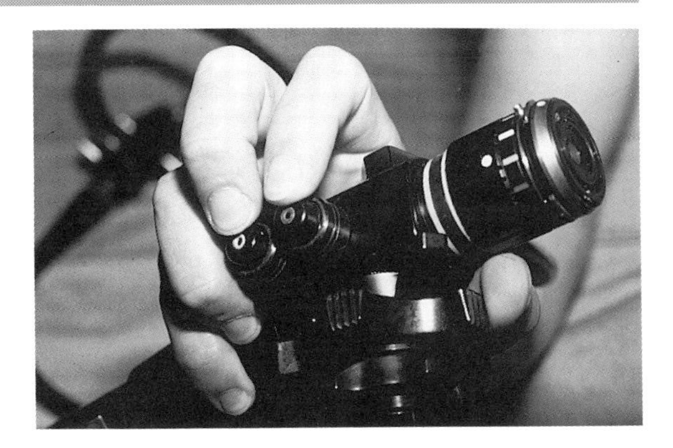

Figure 3.2: The headpiece contains the controls for tip movement, irrigation, insufflation and suction, and the access port for instrumentation.

140°. As with flexible sigmoidoscopy, four-way angulation of the distal end is achieved with approximately 180° up and down and 160° right and left by manipulating the control knobs. Air or carbon dioxide can be insufflated, fluid instilled and liquid debris removed during the procedure. Necessary items for procedures include biopsy forceps, electosurgical snare, grasping forceps and an instrument for brush cytology (Figure 3.2).

Cost is a major consideration and the average colonoscope is priced at around $13 000. If one purchases video equipment along with the colonoscope, the cost may exceed $25 000. Repairs and the limited life-expectancy of the equipment must also be considered when assessing the expense.

Patient preparation

A clean colon is required for endoscopy, so one of the following prepatory routines should be used. At our institution, one gallon of a solution containing primarily sodium sulfate and polyethylene glycol (GoLytely)[3] is administered at a rate of 200 g every 10 minutes. An ingestion of the entire 4 L dose will evacuate the entire gastrointestinal tract in approximately three to five hours. Alternatively, a vigorous cathartic (50 g of castor oil or 250 g of magnesium citrate) the night before examination followed by several tap water enemas two hours before the procedure usually gives an adequate preparation.

Premedication

Whenever total colonoscopy is contemplated, sedation is advised. Distension of the bowel upon insufflation or traction on the bowel from instrumentation may cause abdominal discomfort. General anesthesia is contraindicated, however, because the examiner must know when excessive pain is experienced by the patient because of possible injury to the bowel. Upon arrival at the endoscopy suite, a heparin lock should be started in order to administer sedation. Many varieties of sedation have been recommended. We use a combination of 75 mg of meperidine and 1-2 mg midazolam administered intravenously. Patients are monitored with pulse oximetry and automatic blood pressure cuff. The presence of a skilled nurse is vital to aid in monitoring the patient, to help with equipment preparation and to position the patient.

Technique

The procedure is performed with the patient in the left lateral decubitus position. The anus and rectum are then inspected for hemorrhoids, fistula or fissure, as well as any other abnormalities, and then a careful digital rectal exam is performed to feel for any masses. The rectum is well lubricated and the colonoscope is inserted by placing the index finger of the right hand on the tip of the scope and advancing the instrument into the rectum. The tip of the scope is flexed at a 90° angle in order to visualize the rectal wall. Air should be insufflated in order to negotiate the valves of Houston as well as the anatomical curves of the rectum (Figure 3.3). As with all endoscopy, the instrument should not be advanced unless the lumen can be visualized. Advancement generally proceeds to about 16 or 18 cm without difficulty.

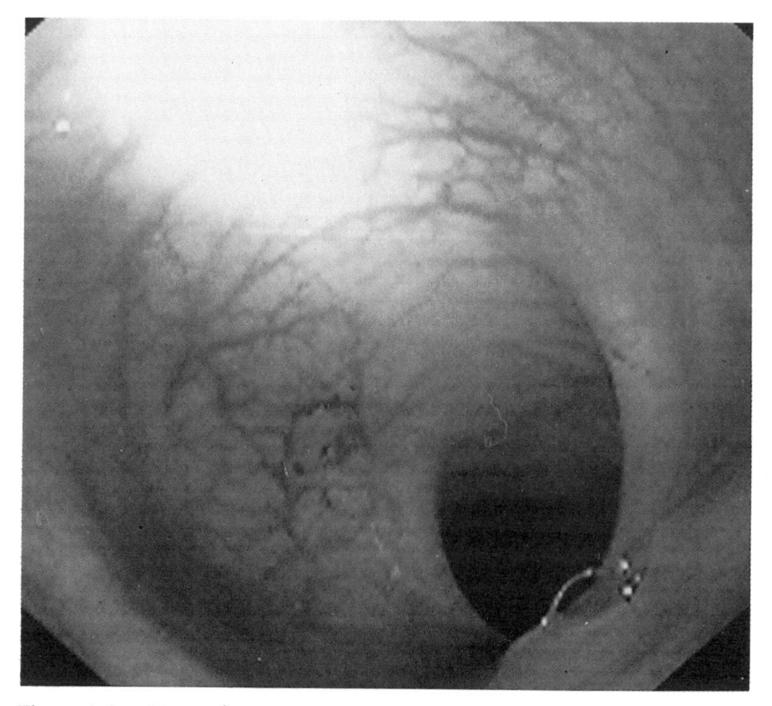

Figure 3.3: Normal rectum.

The rectosigmoid junction is the first area which may be difficult to maneuver. The tip of the colonoscope must be maximally flexed and pulled back toward the endoscopist. Once the sigmoid lumen is visualized, the scope may be advanced. In patients with a short sigmoid colon the examination is simple and easy. Sometimes it is necessary to perform an alpha loop maneuver, so named because the colonoscope configuration resembles that of the Greek letter alpha (Figure 3.4). Counterclockwise rotation during advancement results in the loop. The colonoscope then enters the descending colon. Clockwise torque during withdrawal permits straightening of the sigmoid colon. The purpose of this procedure is to remove the sharp flexure of the proximal

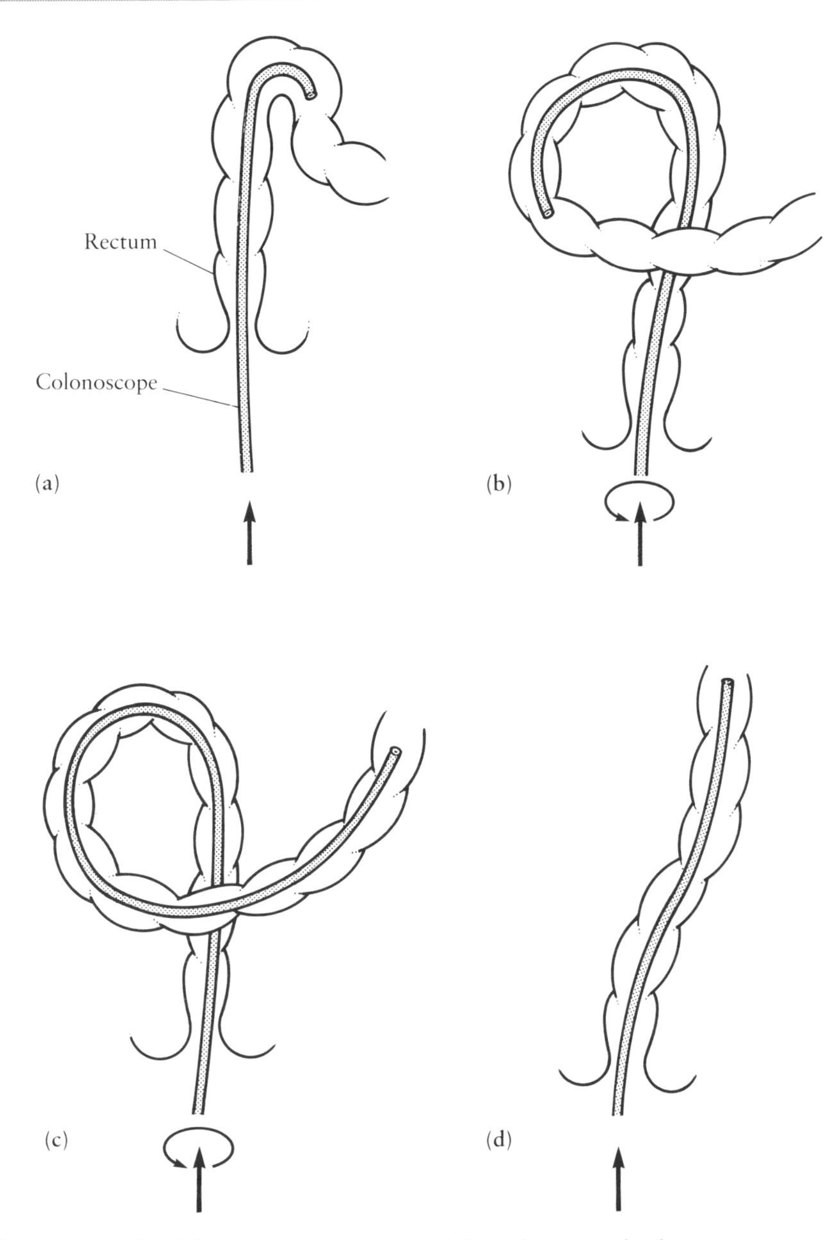

Figure 3.4: The alpha loop maneuver to straighten the sigmoid colon.

sigmoid colon. It can be performed easily except in cases of adhesions or carcinomatous fixation.

Other techniques which help to negotiate the sigmoid and other difficult areas include gentle extra-abdominal pressure of an assistant's open hand on the left lower quadrant and a 'to-and-fro' motion which will help to telescope the colon. This is especially helpful when resistance is encountered. If a barium enema has been performed previously it is useful to have this 'road map' available for review.

When one has passed through the descending colon, the distance between the anal verge and the splenic flexure is approximately 40 cm assuming no looping is present. At the splenic flexure, a blue appearance denotes the spleen which may be seen through the bowel wall because of the spenocolic ligaments which attach it to the colon. To advance the instrument, the splenic flexure may be 'hooked'. In general, the transverse colon is one of the easiest areas to traverse. An unobstructed view of the triangular lumen of the transverse colon is possible due to tensed circular muscles and teniae coli (Figure 3.5). At the hepatic flexure, one may also see the neighboring liver which appears blue.

After negotiating the hepatic flexure, the colonoscope is easily introduced into the cecum through the ascending colon because the ascending colon is usually fixed to the lateral gutter. The orifice of the appendix is noted about 5 cm beneath the ileocecal junction. The bottom of the cecum appears as a blind pouch, and at this point during the procedure it is possible to see the red glow of the colonoscope through the right lower quadrant of the abdomen. One can usually reach the cecum by using less than 90 cm of the instrument. Experienced colonoscopists are accurate in assessing the extent of colonoscopy, and fluoroscopic confirmation is not routinely needed[4].

It is sometimes possible, though often difficult, to enter the ileocecal valve and then traverse up to 25 cm into the terminal ileum. Examination of the terminal ileum can be helpful in the evaluation of patients with inflammatory bowel disease, gastrointestinal bleeding and diarrhea.

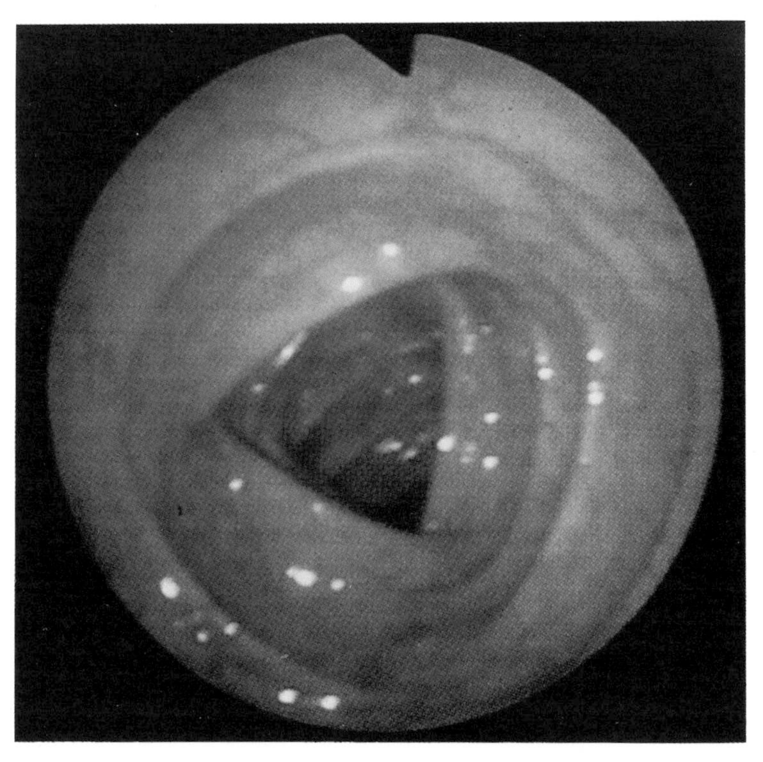

Figure 3.5: Transverse colon — the typical triangular appearance.

Finally, withdrawing the instrument slowly is perhaps one of the most important steps during colonoscopy. It is at this time that the bowel can be carefully reinspected to note any lesions which may have been missed on the way in. The endoscopist should develop a routine for inspection, using the controls to ensure the complete circumference is surveyed. If puddles of fluid obscure the mucosa at any point, they may be either aspirated or moved by rolling the patient.

Complications of colonoscopy

Many possible complications of colonoscopy can occur. The most common serious complications are perforation, hemorrhage and respiratory problems[5]. The less serious complications include transient bacteremia, vasovagal responses, pneumatosis cystoides intestinalis, ileus, and the side-effects of bowel preparation.

Side-effects of bowel preparation

In general, most patients can tolerate standard bowel preparation, but there may be some untoward side-effects. Bowel preparation can cause dehydration in the elderly, and these patients should be encouraged to drink plenty of fluids. Patients with a history of cardiorespiratory problems should be admitted to the hospital for bowel preparation. Individuals with inflammatory bowel disease may develop exacerbations of their disease and even toxic megacolon if one is overzealous in their bowel preparation.

Side-effects of medication

The standard medications used for sedation during colonoscopy, meperidine and midazolam, may cause respiratory depression if used in excessive amounts. The assistant should be monitoring the patient, and the use of pulse oximetry may help alert one to over-sedation. Naloxone hydrochloride is used to reverse the effects of narcotics, and flumazenil can now be used to reverse the effects of the benzodiazepines.

Bacteremia

Transient bacteremia may be induced by colonoscopy. It may be related to the length of the procedure, adequacy of bowel preparation, and amount of manipulation of the bowel. For most patients, the bacteremia is not clinically significant and the routine administration of antibiotics is not recommended. Individuals with valvular heart disease, prosthetic implants or a compromised immune system should receive prophylactic antibiotics before colonoscopy.

Bleeding

Bleeding is the most common complication following polypectomy, representing 53% of all complications in the experience of Nivatvongs[6]. An adequate history should be taken of all patients to determine those at increased risk of bleeding. The rate of bleeding in diagnostic colonoscopy is stated to be 0.05%. For therapeutic colonoscopy with polypectomy, the rate is 1–2.5%[7]. Hemorrhage may occur as an immediate or delayed phenomenon. Bleeding after polypectomy can usually be controlled by reapplying the snare for at least five minutes or by the use of electrocauterization. Bleeding can also result from a tear in the mesentery or from a splenic injury, in which case the bleeding may not be evident until some time later. On rare occasions, uncontrollable hemorrhage necessitates an operation for suture ligation of the bleeding site.

Perforation

The rate of perforation varies from series to series, from 0.3 to 2.14%[8]. Perforation usually occurs following polypectomy, or at the site of pre-existing diverticula. Vigorous manipulation or over-distension with air or gas may precipitate perforation. The most common site of perforation is the sigmoid colon. This may be due to the difficulty of negotiating the sigmoid and also because of the frequency of diverticula in this area.

The classic presentations of transmural burn are fever, localized abdominal pain, tenderness, focal peritoneal signs, distension and leukocytosis. Nonsurgical management may be reasonable if the patient is in a stable condition, shows improvement with antibiotics and has no evidence of peritonitis, distal obstruction or underlying pathology that would demand ultimate resection[9]. This is most often the case in posterior retroperitoneal perforation. Patients must be maintained on intravenous fluids and antibiotics, and must have frequent abdominal examinations. Laparotomy should be undertaken in the patient exhibits signs of peritonitis. If there is little contamination, then the hole or tear may be closed primarily. If sepsis or gross contamination is evident, diversion may be necessary.

Other complications

A postcolonoscopy syndrome has been described which is manifested by abdominal distension, discomfort, and dilated loops of bowel[10]. Patients do not exhibit signs of peritonitis. Treatment consists of observation and medical management. Incarceration of the colonoscope in an inguinal hernia has been reported[11]. Volvulus, hepatic injuries, pneumomediastinum and pneumothorax have all been reported as rare complications.

Colonoscopic polypectomy

Most colon and rectal carcinomas develop from an initially benign adenomatous polyp[12]. Because of the adenoma-to-cancer sequence, the removal of benign colonic polyps may prevent or reduce the potential risk of the development of colorectal cancer[13]. The term 'polyp' is morphologic, and no histologic diagnosis is implied. Polyps of the large intestine include adenomas, hamartomas and inflammatory polyps. The latter two subtypes have no malignant potential whereas adenomas may be considered to be precursors of malignancy. This hypothesis is supported by the fact that patients with familial polyposis die of cancer at a young age unless the colon is removed.

The malignant potential of an adenoma depends on growth pattern, size and the degree of epithelial atypia. The three histologic patterns of adenoma reflect the neoplastic progression; about 5% of tubular adenomas, 22% of tubulovillous adenomas and 40% of villous adenomas become malignant. Cancer is found in 1% of adenomas under 1 cm in diameter, 10% of adenomas 1–2 cm in diameter, and 45% of adenomas larger than 2 cm. Sessile lesions are more apt to be malignant than pedunculated ones. It probably takes at least five years, but more often 10–15 years, for an adenoma to become malignant[14].

Colonoscopic polypectomy should only be undertaken after the examiner has had thorough experience with diagnostic colonoscopy. Visualization of the entire polyp and its base or stalk is necessary in order for the physician to decide whether the polyp can and should be removed colonoscopically.

Pedunculated lesions

Virtually all pedunculated polyps can be removed, regardless of size and location, provided that one is comfortable with the electrosurgical snare techniques. A snare is placed around the stalk of the polyp and then the stalk is transected closer to the adenoma side than to the bowel to avoid potential thermal damage to the bowel wall (Figure 3.6). Many endoscopists limit the management of diminutive polyps to 'cold' (non-coagulating) forceps biopsy in order to obtain a tissue sample. Data have shown that cold snare excision of small polyps is a safe and effective alternative method of treatment in patients without clotting problems[15]. Whichever technique is used, the role of good judgement and excellent technical skill is paramount.

Sessile polyps

Large, sessile, soft, velvety lesions in the rectum are usually villous adenomas; these tumors have a high malignant potential and must be completely excised. Removal of sessile polyps is more involved than that of pedunculated polyps because of the margin of transection and cauterization is always directly on the bowel wall. These large polyps may be removed in a piecemeal excision as described by Shinya, Christie and others[16,17] (Figure 3.7). Although this approach may obviate a formal laparotomy, the pathologist may have a problem in orientation as well as in ensuring that the excision is complete[18]. Multiple endoscopic resections may be necessary to extirpate the lesion fully and it is not surprising that villous adenomas have a high risk of local recurrence. Alternatives to colonoscopic excision include surgical excision of rectal villous adenomas, transanal endoscopic microsurgery (*see* Chapter 6), and the use of lasers in the selected management of benign lesions of the colon as discussed later[19].

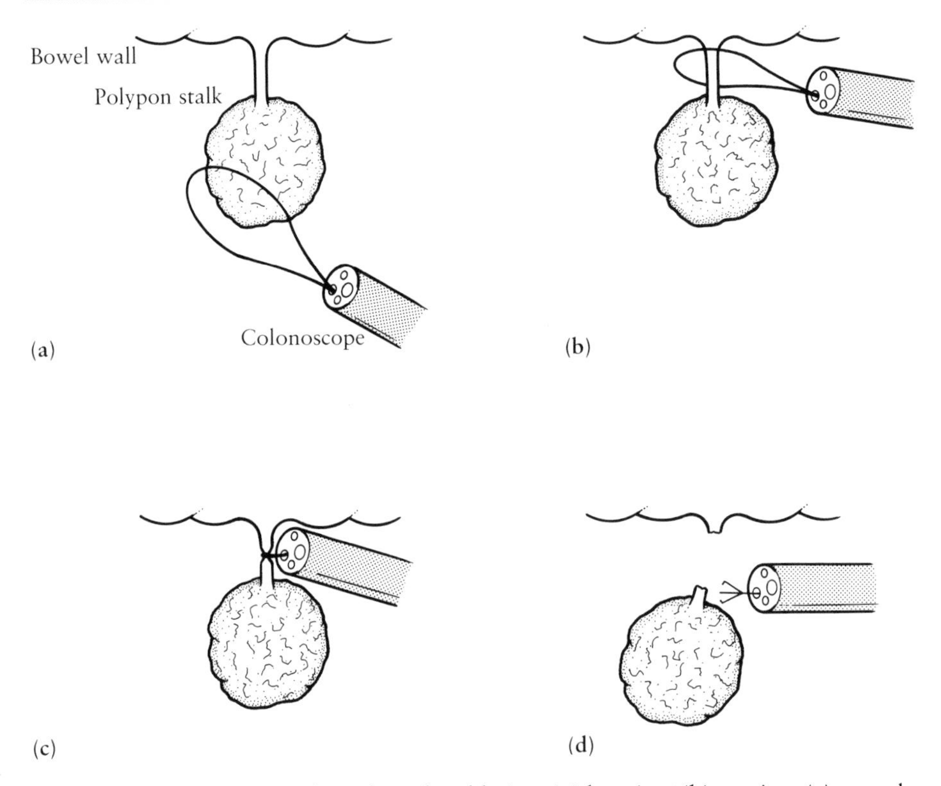

Figure 3.6: Polypectomy of a pedunculated lesion: (**a**) location, (**b**) snaring, (**c**) coagulation, and (**d**) retrieval with three-prong graspers.

Polyps containing invasive carcinoma

It is not surprising that on occasion a polyp with a benign clinical appearance contains either carcinoma in situ or invasive adenocarcinoma. Polyps with carcinoma in situ are thought to be cured by polypectomy alone[20]. Polyps with invasive carcinoma, as defined by infiltration of malignant cells into the submucosa, have the potential for lymph node metastasis, in which case endoscopic polypectomy may not be curative. These polyps are uncommon, representing 2.7% of adenomatous polyps in one series[21]. If favorable histologic features are present, then polypectomy may be adequate therapy. Invasive carcinoma at the margin appears to be the single best indicator of adverse outcome and polyps with such pathology should be surgically reexcised.

Ulcerative colitis

Carcinoma of the colon and rectum is the most feared complication in patients with long-standing, chronic ulcerative colitis. By eight to 10 years after the onset of ulcerative colitis, about 5% of patients have developed colorectal cancer; the cumulative incidence is 20–25% after 20 years and 30–40% by 30

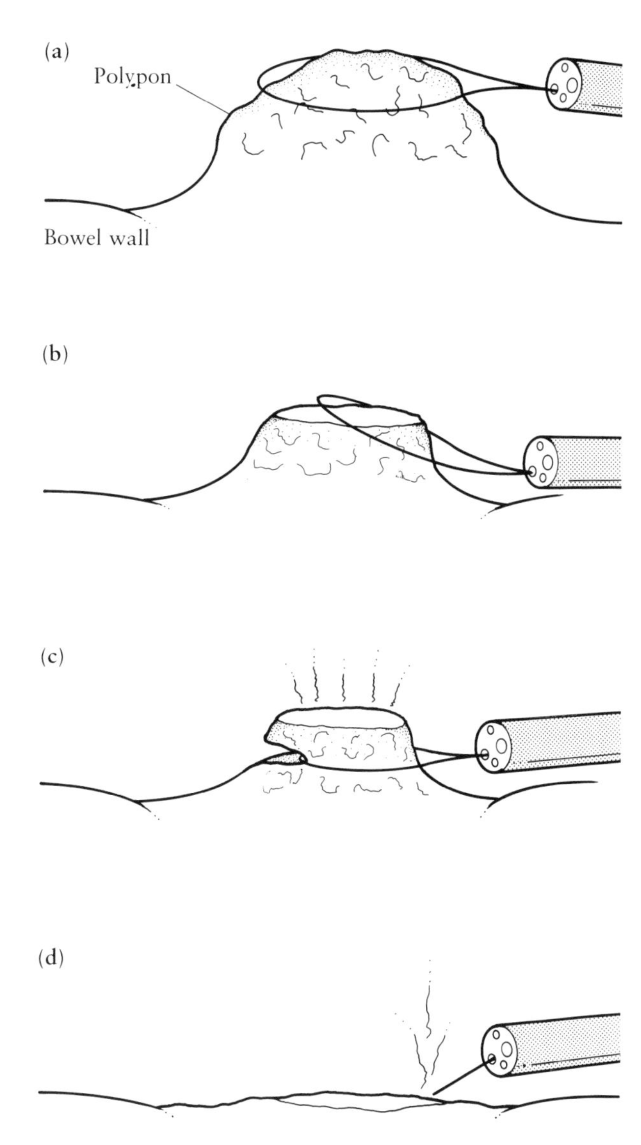

Figure 3.7: Piecemeal excision of a sessile polyp: (**a**) first cut, (**b**) and (**c**) oblique cuts, and (**d**) final hemostasis.

years[22]. Interestingly, the degree of activity for the eight to 10 years of colitis does not appear to be an important variable in the development of carcinoma[23,24]. Even if the patient remains relatively asymptomatic for several years, the increased risk of carcinoma remains. It appears that the increased turnover of mucosal cells predisposes the patient to the development of carcinoma.

Vigilant surveillance is required. The current recommendation for patients with chronic ulcerative colitis is annual colonoscopy with multiple biopsies taken at 10 cm intervals throughout the entire colon[25]. This should provide at least eight biopsy specimens for histologic assessment for dysplasia. If severe dysplasia persists on serial biopsies, the chances of finding cancer in the colon are about 50% and colectomy should be performed promptly. Acute inflammation may cause histologic changes similar to those of dysplasia, making the diagnosis of dysplasia difficult. Therefore target biopsies should be taken from the less inflamed segments of colon. If possible, surveillance should be performed during a quiescent phase of the disease.

Colonoscopy in the preoperative evaluation and postoperative surveillance for patients with colorectal carcinoma

Preoperative evaluation

The incidence of synchronous carcinoma has been reported to be between 2.5% and 7.2%[26,27]. The incidence of benign synchronous polyps is 12–62%[28]. One of the goals in the preoperative assessment of the patient with carcinoma of the colon and rectum is to exclude the presence of synchronous lesions. Colonoscopy is the preferred method for this evaluation. Colonoscopy allows for the removal of synchronous polyps outside of the planned area of resection. Often it is difficult to pass the colonoscope beyond the primary lesion because of narrowing of the lumen. In this instance, intraoperative or postoperative colonoscopy is mandatory to assess the remaining bowel.

Brullet and colleagues performed intraoperative colonoscopy in 67 patients undergoing elective surgery for colorectal cancer[29]. A synchronous carcinoma was found in 9% of patients which necessitated a change of planned surgical procedure. Synchronous polyps were removed in 36% of patients, two of whom had carcinoma in situ. Intraoperative colonoscopy took a mean of 15 minutes of surgical time and only two minor complications occurred. The author concluded that intraoperative colonoscopy allows complete assessment of the colon and identifies synchronous lesions.

Preoperative colonoscopy helps to locate the tumors (Figure 3.8). Small lesions can be difficult for the operating surgeon to find. The operative procedure may be simplified by intraoperative colonoscopy or by preoperative marking of the lesion with an injection of India ink.

Postoperative surveillance

Recurrent disease will develop in about 40% of patients who undergo curative resection[30]. After resection, almost all recurrent tumors are seen in the first five years. Of tumors that recur, 85% do so in the first 30 months after resection, with the rest detected in the next 30 months[31]. Because recurrent disease develops during the first two years, surveillance should be most intensive during that period. Surveillance strategies include history and physical exam, routine liver function studies, carcinoembryonic antigen (CEA) levels, chest roentgenogram and colonoscopy.

The extent of postoperative colonoscopic follow-up is controversial. A recent survey of members of the American Society of Colon and Rectal Surgeons showed that not even 50% of responders could agree on how

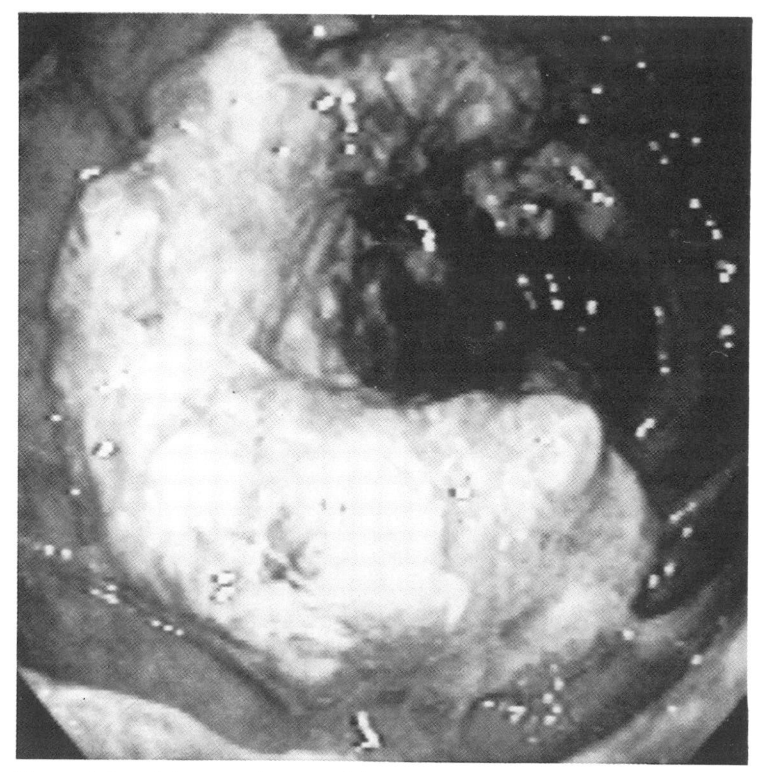

Figure 3.8: Adenocarcinoma of the rectum.

frequently the test should be performed at any time during the five years surveyed[32]. The most controversial finding was the frequency of colonoscopy. The vast majority of colonoscopies are negative.

Most clinicians would agree that patients who do not have preoperative complete colonoscopic evaluation should have this between three and six months after surgery to look for synchronous lesions. Steele and colleagues recommended that, if the intial exam is negative, then it is reasonable to perform another colonoscopy at one year postoperatively and every two or three years thereafter[33].

Brady and colleagues followed 207 asymptomatic patients with a previous history of colorectal carcinoma for between two and eight years[34]. They found that 35% of patients had a neoplastic lesion on initial colonoscopy. Synchronous carcinomas were found in 11 patients, and six recurrent carcinomas at the anastomosis were demonstrated. They concluded that after two annual colonoscopies fail to show neoplasms, surveillance colonoscopy may be scheduled at three to five year intervals.

The biggest improvement in survival may be in the early detection of disease in first-degree relatives of patients with colorectal cancer. Patients with a first-degree relative with colorectal carcinoma are at increased risk for the development of colorectal carcinoma, and therefore all such relatives should be counseled to have regular surveillance[35].

Lasers for obstructing carcinomas

Over the last decade, photoablative laser therapy for advanced gastrointestinal malignancy has seen increasing utilization as a palliative mode of treatment. Traditional surgical methods for obstructing colon cancer include two or three stage procedures for left-sided colon carcinoma resulting in high morbidity and mortality rates from the stoma including prolapse, paracolostomy hernia, abcess, retraction and necrosis. In addition, many patients refuse to undergo a second or third operation, often despite the presence of a nonresected tumor. Patients with distant metastatic disease, extensive local invasion, obstruction and bleeding from nonresectable rectal tumor, and patients with concomitant medical illnesses that would preclude operative intervention, are all candidates for laser ablation to palliate and avoid surgery.

A large body of literature is currently available demonstrating the efficacy of neodymium:yttrium-aluminum-garnet (Nd:YAG) laser therapy for the treatment of obstructing or bleeding esophageal, gastric, and colorectal neoplasms[36–39]. With its power output of 90–100 W and a pulse duration of 0.5–1 seconds, inducing energy densities of more than 1000 joules/cm^2, the Nd:YAG laser produces vaporization of tumor tissue at the surface and coagulation in the deeper layers of the tumor. In this way, ablation of tumor tissue and simultaneous coagulation of potential bleeding vessels can be effected (Figures 3.9).

Preresectional laser therapy

In 1986, the first large series of patients undergoing laser therapy prior to resection was reported by Kiefhaver *et al.*[40]. Of 57 patients with colonic obstruction, 54 obtained recanalization using the Nd:Yag laser. Of these 54 patients, 27 subsequently underwent a left colectomy. Eleven patients received laser therapy alone for their obstructing tumor, with a mean survival of 5.2 months.

Eckhauser and colleagues demonstrated a significant reduction in preoperative and total hospital costs and length of stay for patients receiving preresectional laser therapy[41]. Of 58 patients undergoing laser therapy, there was one laser-related perforation that required urgent subtotal colectomy.

Palliative laser therapy

A large multicenter European study investigated the role of palliative treatment of advanced colorectal malignancy[42]. The study included 181 patients deemed unsuitable for operation because of refusal of surgery, severe multisystem disease or extensive metastatic disease. Laser treatments were performed one to three times per week until resolution of symptoms, and patients were followed at regular intervals every four weeks in a maintenance treatment schedule. Good palliation was observed in 161 of 181 patients (89%). The overall complication rate for the series was 9.4% and included five

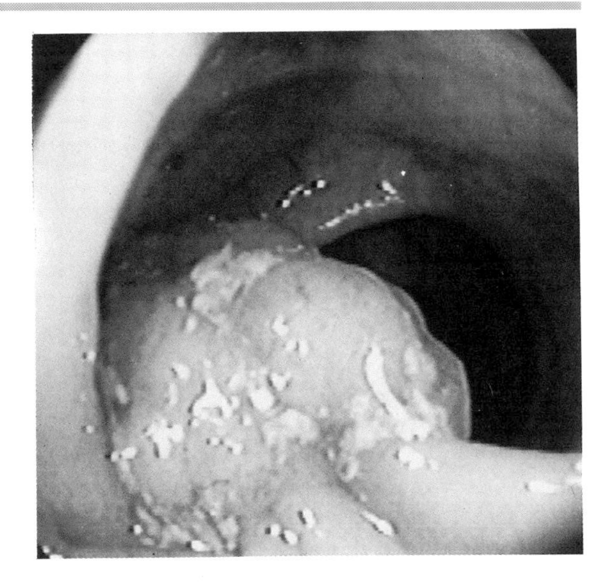

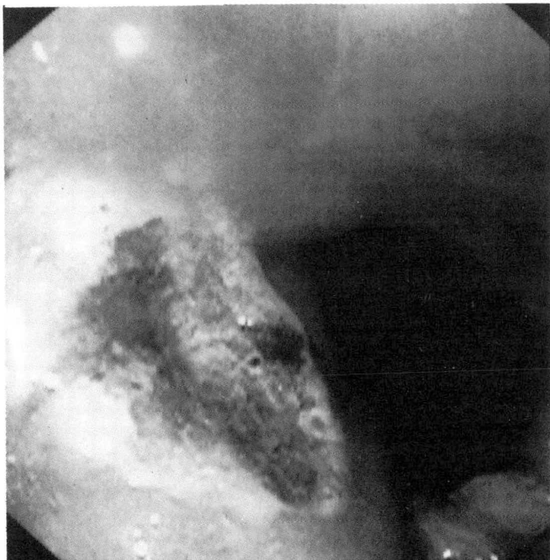

Figure 3.9: Pre- and post-laser ablation of a rectal cancer.

perforations, six strictures and six instances of induced hemorrhage requiring transfusion. The average length of survival was six months.

Colonoscopy as an intraoperative aid in laparoscopic assisted colectomy

The technique of laparoscopic assisted colectomy will be discussed elsewhere in this text. The laparoscopic surgeon may use colonoscopy as an intraoperative aid during laparoscopic assisted colectomy. When an intracorporeal anastomosis is performed, it may be difficult to locate the malignancy precisely, especially with small masses. Intraoperative colonoscopy can accurately define the lesion and assure that the surgeon is able to take appropriate margins of normal colon with the specimen (Figure 3.10). Additionally, flexion of the scope may help to raise and retract an unduly mobile sigmoid colon.

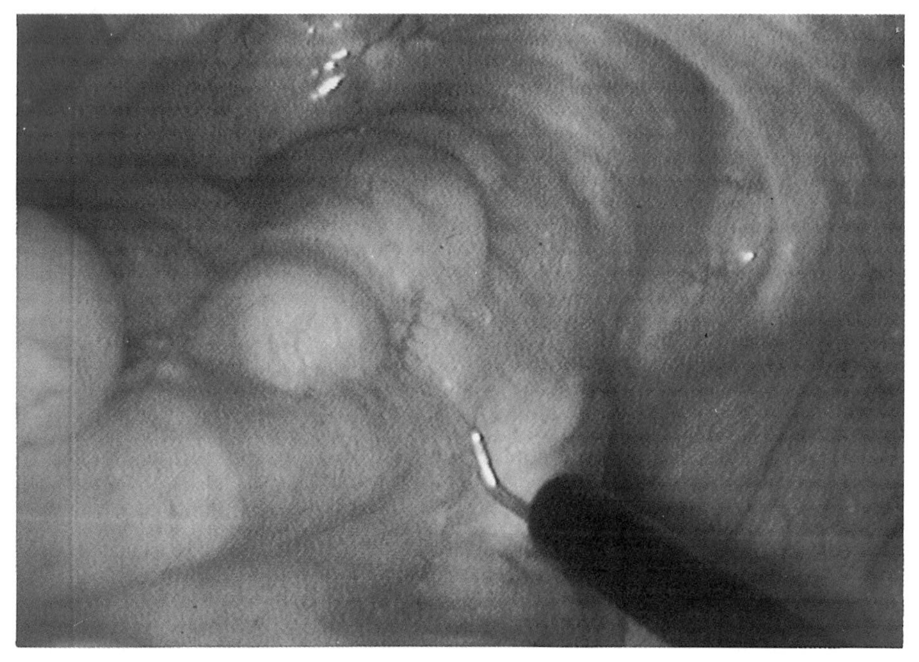

Figure 3.10: Laparoscopic view of the colonoscope illuminating a sigmoid tumor; the electrosurgery probe will be used to mark the tumor on the serosa of the bowel.

Conclusion

Colonoscopy is a valuable tool in the evaluation, diagnosis and treatment of malignant colorectal conditions. Colonoscopic polypectomy can be performed safely by well trained endoscopists and may detect carcinoma at an early stage. Total colonoscopy is essential in patients with ulcerative colitis because of the increased risk of malignancy. The indications for colonoscopy are increasing in number, partly because of laser palliation of advanced malignancy and also because of laparoscopic assisted colectomy. General surgeons need to be familiar with the indications, techniques, and also potential complications of colonoscopy.

References

1 American Cancer Society (1992) *Cancer facts and figures*. American Cancer Society, Atlanta.

2 Wolff WI (1989) Colonoscopy: history and development. *Am J Gastroent.* **84**:1017–25.

3 Dunphy JE, Moore FD, (1973) In discussion of paper by Wolff WI and Shinya H. *Ann Surg.* **178**:376–7.

4 Anderson ML, Heigh RI, McCoy GA *et al.* (1992) Accuracy of assessment of the extent of examination by experienced colonoscopists. *Gastrointest Endosc.* **38**:560–3.

5 Ghazi A and Grossman M (1982) Complications of colonoscopy and polypectomy. *Surg Clin N Am.* **62**:889–96.

6 Nivatvongs S (1988) Complications in colonoscopic polypectomy: lessons to learn from an experience of 1576 polyps. *Am Surg.* **54**:61.

7 Davis R and Graham D (1979) Endoscopic complications: the Texas experience. *Gastrointest Endosc.* **25**:146–9.

8 Schwesinger W, Levine B and Tamos R (1979) Complications of fiberoptic colonoscopy. *Surg Gynecol Obstet.* **148**:270–81.

9 Christie JP and Marazzo J III (1991) 'Miniperforation' of the colon – not all postpolypectomy perforations require laparotomy. *Dis Colon Rectum.* **34**:132.

10 Mendoza CB and Watne AL (1982) Value of intraoperative colonscopy in vascular ectasia of the colon. *Am Surg.* **48**:153.

11 Koltun WA and Coller JA (1991) Incarceration of colonoscope in an inguinal hernia: 'Pulley' technique of removal. *Dis Colon Rectum.* **34**:191.

12 Shinya H and Wolff WI (1979) Morphology, anatomic distribution and cancer potential of colonic polyps: analysis of 7000 polyps endoscopically removed. *Ann Surg.* **190**:679–83.

13 Morson B (1974) The polyp–cancer sequence in the large bowel. *Proc R Soc Med.* **67**:451–7.

14 Way LW (1985) *Current surgical diagnosis and treatment, 7th edn.* Lange, Los Altos, California. p. 602.

15 Tappero G, Gaia E, De Giuli P. *et al.* (1992) Cold snare excision of small colorectal polyps, *Gastrointest Endosc.* **38**:310–13.

16 Christie JP and Shinya H (1982) Technique of colonoscopic polypectomy. *Surg Clin N Am.* **62**:869.

17 Shinya J. (1982) *Colonoscopy: diagnosis and treatment of colonic diseases.* Igaku-Shoin, New York.

18 Nivatvongs S, Snorer DC and Faug DT (1984) Piecemeal snare excision of large sessile colon and rectal polyps: Is it adequate? *Gastrointest Endosc.* **30**:18.

19 Buess G, Mentges B, Manncke K *et al.* (1992) Techniques and results of endoscopic microsurgery of early rectal cancer. *Am J Surg.* **163**:63–9.

20 Shatney CH, Lober PH, Gilbertson VA *et al.* (1974). The treatment of pedunculated adenomatous colorectal polyps with focal cancer. *Surg Gynecol Obstet.* **139**:845–50.

21 Cranley JP, Petras RE, Carey WD *et al.* (1986) When is endoscopic polypectomy adequate therapy for colonic polyps containing invasive carcinoma? *Gastroenterol.* **91**:419–27.

22 Way L W (1991) *Current surgical diagnosis and treatment, 9th edn.* Appleton and Lange, Norwalk, Connecticut. pp. 668–9.

23 Waye JD and Hunt RH (1982) Colonoscopic diagnosis of inflammatory bowel disease. *Surg Clin N Am.* **62**:905–13.

24 Gyde SN, Prior P, Allan RN *et al.* (1988) Colorectal cancer in ulcerative colitis: a cohort study of primary referrals from three centres. *Gut.* **29**:206–17.

25 Yardley JH, Bayless TM and Diamond MP (1979) Cancer in ulcerative colitis. *Gastroenterol.* **76**:221.

26 Barillari P, Ramacciato G, De Angelis R *et al.* (1990) Effect of preoperative colonoscopy on the incidence of synchronous and metachronous neoplasms. *Acta Chir Scand.* **156**:163–6.

27 Sugrue M, Black R, Watts J *et al.* (1991) Perioperative colonoscopy detects synchronous tumours in patients with colorectal cancers. *Aust NZ J Surg.* **61**:25–8.

28 Vignati PV and Roberts PL (1993) Preoperative evaluation and postoperative surveillance for patients with colorectal carcinoma. *Surg Clin N Am.* **73**:67–84.

29 Brullet E, Montane JM, Bombardo J *et al.* (1992) Intraoperative colonoscopy in patients with colorectal cancer. *Br J Surg.* **79**:1376–8.

30 Moertel CG, Fleming TR, Macdonald JS *et al.* (1990). Levamisole and fluorouracil for adjuvant therapy of resected colon carcinoma. *N Engl J Med.* **322**:352–8.

31 Sugarbaker PH, Gianola FJ, Dwyer A *et al.* (1987) A simplified plan for follow-up of patients with colon and rectal cancer supported by prospective studies of laboratory and radiologic test results. *Surgery.* **102**:79–87.

32 from General Surgery and Laparoscopy News. New York, McMahon Group. Aug. 1993.

33 Steel G Jr (1985) Follow-up plans after 'curative' resection of primary colon or rectum cancer. In: Steel G Jr and Osteen RT (Eds) *Colorectal cancer*. Marcel Dekker, New York. p. 271.

34 Brady PG, Straker RJ and Goldschmid S (1990) Surveillance colonoscopy after resection for colon carcinoma. *Southern Med J*. **8**:765–8.

35 Guillem JG, Forde KA, Treat MR *et al.* (1992) Colonoscopic screening for neoplasms in asymtomatic first-degree relatives of colon cancer patients. A controlled, prospective study. *Dis Colon Rectum*. **35**:523–9.

36 Brunetaud JM, Maunory V, Ducrotte P *et al.* (1987) Palliative treatment of rectosigmoid carcinoma by laser endoscopic photoablation. *Gastroenterol.* **92**:663–8.

37 Eckhauser ML (1985) Endoscopic laser vaporization of obstructing left colonic cancer to avoid decompressive colostomy. *Gastrointest Endosc*. **33**:105–6.

38 Fleischer D and Kessler F (1983) Endoscopic Nd:YAG laser therapy for carcinoma of the esophagus: A new form of palliative treatment. *Gastroenterol.* **85**:600–5.

39 Schwesinger WH and Chumley DL (1988) Laser palliation for gastrointestinal malignancy. *Am Surg*. **54**:100–4.

40 Kiefhaber P, Keifhaber K and Huber F (1986) Preoperative neodymium:YAG laser treatment of obstructive colon cancer. *Endoscopy*. **18**: 44–6.

41 Eckhauser ML, Marshall JB and Imbembo AL (1989) The role of pre-resectional laser recanilization for obstructing carcinomas of the colon and rectum. *Surgery*. **106**:710–17.

42 Mathus-Vliegen EMH and Tytgat GNJ (1986) Laser ablation and palliation in colorectal malignancy. *Gastrointest Endosc*. **32**:393–6.

4

Minimal Access Management of Anorectal Problems

PHILIP H GORDON

Introduction

Unlike most procedures described in this book, minimal access procedures for anorectal problems do not involve a laparoscope. The editors believe it is appropriate to include a chapter on anorectal disorders which can be managed without necessarily performing an operation, or where the recommended operations fall into the category of being minimally invasive. With this in mind, options for the management of common anorectal disorders are discussed.

Hemorrhoids

For centuries the human race has been plagued by hemorrhoids and yet the whole subject is still clouded by misconception and folklore. In his early writings, Maimonides pointed out that the composition of one's foods should always produce softening of the stools[1], and broth made from the flesh of fat chickens was considered to be particularly beneficial. In his treatise on hemorrhoids, a host of concoctions in the form of suppositories, ointments and enemas were recommended for the alleviation and even prevention of the symptoms of hemorrhoidal disease. Currently available preparations are very reminiscent of such historical concoctions. Even then Maimonides regarded the operative excision of hemorrhoids with scepticism because, as he wisely recognized, surgery does not remove the underlying causes that produced hemorrhoids. It is the aim of this chapter to dispel such myths and to discuss optional forms of therapy.

According to the National Center for Health Statistics[2] there were 10 million people in the USA complaining of hemorrhoids in 1990 (a prevalence of 4.4%). Approximately one third of these individuals presented to physicians for evaluation and an average of 1.5 million prescriptions were written annually for hemorrhoidal preparations.

Treatment recommendations usually depend upon the severity of hemorrhoidal disease. From a descriptive point of view, first-degree internal hemorrhoids are said to be present when the hemorrhoids are seen to be bulging into the lumen of the anal canal and produce painless bleeding. Second-degree internal hemorrhoids are those which protrude at the time of a bowel movement but which reduce spontaneously. Third-degree internal hemorrhoids are said to be present if protrusion occurs spontaneously or at the time of a bowel movement and require manual replacement. Fourth-degree internal hemorrhoids are those which are permanently prolapsed and irreducible despite attempts at manual replacement.

Management options

External hemorrhoids

External hemorrhoids are swellings covered with squamous epithelium which is distal to the dentate line. Treatment is not indicated unless there is an acute thrombosis causing severe pain or repeated episodes of acute thromboses, in which case excision under local anesthesia can easily be accomplished as an outpatient procedure in the office or outpatient department.

Internal hemorrhoids

Bulk-forming agents The rationale of adding bulk to the diet is to eliminate straining at defecation. In addition to the intake of adequate fruits, vegetables and cereals, bulk in the diet can be supplemented by raw unprocessed wheat or oat bran. An alternative measure is to take psyllium seed, two teaspoons per day. Adequate volume of fluids must be consumed each day. A high-fiber diet reduces symptoms of hemorrhoids and is ideal for first and some second-degree hemorrhoids[3,4].

Rubber-band ligation Barron popularized rubber-band ligation of bleeding and prolapsed internal hemorrhoids and reported excellent results in 150 patients[5]. Rubber-band ligation has proved to be simple, quick, and an effective means of treating grade 1 and 2 hemorrhoids and selected cases of grade 3 and 4[6–9]. This option has become the author's preferred method for the nonoperative treatment of internal hemorrhoids.

The procedure is performed in the office. Sedation is unnecessary. Two rubber-bands are used on each drum in case one breaks. The procedure is performed through an anoscope using a rubber-band ligature. The bands should be placed on the mucosa well above the dentate line (Figure 1). Some authors have recommended band placement on rectal mucosa above the internal hemorrhoids[10]. Generally the ligation is performed at one site at a time. Subsequent ligation is usually performed three to six weeks later if the patient remains symptomatic. Some authors have recommended ligation of two or three sites at one sitting[6,7].

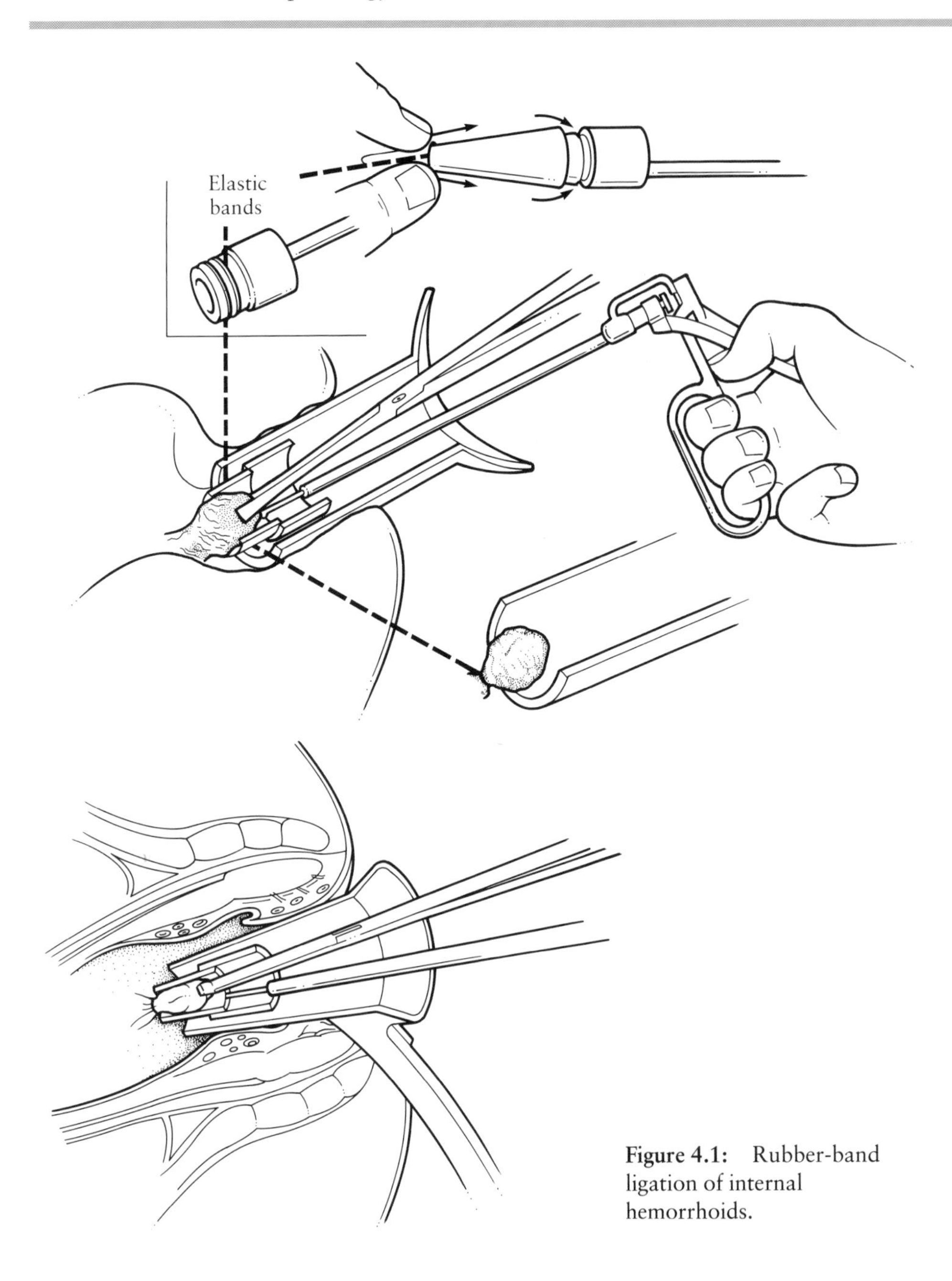

Figure 4.1: Rubber-band ligation of internal hemorrhoids.

Rubber-band ligation may be associated with varying degrees of discomfort. Warm sitz baths will relieve the discomfort and an appropriate non-codeine containing analgesic should be prescribed. Immediate severe pain is an indication that a band is too close to the dentate line and requires immediate removal.

There has been concern about the safety of rubber-band ligation because of reports of death due to acute perianal sepsis[11,12]. The clue to severe anal and perianal infection after rubber-band ligation is a triad of symptoms: delayed anal pain, urinary retention and fever[13]. Continual awareness of this rare but potentially life-threatening complication is essential, and immediate aggressive treatment is mandatory if death is to be prevented[14,15]. This should include administration of triple antibiotics, drainage of an abscess or excision of necrotic tissues, if present.

Other options The infrared photocoagulator is a relatively new apparatus which produces infrared radiation. The unit has an infrared probe which is applied just proximal to the internal hemorrhoids via an anoscope. It is recommended that three of four burns are applied on each hemorrhoid for one or two seconds. Unfortunately each application results in some pain. Infrared photocoagulation produces as good results in first- and second-degree hemorrhoids as sclerotherapy and rubber-band ligation[16,17].

Bipolar (Bicap) coagulation was introduced only recently. This is simply an electrocautery device in which the heat does not penetrate as deeply as with monopolar electrocoagulation. Its effect is similar to infrared photocoagulation, and the device is simple to use on an outpatient basis.

With direct current therapy (Ultroid), current is applied through a probe placed via an anoscope onto the mucosa at the apex of the hemorrhoid. The current is set at the maximal tolerable level and continued for 10 minutes. Because it is time-consuming compared with other methods, it has never become popular. Both bipolar and direct current therapy can be used for first- and second-degree hemorrhoids, but some authors found these to be effective for third-degree hemorrhoids as well[18].

The rationale of injecting chemical agents into hemorrhoids is that it will create fibrosis so that prolapse cannot occur. Solutions that have been used include phenol in oil, quinine urea and sodium morrhuate. It is important that the injection be made into the submucosa above the internal hemorrhoid at the anorectal ring and not intravascularly. Sclerotherapy used to be the treatment of choice for first- and second-degree hemorrhoids, particularly in the United Kingdom[4]. One major drawback of sclerotherapy is the length of time it takes for the nursing staff to lean and sterilize the syringes after use. Sclerotherapy usually produces dull pain, lasting up to 48 hours. Although misplacement of the injection rarely occurs it may lead to mucosal ulceration and necrosis.

The rationale for manual dilatation of the anus is based on the belief that hemorrhoids constitute a reversible condition caused by a fibrous narrowing (pecten band) of the lower anal canal leading to abnormal straining which causes venous congestion and eventually hemorrhoids. The procedure is performed for third-degree hemorrhoids. The anal canal is maximally stretched under intravenous sedation or general anesthesia until the band gives way. It is usually necessary to stretch the anal canal and the lower rectum until four fingers from each hand are inserted[19]. An anal dilator is provided for patients to use at home for the next six months to prevent a recurrence of anal stenosis. Lord claimed that pain and complications are low and he has had no problems with anal incontinence[19]. In a trial comparing the results of maximal anal dilatation and hemorrhoidectomy, Lewis *et al.*[20] found that maximal anal dilatation had good short-term results, but that in the long term some patients develop symptoms which require hemorrhoidectomy. Maximal anal dilatation is performed by many surgeons in the UK but rarely used in the USA because of the concern of anal incontinence and mucosal prolapse. Another disadvantage of maximal anal dilatation is that the associated external hemorrhoids and skin tags are not treated.

Cryotherapy is based on the concept that freezing can destroy hemorrhoidal tissues. The freezing temperature is achieved by a special probe through which nitrous oxide at $-60°$ to $-80°$ or liquid nitrogen at $-196°$ is circulated. Tissue is frozen white for two to four minutes. After it thaws, necrosis and slough occur leaving an ulcer. The size and depth of the ulcer are not controlled[21]. A study by Smith and colleagues[22] showed that profuse discharge associated with a foul smell and irritation from the necrosis is the rule. It is not painless, and takes a long time to heal. If not done properly, destruction of the anal sphincter muscle can cause anal stenosis and incontinence. This technique has now fallen into disrepute and should be abandoned.

Some authorities believe that increased internal sphincter tone accounts for hemorrhoidal disease, and have advocated lateral internal sphincterotomy[23,24]. This operation can be done under local, regional or general anesthesia. A greater or lesser degree of incontinence occurs in 25% of patients, though in most instances it is not serious. Prolapse of redundant mucosa is common and usually requires further treatment. Recurrence of symptoms has been reported to be as low as 5%[23]. In a series by Schouten and van Vroonhoven[24], hemorrhoids associated with high anal pressure (> 125 cm H_2O) were treated by a lateral internal sphincterotomy under local anesthesia on an outpatient basis. Evaluation of the results six months after the operation showed that 78% of patients with first- and second-degree hemorrhoids, and 65% of patients with third- and fourth-degree hemorrhoids, had excellent or satisfactory results. De-Roover *et al.*[25] reported excellent results of lateral internal sphincterotomy for fourth-degree hemorrhoids.

Lasers may also be used to create fixation of hemorrhoidal tissue above the dentate line. Either CO_2 or Nd:YAG lasers can be used, though they are too expensive to use as an office procedure. Heat and localized pain may result, and complications are similar to those with lesser fixation techniques.

Fissure-in-ano

Introduction

Fissure-in-ano is a very common anal disorder which causes suffering out of all proportion to the size of the lesion. The condition is frequently easily treated with bulk-forming agents but chronicity is due to an abnormality in the internal sphincter[26–28]. It is the latter abnormality which must be considered in making a rationale recommendation for therapy.

Management options

Acute fissure

The aim of treatment of an acute fissure-in-ano is to break the cycle of a hard stool, pain and reflex spasm. This goal can often be accomplished with simple measures such as warm baths to help relieve the sphincter spasm[29] and stool softeners. Bulk-forming foods (eg adequate amounts of unprocessed bran) may be helpful. Alternatively stool softeners, such as psyllium seed preparations, can be used. In a double-blind placebo controlled trial, Jensen[30] found that the use of unprocessed bran in doses of 5 g three times daily resulted in a decreased recurrence rate. There is no proof that the host of topical anorectal preparations that have been suggested for the treatment of fissure-in-ano are in fact effective.

Chronic fissure

Many operative techniques have been suggested for the treatment of chronic fissure. I have adopted the technique described by Sir Alan Parks[31], but I perform the operation under local anesthesia as an outpatient procedure in the office unless there are extenuating circumstances such as an allergy to the local anesthetic. This technique certainly belongs in the category of minimal access procedures.

With the patient in the prone jackknife position, the perianal region is prepared with a disinfectant solution and draped in the usual fashion (Figure 4.2). With a fine needle, an anesthetic solution of 0.5% lignocaine in 1 : 200,000 epinephrine is first infiltrated in the area of the fissure. The anesthetic solution is then infiltrated into the left lateral aspect near the anal verge, ensuring that the solution is directed to the level of the dentate line. A Pratt bivalve is inserted into the anal orifice. Should there still be some discomfort, the entire perianal region may be anesthetized. A short incision is made just distal to the intersphincteric groove, which can usually be palpated quite easily. The anoderm is lifted off the underlying internal sphincter to the level of the dentate line and the intersphincteric plane is developed. The full thickness of the internal sphincter is divided from its lower edge to the level of the dentate line using either a pair of Metzenbaum scissors or a scalpel. Hemostasis is obtained with cautery and the wound can be closed with a couple of interrupted sutures of 3–0 chromic catgut.

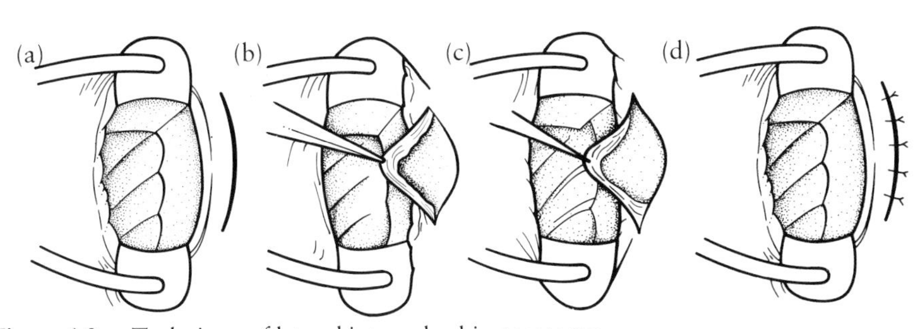

Figure 4.2: Technique of lateral internal sphincterotomy.

Postoperatively, patients are discharged home on a regular diet, advised to take sitz baths, and use a psyllium seed preparation as a stool softener; a non-constipating oral analgesic is prescribed. Patients should be seen again one month after the procedure.

The great advantage of this method is that it avoids an intraanal wound. The internal sphincter is divided under direct visual control, a point worth emphasizing, because the thickness and length of the internal sphincter may vary from patient to patient. Bleeding sites can be seen and directly controlled. For these reasons this is my preferred technique.

A number of technical variations have been described but all have the same purpose, to divide the lower half of the internal sphincter.

Other options

The classic excision of a fissure-in-ano is still used by many surgeons and is usually associated with division of varying amounts of sphincter muscle. The main criticism of this operation is that it leaves the patient with a large and rather uncomfortable external wound that may be difficult to handle on an outpatient basis as well as requiring a long time to heal. For these reasons, few surgeons consider it a viable option.

A method employing the use of excision of the fissure combined with an advancement flap of anoderm has been referred to as the V–Y anoplasty. Using this technique, the fissure and the adjacent crypt bearing hemorrhoidal tissue are completely excised. A triangular skin flap based outside the anal canal is elevated in continuity with the excised fissure. One must ensure that there is a broad base with adequate blood supply to the flap. The flap is adequately mobilized to avoid tension on the suture line. Meticulous attention is paid to hemostasis, in order to prevent hematoma formation which increases tension and the chance of infection. The flap is then advanced and the defect of the skin and anal canal is closed. Very good results have been reported with this technique[32] but, because it involves considerable dissection and requires an increased operative time, the procedure is probably of greater magnitude than is necessary to treat the problem.

Manual dilatation of the anus involves the forceful stretching of the anal sphincter with as many as six or eight fingers. Because this technique has the potential to cause considerable injury to the sphincter mechanism resulting in alteration in continence, I personally find no place in the surgical armamentarium for this procedure.

Results

Wide variations in results have been reported, with recurrence rates ranging from 10 to 30% (mostly in the upper range) after manual dilatation of the anus[33–37], and from 0 to 15% (the majority being in the 1–3% range) after lateral internal sphincterotomy (Table 4.1). Similarly incontinence is reported to occur in up to 34% of patients after manual dilatation of the anus[33–35,37,39] compared with 0–15% (the majority being in the 0–3% range) of patients after lateral internal sphincterotomy (Table 4.1). Amongst the various operative options available for the treatment of fissure-in-ano, the procedure which has

Author	No. of patients	Impaired control: Flatus (%)	Feces (%)	Fecal soiling (%)	Unhealed or recurrence (%)
Hawley[34]	24	?	0	0	0
Hoffmann and Goligher[38]	99	6	1	7	3
Millar[39]	99	2	0	1	0
Notaras[40]	82	2	1	5	10
Clery[41]	217	5	0	5.5	1
Hunter[42]	74	27	27	34	12
Rudd[43]	200	0	0	0	0.5
Bailey *et al.*[44]	418	1	1.2	?	1
Oh[45]	300	1	0.6	2	1.6
Collopy and Ryan[35]	86	15	7	7	15
Marby *et al.*[36]	78	0	0	0	29
Rosenthal[46]	125	Few	Few	0	0.8
Abcarian[47]	150	0	0	0	1.3
Bell[48]	56	?	?	?	1.8
Marya *et al.*[49]	100	0	0	0	2
Vafai and Mann[50]	300	15	0	11	3
Ravikumar *et al.*[51]	60	0	0	5	3.3
Hsu and Mackeigan[52]	89	?	?	?	5.6
Jensen *et al.*[53]	30	0	0	3.3	3.3
Gordon and Vasilevsky[54]	133	2.3	0.8	0	1.5
Gingold[55]	86	0	0	0	3.6
Lewis *et al*[56]	350	17*		2.6	6

*Impaired control for flatus and feces were combined, but only a third of these results were permanent.

Table 4.1: Results of lateral internal sphincterectomy.

gained the greatest favor is the lateral internal sphincterotomy. There are only a few complications that may occur after internal sphincterotomy (Table 4.2).

Advantages of lateral internal sphincterotomy

My own experience, which is similar to what others have reported in the literature, strongly suggests that lateral internal sphincterotomy is a good operation for patients with a chronic fissure-in-ano. It has several definite advantages:

- there is no need for the patient to be hospitalized
- the operation can be performed under local anesthesia
- postoperative discomfort is of short duration and wounds heal quickly
- fecal soiling is not a problem
- recurrence following this mode of therapy is uncommon.

Author	No. of patients	Prolapsed thrombosed hemorrhoids	Hemorrhage	Ecchymoses or hematoma	Perianal abscess	Fistula-in-ano
Hoffmann and Goligher[38]	99	2	1	22	1	1
Millar[39]	99	1	0	6	1	1
Notaras[40]	82	1	0	0	0	0
Clery[41]	217	1	3	0	2	1
Rudd[43]	200	0	3	0	1	0
Marby *et al.*[36]	78	0	1	4	0	1
Rosenthal[46]	125	0	0	5	1	2
Abcarian[47]	150	0	0	0	1	1
Marya *et al.*[49]	100	0	0	5	0	0
Vafai and Mann[50]	300	1	1	5	5	3
Ravikumar *et al.*[51]	60	0	5	3	0	0
Hsu and Mackeigan[52]	89	0	0	0	1	0
Gordon and Vasilevsky[54]	133	1	0	0	0	0
Gingold[55]	86	0	0	0	0	0
Weaver *et al.*[57]	39	0	0	1	0	0
Lewis *et al.*[56]	350	0	0	1	8	4
Total	2207	7 (0.3%)	14 (0.5%)	52 (2.4%)	21 (1%)	14 (0.6%)

Table 4.2: Immediate or early complications of lateral internal sphincterotomy (From Gordon[58], by permission of Quality Medical Publishing, St Louis, MO.)

Thus less time is lost from work and fewer follow-up visits are required. Because of excellent results, and the fact that the procedure can safely and effectively be performed on an outpatient basis, I believe that lateral internal sphincterotomy is the treatment of choice for patients with a chronic anal fissure.

Anorectal suppuration and fistula-in-ano

Introduction

Infection of the anal glands is probably the commonest cause of fistulous abscess[59]. An understanding of the anatomy of the pelvic floor is critical to appreciate the origin and ramifications of abscesses and fistulae. The commonest course for an abscess or fistula to pursue is from the midanal canal downward in the intersphincteric plane to the anal verge. Infection may overcome the barrier of the external sphincter muscles, thereby penetrating the ischioanal fossa, or it may extend upward in the intersphincteric plane either remaining in the rectal wall or extending extrarectally (Figure 4.3).

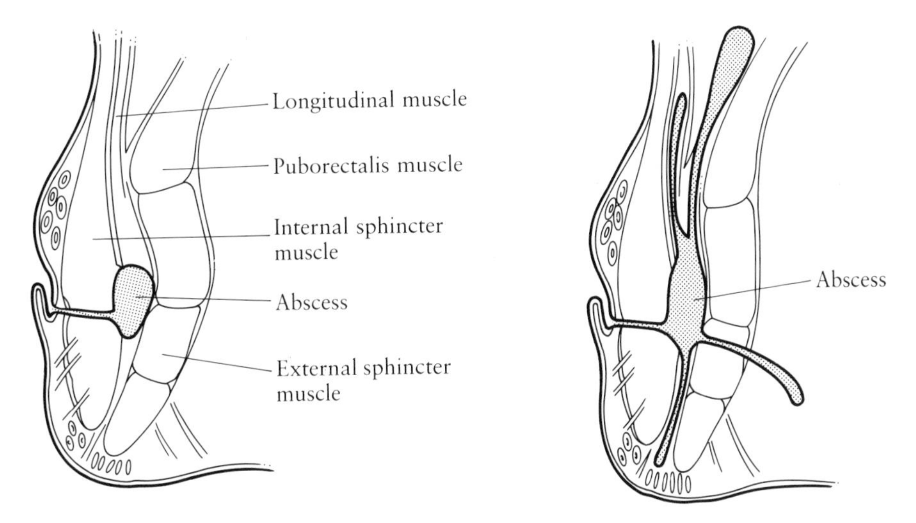

Figure 4.3: Avenues of extension of an abscess or fistula-in-ano.

In addition to tracking upward and downward, pus may pass circumferentially around the anus. This passage can occur in one of three tissue planes, the commonest of which is the ischioanal fossa. This variety commences in the posterior midline of the anal canal, penetrates the sphincter mass and then descends with two limbs, one in each ischioanal fossa. This circumferential spread is referred to as 'horseshoeing'. In addition, circumferential spread may occur in the intersphincteric plane or in the pararectal tissues above the levator muscle.

Management

Acute anorectal suppuration

A simple classification of anorectal suppuration that I have used is as follows:

- perianal
- ischioanal
- intersphincteric
- supralevator.

In a review of 117 consecutive patients with anorectal suppuration seen by the author, the distribution of abscesses encountered was as follows: perianal, 19%; ischioanal, 61%; intersphincteric, 18%; and supralevator, 2%[60]. In a study of the anatomical locations of anorectal suppuration in 506 patients, Prasad and coworkers[61] found the following distribution: perianal, 48%; ischiorectal, 22%; intersphincteric, 12%; supralevator, 9% intermuscular, 5%; submucosal, 4%. The distribution of perianal and ischioanal abscesses reported by the above authors was an almost complete reversal of that seen by Vasilevsky and Gordon[60]. Nevertheless, the vast majority are of the perianal and ischioanal variety.

Abscesses in the anorectal region must be adequately drained. There is no role for antibiotics as the primary form of therapy. Adjunctive antibiotic therapy may be indicated in special circumstances such as in patients with rheumatic or acquired valvular heart disease, those who are immunosuppressed, and diabetic patients with extensive cellulitis.

A simple perianal abscess can almost always be drained under local anesthesia in the office or outpatient department. The skin is usually prepared with an antiseptic solution. At the most tender point, a 2 cm area of skin is anesthesized with 0.5% lignocaine in 1 : 200,000 epinephrine. A cruciate incision is made which will readily allow free drainage of the pus. Skin edges must be excised because, if only an incision is made, edges will readily fall together and seal, and the abscess may recur. In general, no packing is inserted as this only impedes the drainage of pus. Minor bleeding can easily be controlled by electrocoagulation. If cautery is unavailable, packing for a few hours may be necessary to control bleeding (Figure 4.4).

The majority of ischioanal abscesses may also be incised and drained under local anesthesia as an outpatient procedure. Patients with intersphincteric abscesses require a general or regional anesthetic since adequate exposure cannot otherwise be obtained. Treatment consists of laying open the abscesses with division of the fibers of the internal sphincter, from its lower end up to the level of the dentate line, or higher if the cavity extends higher. Patients with supralevator abscesses certainly do not qualify for treatment as minimally invasive as it must first be determined what the etiology of the abscess is prior to treatment. Such an abscess may arise in one of three ways. It may be due to the upward extension of an intersphincteric abscess, or an upward extension of an ischioanal abscess, or it may result from pelvic disease such as perforated diverticulitis, Crohn's disease or appendicitis. Therapy depends on the pre-

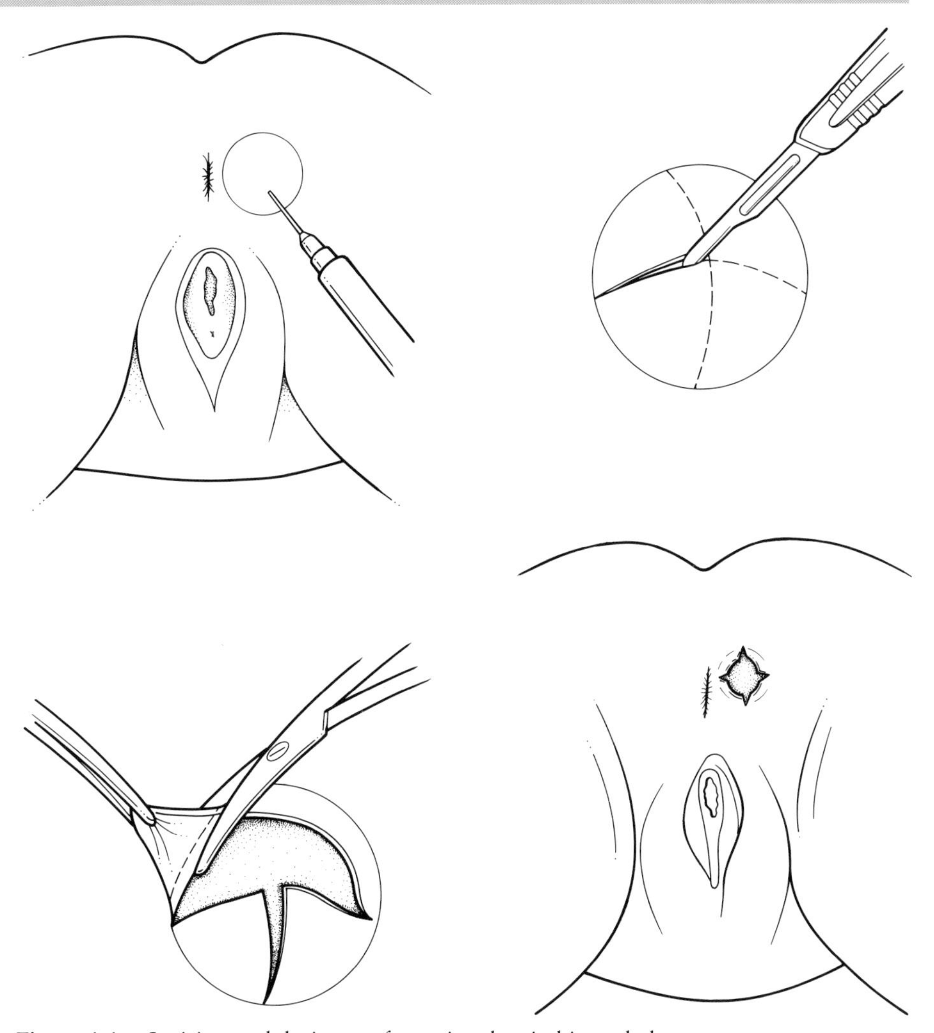

Figure 4.4: Incision and drainage of a perianal or ischioanal abscess.

sumed origin of this abscess. If the supralevator abscess is secondary to an upward extension of an intersphincteric abscess, it should be drained into the rectum by division of the internal sphincter. The cut edges are run with an absorbable suture, such as 3–0 chromic catgut, to control hemostasis. No packing is used. This abscess should not be drained through the ischioanal fossa because a suprasphincteric fistula may result and become a difficult problem to manage. If a supralevator abscess arises secondary to the upward extension of an ischioanal abscess, however, it should be drained through the ischioanal fossa. Attempts at draining this kind of abscess into the rectum will result in an extrasphincteric fistula, making the problem much more difficult to handle. When draining supralevator abscesses of pelvic origin, one must take the original disease into consideration. These abscesses can be drained by three routes: into the rectal lumen, through the ischioanal fossa, or through the abdominal wall. The choice of procedure would seem to depend upon the area to which the abscess points most closely, and the general condition of the patient.

Patients who have had abscesses drained under local anesthesia should be advised to continue a regular diet, to take sitz baths three or four times daily, and to take a stool softener such as a psyllium seed preparation. Analgesics should be prescribed as necessary. These patients should be given a follow-up appointment for one month but advised to return promptly if the pain does not diminish. Patients with intersphincteric abscesses drained under general anesthesia are discharged after they have had their first bowel movement. They are followed up weekly once every two weeks until the wound is completely healed.

Fistula-in-ano

A detailed description of the classification of fistula and the principles in details of operative management are out of the scope of this chapter, but the interested reader is referred to a comprehensive dissertation which has recently been published[58]. However, some patients with a simple intersphincteric or low transsphincteric fistula may be treated with a fistulotomy on an outpatient or short-stay basis.

Results

There is still controversy about whether primary fistulotomy should be employed in the treatment of anorectal abscesses. Those who favor a more conservative approach believe that performing a fistulotomy in the presence of acute inflammation is potentially hazardous. Since a fistulous opening may not be seen, overzealous attempts to find one may result in the creation of a false passage while inadvertently neglecting the true opening, leading to persistent suppuration[62].

The fact that a significant number of patients will not develop fistulas makes primary fistulotomy unnecessary in those cases. Vasilevsky and Gordon[60] found that, following the drainage of anorectal abscesses, 11% of patients developed recurrent abscesses while 37% of patients were left with an anal fistula, giving an overall recurrence or persistence rate of 48%. However, in the subset of patients in that study who were having their abscesses drained for the first time, only 5% developed a recurrent abscess, and 31% went on to develop an anal fistula: thus only 36% of these patients required a definitive operation. It would appear that primary fistulotomy is not necessary, especially for patients with an anorectal abscess who are being treated for the first time. In addition, the majority of perianal and ischioanal abscesses can be drained using local anesthesia, which obviates the need for a general or spinal anesthesia. The use of local anesthetics also removes the temptation to do a fistulotomy. Since 35–65% of patients will never have a further problem, a primary lay-open technique would be unnecessary in these patients[58,63].

Pilonidal disease

Recommendations for the treatment of pilonidal disease have varied considerably. It has always been the author's philosophy that a conservative approach is more than adequate therapy, and consequently treatment of this condition easily qualifies for inclusion in a chapter on minimal access surgery.

Management

Abscess

Drainage of a pilonidal abscess can almost always be done under local anesthesia in the emergency room or outpatient department. A longitudinal incision is made lateral to the midline, as it has been suggested that midline wounds do not heal so well. The abscess cavity is unroofed and hair, if present, is removed. The patient is instructed to clean the wound in the shower or bath twice a day. Office follow-up every one or two weeks is recommended in order to shave the hair around the wound and ensure that healing progresses satisfactorily. Antibiotics are not indicated. A prospective study by Jensen and Harling[53] showed that proper incision and drainage and postoperative care will relieve symptoms in all patients, with a cure rate of 60%.

Chronic pilonidal sinuses

Marsupialization Marsupialization consists of opening the sinus track in the midline and joining secondary multiple tracks if present. The debris and granulation tissues are curetted. The fibrosis in the track is saved and sutured to the edges of the wound. This technique not only minimizes the size and depth of the wound, but also prevents the wound from premature closure. In addition, it is easy to pack and clean the wound (Figure 4.5). In so doing, the size of the wound may be reduced by as much as 50–60%. The wound still takes about six weeks to heal. The procedure is simple and can generally be performed on an outpatient basis[64,65], and consequently it has become my procedure of choice.

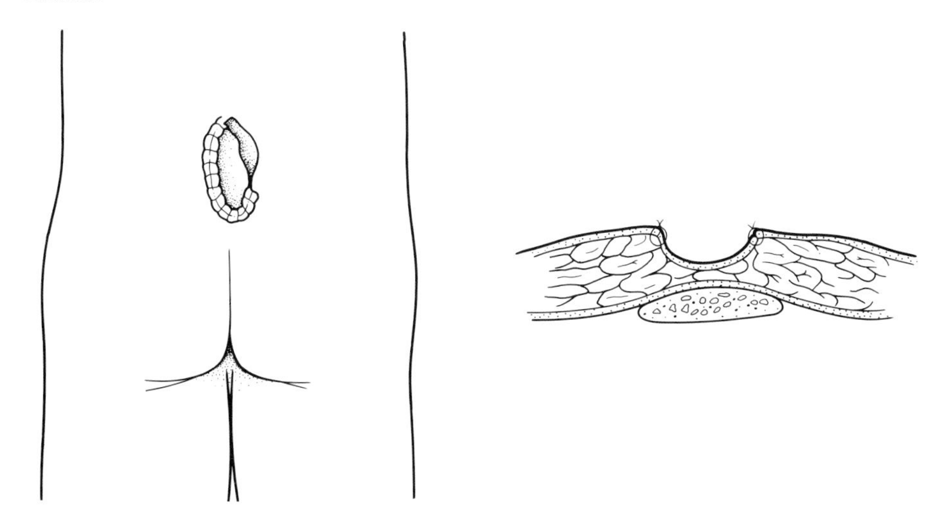

Figure 4.5: Marsupialization. The fibrous track or wall is sutured to the edge of the skin all around with continuous absorbable suture.

Other options Phenol injection into the sinus track has been advocated by some authors who obtained excellent results[66]. The phenol serves to destroy epithelium, sterilize the track and remove the embedded hair. 1–2 mL of 80% phenol are injected, taking great care to protect the patient's skin. The injection can be repeated every four to six weeks as necessary. The region should be kept clean and shaved.

Bascom described a different option for the treatment of pilonidal disease. He emphasizes that midline wounds should be avoided by using a longitudinal incision off the midline to enter the abscess cavity[67]. In a follow-up of 149 patients (mean follow-up 3.5 years, longest nine years), the cure rate was 84%[68]. Advantages of this technique are minimal access approach and the small wounds involved. It can be done on an outpatient basis and total healing is rapid (usually within three weeks).

Wide local excision when performed is carried down to the sacrococcygeal fascia. The wound is kept open with gauze[69]. Some authors advocate a wide local excision with primary closure of the wound to minimize the healing time. In a randomized trial with a three-year follow-up, Kronborg *et al.*[70] found that excision with primary closure of the wound had a shorter healing time than excision with open wound; the recurrence rate varied from 0 to 38%[64]. This radical technique has no advantages over marsupialization and is seldom necessary.

Extensive operations, including excision and z-plasty and the advancing flap operation, have been described but are out of the purview of a chapter on minimal operations[71].

Conclusion

In recent years there has been growing interest in the performance of outpatient procedures. With health costs continuing to rise, physicians, hospitals and third-party carriers are seeking ways to save health care dollars without jeopardizing patient safety. Recommendations for outpatient procedures should be predicated on considerations of the complexity and risks of the procedure, the facilities resources, the availability of quality aftercare, and the physical and emotional state of the patient. The procedures described in this chapter fall within these goals.

References

1 Maimonides M (1969) Treatise on hemorrhoids. (Trans. by Rosner F and Muntner S.) J.B. Lippincott, Philadelphia.

2 Johanson JF and Sonnenberg A (1990) Prevalence of hemorrhoids and chronic constipation. An epidemiologic study. *Gastroent.* **98**:380–6.

3 Moesgaard F, Nielsen ML, Hansen JB *et al.* (1982) High fiber diet reduces bleeding and pain in patients with hemorrhoids. *Dis Colon Rectum.* **25**:454–6.

4 Senapati A and Nicholls RJ (1988) Randomized trial to compare the results of injection sclerotherapy with a bulk laxative alone in the treatment of bleeding hemorrhoids. *Int J Colorect Dis.* **3**:124–6.

5 Barron J (1963) Office ligation treatment of hemorrhoids. *Dis Colon Rectum.* **6**:109–13.

6 Wroblewski DE, Corman ML, Veidenheimer MC *et al.* (1980) Long-term evaluation of rubber ring ligation in hemorrhoidal disease. *Dis Colon Rectum.* **23**: 478–82.

7 Lau WY, Chow HP, Poon GP *et al.* (1982) Rubber band ligation of three primary hemorrhoids in a single session. A safe and effective procedure. *Dis Colon Rectum.* **25**: 336–9.

8 Jensen SL, Harling H, Arseth P *et al.* (1989) The natural history of symptomatic hemorrhoids. *Int J Colorect Dis.* **4**:41–4.

9 Marshman D, Huber PJ Jr, Timmerman W *et al.* (1989) Hemorrhoid ligation. A review of efficacy. *Dis Colon Rectum.* **32**:369–71.

10 Nivatvongs S and Goldberg SM (1982) An improved technique of rubber band ligation of hemorrhoids. *Am J Surg.* **144**:379–80.

11 O'Hara VS (1980) Fatal clostridial infection following hemorrhoidal banding. *Dis Colon Rectum.* **23**:570–1.

12 Russell TR and Donohue JH (1985) Hemorrhoidal banding: a warning. *Dis Colon Rectum.* **28**:291–3.

13 Shemesh EI, Kodner IJ, Fry RD *et al.* (1987) Severe complications of rubber band ligation of internal hemorrhoids. *Dis Colon Rectum.* **30**:199–200.

14 Quevedo-Bonilla G, Farkas AM, Abcarian H *et al.* (1988) Septic complications of hemorrhoidal banding. *Arch Surg.* **123**:650–1.

15 Scarpa FJ, Hillis W and Sabetta JR (1988) Pelvic cellulitis: a life-threatening complication of hemorrhoidal banding. *Surgery.* **103**:838–5.

16 Templeton JL, Spence RAJ, Kennedy TL *et* al. (1983) Comparison of infrared coagulation and rubber band ligation for first- and second-degree hemorrhoids: a randomized prospective clinical trial. *Br Med J.* **286**:1387–9.

17 Ambrose NS, Morris D, Alexander-Williams J *et al.* (1985) A randomized trial of photocoagulation or injection sclerotherapy for the treatment of first- and second-degree hemorrhoids. *Dis Colon Rectum.* **28**:238–40.

18 Hinton CP and Morris DL (1990) A randomized trial comparing direct current therapy and bipolar diathermy in the outpatient treatment of third-degree hemorrhoids. *Dis Colon Rectum*. **33**:931–2.

19 Lord PH (1972) A new approach to hemorrhoids. *Progr Surg*. **10**:109–24.

20 Lewis AAM, Rogers HS and Leighton M (1983) Trial of maximal anal dilatation, cryotherapy, and elastic band ligation as alternatives to hemorrhoidectomy in the treatment of large prolapsing hemorrhoids. *Br J Surg*. **70**:54–6.

21 Smith LE (1992) Hemorrhoidectomy with lasers and other contemporary modalities. *SCNA*. **72**:665–79.

22 Smith LE, Goodreau JJ and Fouty WJ (1979) Operative hemorrhoidectomy versus cryodestruction. *Dis Colon Rectum*. **22**:10–16.

23 Allgower M (1975) Conservative management of hemorrhoids. Part III: partial internal sphincterotomy. *Clin Gastroenterol*. **4**:608–18.

24 Schouten WR and van Vroonhoven TJ (1986) Lateral internal sphincterotomy in the treatment of hemorrhoids. A clinical and manometric study. *Dis Colon Rectum*. **29**:869–72.

25 De-Roover DM, Hoofwijk AG and van Vroonhoven T J (1989) Lateral internal sphincterotomy in the treatment of fourth-degree hemorrhoids. *Br J Surg*. **76**:1181–3.

26 Nothmann BJ and Schuster MM (1974) Internal anal sphincter derangement with anal fissures. *Gastroent*. **67**:216–20.

27 Abcarian H, Lakshmanan S, Read DR *et al*. (1982) The role of internal sphincter in chronic anal fissures. *Dis Colon Rectum*. **25**: 525–8.

28 Chowcat NL, Araujo JGC and Boulos PB (1986) Internal sphincterotomy for chronic anal fissure: long term effects on anal pressure. *Br J Surg*. **73**:915–16.

29 Dodi G, Bogoni F, Infantino A *et al*. (1986) Hot or cold in anal pain? A study of the changes in internal anal sphincter pressure profiles. *Dis Colon Rectum*. **29**:248–51.

30 Jensen SL (1987) Maintenance therapy with unprocessed bran in the prevention of acute anal fissure recurrence. *J Roy Soc Med*. **80**:296–8.

31 Parks AG (1967) The management of fissure-in-ano. *Hosp Med*. **1**:737–8

32 Samson RB and Stewart WRC (1970) Sliding skin grafts in the treatment of anal fissure. *Dis Colon Rectum*. **13**:372–5.

33 Watts JM, Bennett RC and Goligher JC (1964) Stretching of anal sphincters in treatment of fissure-in-ano. *Br Med J.* **2**:342–3.

34 Hawley PR (1969) The treatment of chronic fissure-in-ano: a trial of methods. *Br J Surg.* **56**:915–18.

35 Collopy B and Ryan P (1979) Comparison of lateral subcutaneous sphincterotomy with anal dilatation in the treatment of fissure-in-ano. *Med J Aust.* **2**:461–2, 487.

36 Marby M, Alexander-Williams J, Buchmann P *et al.* (1979) A randomized controlled trial to compare anal dilatation with lateral subcutaneous sphincterotomy for anal fissure. *Dis Colon Rectum.* **22**:308–11.

37 Jensen SL, Lund F, Nielson OV *et al.* (1984) Lateral subcutaneous sphincterotomy vs anal dilatation in the treatment of fissure-in-ano in outpatients: a prospective randomized study. *Br. Med J.* **289**:528–30.

38 Hoffmann DC and Goligher JC (1970) Lateral subcutaneous internal sphincterotomy in treatment of anal fissure. *Br Med J.* **3**:673–5.

39 Millar DM (1971) Subcutaneous lateral internal anal sphincterotomy for anal fissure. *Br J Surg.* **58**:737–9.

40 Notaras MJ (1971) The treatment of anal fissure by lateral subcutaneous internal sphincterotomy – a technique and results. *Br J Surg.* **58**:96–100.

41 Clery AP (1975) Subcutaneous lateral internal anal sphincterotomy for fissure. A report on 217 cases. *J Irish Med Assoc.* **68**:482–5.

42 Hunter A (1975) Lateral subcutaneous anal sphincterotomy. *Dis Colon Rectum.* **18**:665–8.

43 Rudd WH (1975) Lateral subcutaneous internal sphincterotomy for chronic anal fissure; an outpatient procedure. *Dis Colon Rectum* **18**:319–23.

44 Bailey R, Rubin R and Salvati E (1978) Lateral internal sphincterotomy. *Dis Colon Rectum.* **21**:584–6.

45 Oh C (1978) A modified technique for lateral internal sphincterotomy. *Surg Gynecol Obstet.* **146**:623–5.

46 Rosenthal D (1979) Fissure-in-ano. Management in the military community. *Milit Med.* **144**:505–8.

47 Abcarian H (1980) Surgical correction of chronic anal fissure: results of lateral anal internal sphincterotomy vs fissurectomy – midline sphincterotomy. *Dis Colon Rectum.* **23**:31–6.

48 Bell GA (1980) Lateral internal sphincterotomy in chronic anal fissure – a surgical technique. *Am Surg.* **46**:572–5.

49 Marya SK, Mittal SS and Singla S (1980) Lateral subcutaneous internal sphincterotomy for acute fissure-in-ano. *Br J Surg.* **67**:299.

50 Vafai M and Mann CV (1981) Closed lateral internal sphincterotomy without removal of sentinel pile for fissure-in-ano. *Coloproctology.* **3**:91–3.

51 Ravikumar TS, Sridhar S and Rao RN (1982) Subcutaneous lateral internal sphincterotomy for chronic fissure-in-ano. *Dis Colon Rectum.* **25**:798–801.

52 Hsu TC and Mackeigan JM (1984) Surgical treatment of chronic anal fissure. *Dis Colon Rectum.* **27**:475–8.

53 Jensen SL and Harling H (1988) Prognosis after simple incision and drainage for a first-episode acute pilonidal abscess. *Br J Surg.* **75**:60–1.

54 Gordon PH and Vasilevsky CA (1985) Lateral internal sphincterotomy: rationale, technique and anesthesia. *Can J Surg.* **28**:28–30.

55 Gingold BS (1987) Simple in-office sphincterotomy with partial fissurectomy for chronic anal fissure. *Surg Gynecol Obstet.* **165**:46–8.

56 Lewis TH, Corman ML, Prager ED *et al.* (1988) Long-term results of open and closed sphincterotomy for anal fissure. *Dis Colon Rectum.* **31**:368–71.

57 Weaver RM, Ambrose NS, Alexander-Williams J *et al.* (1987) Manual dilatation of the anus vs lateral subcutaneous sphincterotomy in the treatment of chronic fissure-in-ano. Results of the prospective randomized clinical trial. *Dis Colon Rectum.* **30**:420–3.

58 Gordon PH (1992) Anorectal abscesses and fistula-in-ano. In: Gordon PH and Nivatvongs S. (eds) *Principles and Practice of Surgery for the Colon, Rectum, and Anus.* Quality Medical Publishing, St Louis, MO. pp. 221–65.

59 Parks AG (1961) Pathogenesis and treatment of fistula-in-ano. *Br Med J.* **1**:463–9.

60 Vasilevsky CA and Gordon P H (1984) The incidence of recurrent abscess or fistula-in-ano following anorectal suppuration. *Dis Colon Rectum.* **27**:126–30.

61 Prasad ML, Read DR and Abcarian H (1981) Supralevator abscesses; diagnosis and treatment. *Dis Colon Rectum.* **24**:456–61.

62 Lockhart-Mummary HE (1975) Treatment of abscesses. *Dis Colon Rectum.* **18**:650–1.

63 Sainio P (1984) Fistula-in-ano in a defined population; incidence and epidemiological aspects. *Ann Chir Gynaecol.* **73**:219–24.

64 Duchateau J, De Mol J, Bostoen H *et al.* (1985) Pilonidal sinus. Excision – marsupialization – phenolization? *Acta Chir Belg.* **85**:325–8.

65 Bissett IP and Isbister WH (1987) The management of patients with pilonidal disease – a comparative study. *Aust NZ J Surg.* **57**:939–42.

66 Hegge HGJ, Vos GA, Patka P *et al.* (1987) Treatment of complicated or infected pilonidal sinus disease by local application of phenol. *Surgery.* **102**:52–4.

67 Bascom J (1980) Pilonidal disease: Origin from follicles of hairs and results of follicle removal as treatment. *Surgery.* **87**:567–72.

68 Bascom J (1983) Pilonidal disease: Long-term results of follicle removal. *Dis Colon Rectum.* **26**:800–7.

69 Eftaiha M and Abcarian H (1977) The dilemma of pilonidal disease: Surgical treatment. *Dis Colon Rectum.* **20**:279–86.

70 Kronborg O, Christensen K and Zimmermann-Nielsen C (1985) Chronic pilonidal disease: a randomized trial with a complete three-year follow-up. *Br J Surg.* **72**:303–4.

71 Nivatvongs S (1992) Pilonidal disease. In: Gordon PH and Nivatvongs S *Principles and Practice of Surgery for the Colon, Rectum, and Anus.* Quality Medical Publishing, St Louis, MO. pp. 267–79.

5

Management of Rectal Prolapse, Incontinence and Rectocele

SANTHAT NIVATVONGS

Management of rectal prolapse

Rectal prolapse is one of the most challenging problems in surgery. While it is not life-threatening, the soiling and obstructive defecation which it brings about are extremely incapacitating. Since the etiology of rectal prolapse is often unknown, it is not surprising that it is difficult to treat. Whatever technique is performed, however, rectal prolapse can be relieved (at least temporarily) and there are more than 150 procedures available to alleviate it.

The standard approaches have been transabdominal, such as with rectosigmoid colon resection (with or without rectopexy) and the sling operations. Both techniques give good long-term results with acceptable morbidity and mortality. However, the operations are major and suitable only for patients in good health. There are now other procedures that are suitable for most patients with rectal prolapse, even the very old and sick. In order to put these operations into perspective, a number of approaches will be discussed.

Transperineal repair

All patients with rectal prolapse require at least a proctosigmoidoscopy to rule out neoplasm which may be present. High-risk patients, such as the elderly or those with a personal or family history of cancer, should have a complete colonic investigation, ideally with colonoscopy. Barium enema should be used with caution since it may cause strangulation due to difficulty evacuating the barium.

A mechanical bowel preparation along with oral or systemic antibiotics, as for a colon resection, should be instituted.

Transperineal rectosigmoidectomy

This procedure was first described by Auffret of Paris in 1882[1], when he encountered a patient with rectal prolapse which progressed to strangulation. He was forced to excise the prolapse which measured 70 cm in length. Although the patient died the next day, his description lived on. In 1933, Miles of London[2] reported his experience of transperineal rectosigmoidectomy in 31 patients; there was one death and one recurrence five years after the operation. This operation gained popularity, particularly at St Mark's Hospital in London. However, enthusiasm faded when subsequent studies showed a recurrence rate of 27% in the first year and as high as 50% after three years of follow-up. In 1971 the excellent results of Altemeier and colleagues[3] stimulated the enthusiasm for this procedure in the USA. Over a 19-year period, there were only three recurrences in their series of 106 consecutive patients with rectal prolapse.

Technique This technique is suitable for an overt rectal prolapse that protrudes at least 3 cm from the anal verge. The lithotomy or prone position can be used. A Foley catheter is placed into the bladder before the operation. Endotracheal general anesthesia is preferred but a spinal, caudal, or, if necessary, local anesthesia can also be employed.

After the anorectum has been thoroughly irrigated with dilute povidone–iodine (Betadine) solution, the prolapse is pulled down to its maximum using Babcock clamps. The dentate line is easily recognized by its distinct anoderm. A circular incision is made 2 cm proximal to the dentate line (Figure 5.1**a**), using electrocautery (coagulation current). The incision cuts through the mucosa, submucosa, muscle and serosa of the everted rectum. The serosal layer

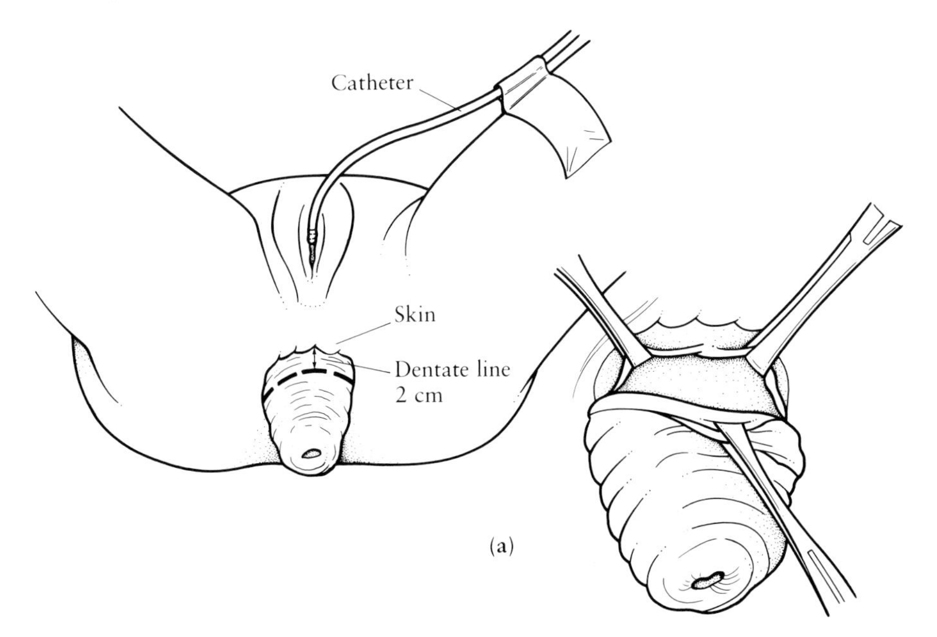

Figure 5.1: Transperineal rectosigmoidectomy. (**a**) A circular incision is made on the prolapsed rectum 2 cm proximal to the dentate line.

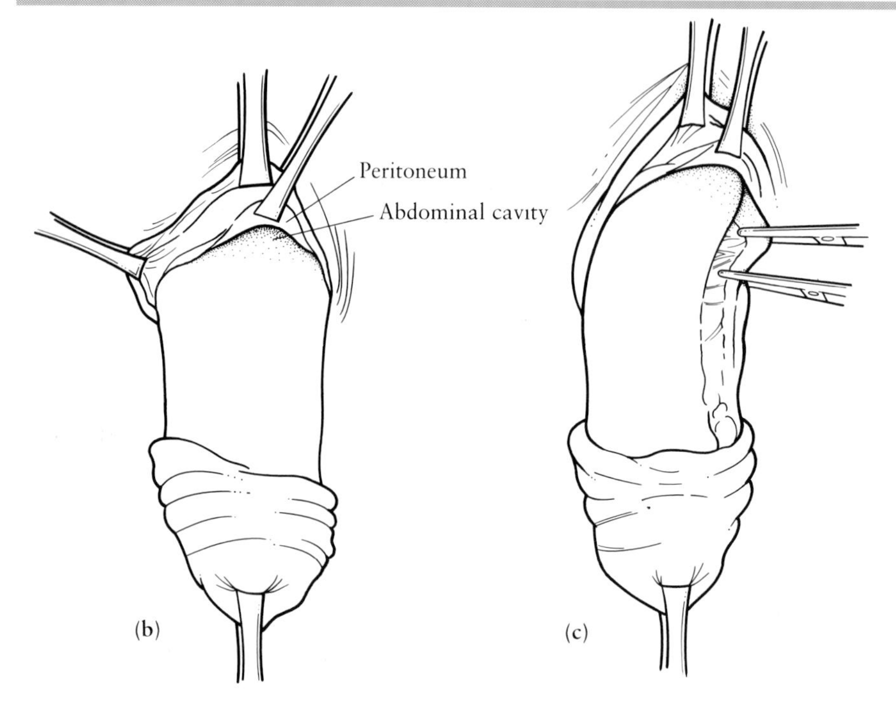

Figure 5.1: *continued* (**b**) The peritoneal attachment is dissected from the anterior rectal wall and opened into the peritoneal cavity. (**c**) The mesorectum or mesosigmoid is clamped and divided laterally and posteriorly.

of the inner rectal tube is now exposed. It is dissected free from the surrounding tissues. At this point, the anterior peritoneal attachment is dissected from the rectum and is cut open thereby entering the abdominal cavity (Figure 5.1**b**). With the patient in slight Trendelenburg position, the small bowel will fall back into the abdominal cavity. The attachment here is the mesorectum, and higher up the mesocolon of the sigmoid laterally and posteriorly. It is clamped, divided, and tied with 2–0 or 3–0 chromic catgut (Figure 5.1**c**). Other flimsy attachments can be cut with scissors or using electrocautery. The dissection is carried on until the rectal tube no longer comes down and there is no slack of the sigmoid colon; this can be determined by palpating with the index finger. Care must be taken not to cut the mesorectum or the sigmoid mesocolon too far proximal from the anal verge, otherwise the blood supply to the anastomotic line will not be sufficient. The previously cut anterior peritoneum is now sutured to the anterior wall of the rectum or sigmoid colon, using running 3–0 chromic catgut (Figure 5.1**d**). If the patient has good anal continence, a sphincter repair is unnecessary. On the other hand, if the patient has fecal incontinence, it is reasonable to approximate the puborectalis and external sphincter using 3–0 Vicryl or Dexon sutures (Figure 5.1**e**). The rectal tube or the sigmoid colon is transected at the level of the anal verge (Figure 5.1**f**). This is then anastomosed to the distal cut end in the anus, using running 3–0 Vicryl of Dexon sutures (Figure 5.1**g–i**). No drain or packing is required.

Williams[4] reported a recurrence rate of 10% which developed three to 48 months after surgery, among 114 patients but the length of follow-up was not

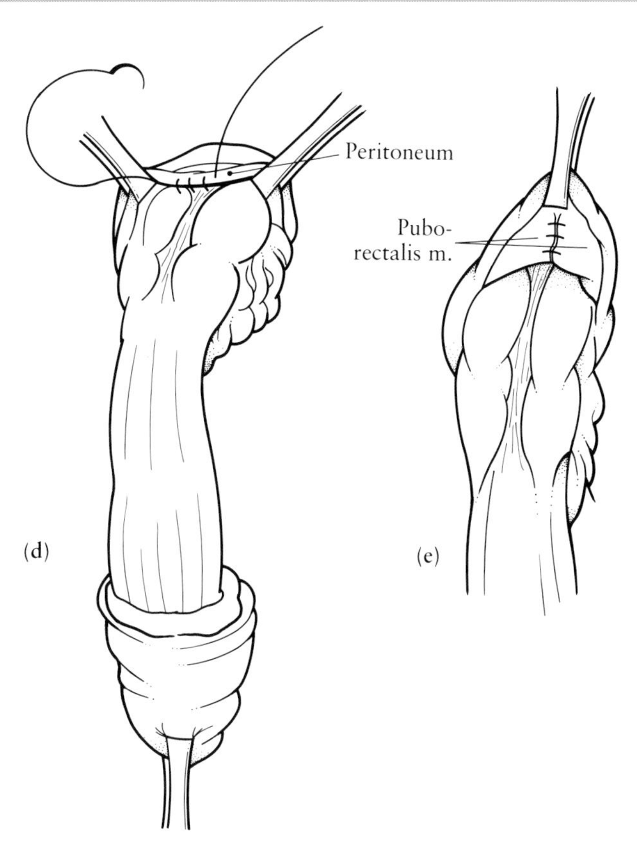

Figure 5.1: *continued* (**d**) The previously opened peritoneum is sutured to the anterior wall of rectum or sigmoid colon as high as possible. (**e**) Approximation of puborectalis.

stated and there was no mortality. Complications developed in 12%, mostly medical in nature. Most other series also showed consistently low morbidity and mortality rates; however, the long-term follow-up data for recurrences were lacking[5,6].

Anorectal mucosectomy and plication of anorectum (modified Delorme's procedure)

In 1900, Delorme[7] described a technique of repair of rectal prolapse by peeling the mucosa and submucosa of the prolapsed rectum all around, from a point just proximal to the dentate line to the end of the prolapse. The denuded rectal wall was then plicated to shorten the anorectum, resulting in reduction of the prolapse into the anal canal. This operation has never become popular, although during the past two decades there have been sporadic reports of Delorme's procedure (with some modifications) being used as a primary treatment for complete rectal prolapse.

Uhlig and Sullivan[8] and Berman and colleagues[9] applied Delorme's concept of shortening the rectum with mucosectomy and plication but modified the technique from extraanal to intraanal mucosectomy. The technique described here is a further modification of the intraanorectal mucosectomy and plication

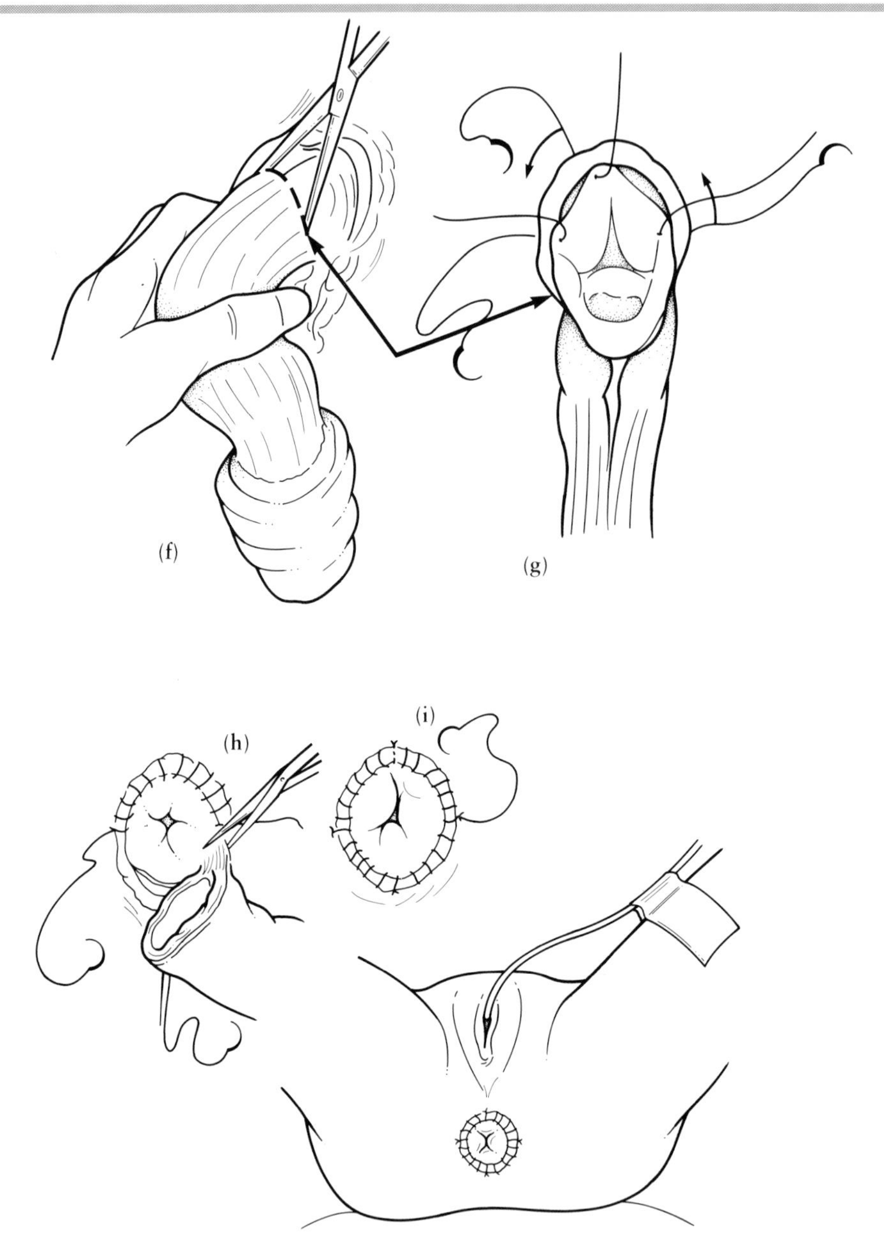

Figure 5.1: *continued* (**f**) Anterior wall of the protruding rectum is cut 1 cm distal to the anal verge. (**g**) Stay sutures of 3–0 Vicryl or Dexon are placed in four quadrants. (**h,i**) Anastomosis using running 3–0 Vicryl or Dexon. (Reproduced from Nivatvongs 1991[10], by permission.)

to simplify the procedure[10]. This technique is suitable for rectal prolapse that protrudes to the anus, but not through it more than 3 cm.

Technique A Foley catheter is inserted into the bladder before turning the patient to the prone position. The anorectum is thoroughly irrigated with dilute povidone–iodine solution. The anal canal is injected submucosally all around using 0.25% bupivacaine (Marcaine) containing 1 : 200,000 epinephrine to decrease bleeding. A Pratt anal speculum is inserted into the anal canal for exposure. Using electrocautery (coagulation current) or scissors, the mucosa and submucosa 1 cm above the dentate line is cut circumferentially (Figure 5.2**a**). The submucosal tube is dissected from the underlying internal sphincter and carried up to the anorectal ring. The Pratt anal speculum is removed and two Gelpi retractors are placed at the dentate line at right angles to each other (Figure 5.2**b**). In patients with deep buttocks, a Lone Star self-retaining hook retractor (Lone Star Medical Products, Houston, Texas) is most useful. This allows the submucosal tube and the rectum to prolapse so that the proximal dissection can be carried out. A small Richardson retractor or a right angle retractor should be available to facilitate the exposure. The dissection is carried out proximally until the rectum no longer comes down and feels tight on traction.

At this point, the submucosal tube is transected at its upper part (Figure 5.2**c**). Usually the dissection can go up to 10–15 cm from the anal verge. A Pratt anal speculum is again inserted into the anal canal to expose the upper cut end of the mucosa. A stitch of 3–0 Vicryl or Dexon is placed at the upper end as the first bite. In subsequent bites, the denuded muscle wall of the rectum is taken in a left–right fashion (Figure 5.2**d**) until the last bite takes the distal cut end just above the dentate line. Eight such stitches are placed and tied, resulting in an anastomosis between the upper and the lower cut ends. Additional sutures are placed to complete the anastomosis. At completion, the prolapsed rectum is shortened by its pleated wall (Figure 5.2**e**). No packing is placed in the anorectum.

The morbidity and mortality rates have been consistently low and the recurrence rate was 0–17% in the short- and intermediate-term follow-up times[11–14].

Encirclement of anus

A simple palliative procedure for rectal prolapse, first described by Thiersch in 1891[15] involves encirclement of the anal orifice with a silver wire. This procedure was plagued with complications, however, especially fecal impaction, infection, pain and wire breakage. Although the original Thiersch operation has now been abandoned by most surgeons, its concept has remained in a modified form, using a silastic sheet or a Marlex mesh.

One must keep in mind that encirclement of the anus does not remove the prolapse and should be reserved for facilitating general care and hygiene in very sick patients.

Technique The procedure can be performed under local anesthesia. The patient is placed in the prone-jackknife or lithotomy position. Perianal incisions 2 cm long are made in the left posterior and right anterior quadrants about 2–3 cm from the anal verge (Figure 5.3**a**). A subcutaneous tunnel lateral to the external sphincter muscle is created around the anal canal. A strip of silastic

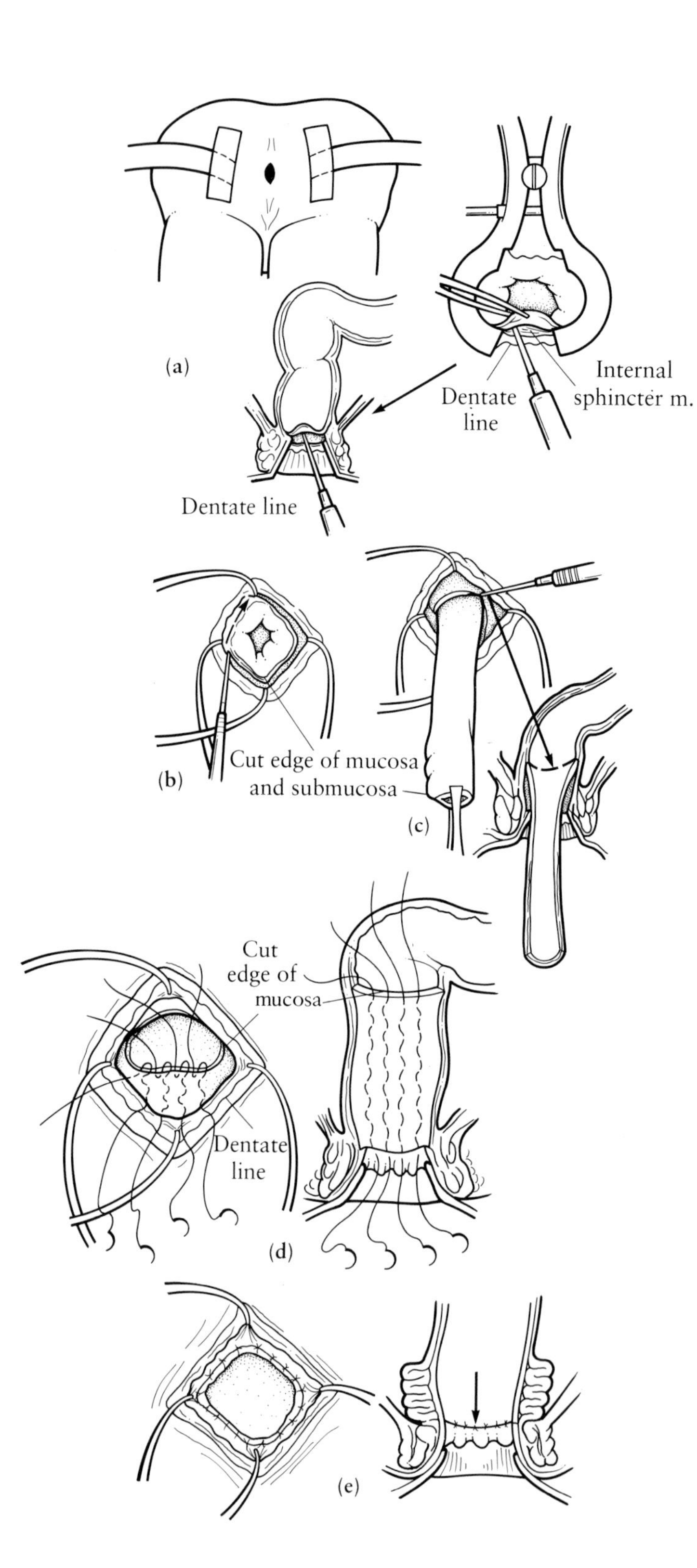

Figure 5.2: Modified Delorme procedure. (**a**) Patient is placed in prone position. Using a Pratt speculum for exposure, a circumferential incision is made 1 cm proximal to the dentate line. The submucosa is dissected from the underlying internal sphincter. (**b**) At the level of anorectal ring, the Pratt speculum is replaced by Gelpi retractors placed at right angle at the dentate line. (**c**) The dissection is carried proximally until the submucosal tube resists the pulling down. It is then cut. (**d**) Using 3–0 Vicryl or Dexon sutures, the mucosa and submucosa at the upper cut end is brought down to the lower cut end, taking along the denuded anorectal wall. Eight such sutures are placed all around. (**e**) At completion of the anastomosis, the anorectum is plicated. (Reproduced from Nivatvongs 1991[10], by permission.)

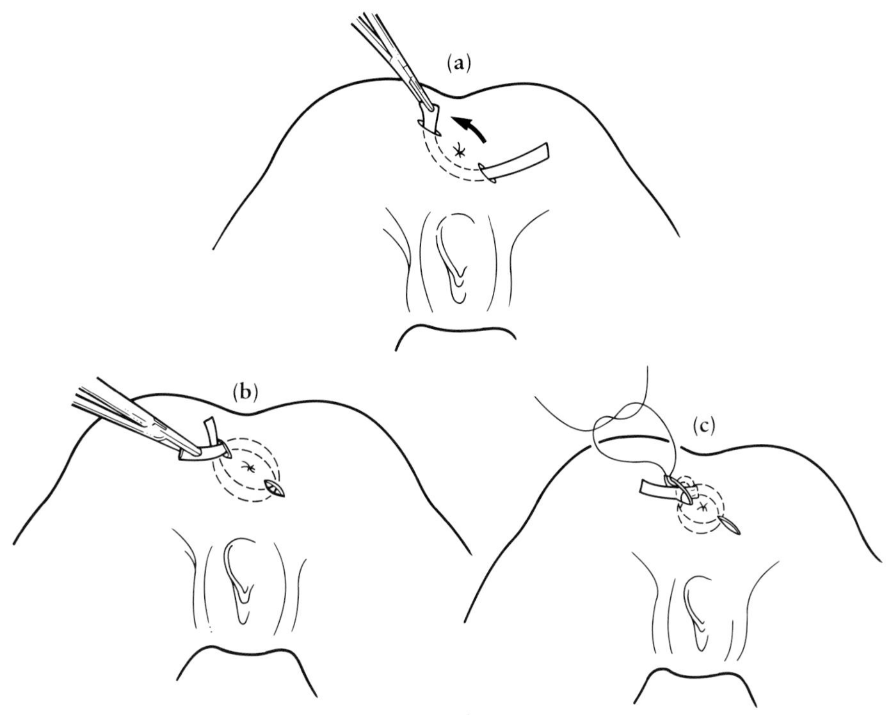

Figure 5.3: Encirclement of anus. (**a**) Incisions are made and subcutaneous tunnel created around the anal canal. (**b**) A strip of silastic sheet placed around the anal canal. (**c**) The silastic sheet is tightened and the ends sutured or stapled. (From Labow *et al.* 1980[46], by permission.)

sheet, 1.5 cm wide and 15 cm long, is inserted and encircled around the anus until it is snug to the base of the index finger (Figure 5.3**b**). The ends of the sheet are sutured together or stapled (Figure 5.3**c**).

Laparoscopic rectopexy and laparoscopic rectosigmoid colon resection

Although laparoscopic cholecystectomy has become the procedure of choice for cholelithiasis, laparoscopic colectomy still has to find its place in the treatment of diseases of the colon and rectum. It has been shown that laparoscopic colectomy with intra- and extracorporeal anastomosis is feasible, with reasonable morbidity and mortality[16,17].

Berman[18] reported a case of laparoscopic rectopexy for rectal prolapse. He secured the mesh to the sacrum with a thumb-tack, and sewed the sling to the rectal wall with a stapler.

Technique

Berman[18] used four 12 mm laparoscopic ports (placed at the suprapubic, bilateral abdominal and supraumbilical positions) in addition to the central umbilical camera port. The sigmoid colon and the rectum were mobilized with coagulation scissors. The rectum was mobilized all the way to the levator ani muscle. The lateral stalks were divided with electrocautery. A strip of Marlex mesh, approximately 4 × 10 cm, was rolled up and introduced into the abdomen through the suprapubic port. The Marlex mesh was secured to the sacrum below the promontory with a specially made laparoscopic sacral tacker (Figure 5.4**a**). Because this is an unsuitable angle to place the thumb-tack, Berman used a 12 cm vaginal trocar which allowed excellent perpendicular alignment of the tacker. The tack should be placed in the midportion of the sacrum. The rectum is now held on lightly with Babcock forceps, and the mesh is secured to the rectal wall using a stapler or sutures (Figure 5.4**b**). Simple sutured rectopexy and mesh repairs with sutures may also be performed.

Whether laparoscopic rectopexy is appropriate for rectal prolapse remains to be seen. Its efficacy must be judged against the less invasive and less complicated perineal rectosigmoidectomy and Delorme procedures. As stated by Thorson and colleagues 'the mere feasibility of laparoscopic colon and rectal surgery does not necessarily equate with appropriateness of the decision to use the technique'[17].

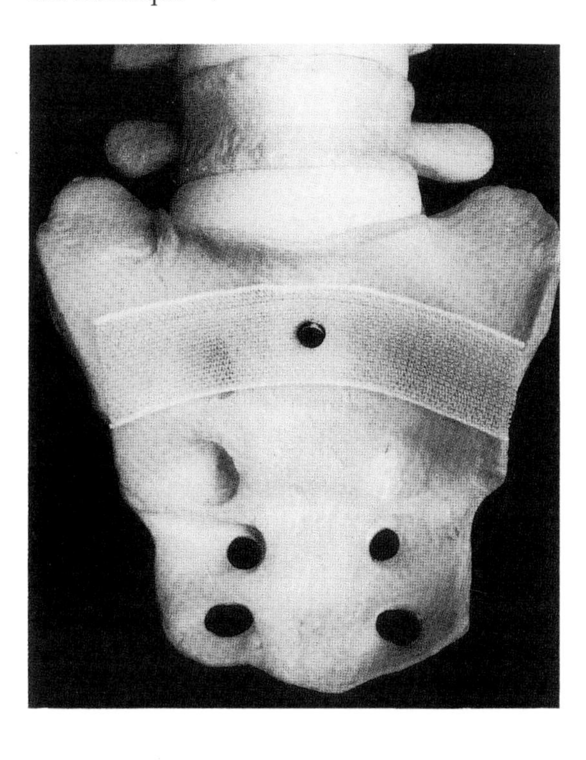

Figure 5.4: Laparoscopic rectopexy. (**a**) Model showing mesh fixation by titanium tack below the sacral promontory.

Management of anal incontinence

Anal continence relies on a complex mechanism incorporating the anorectum, pelvic floor muscles and the external sphincter, which prevents the anorectal content from leaking or premature evacuation until a desired time. Its real and complete mechanism is poorly understood. Surgical procedures can improve

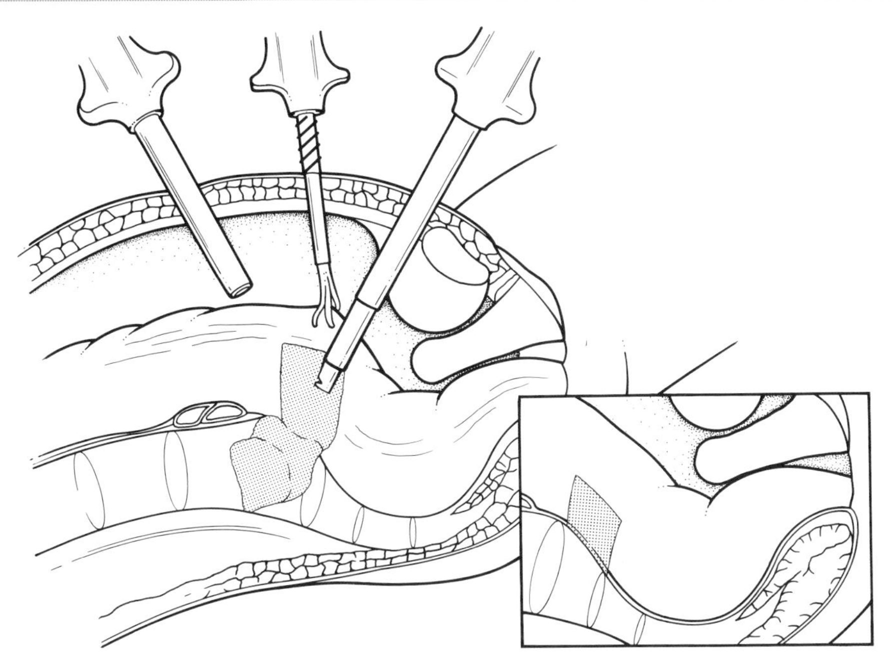

Figure 5.4: *continued* (**b**) The mesh is secured to the rectum by sutures or staples. (Reproduced from Berman 1992[18] by permission.)

anatomic deviations but may not enhance the physiologic deficiency. It is obvious, then, that surgical treatment should not be performed in every patient with anal incontinence. This chapter will deal only with those procedures that are of practical value to these patients.

Patient selection is the most important factor for success. Patients who are incontinent for gas, or who leak mucus or liquid stool, are not candidates for surgical treatment. Patients with incontinence associated with irritable bowel syndrome should not undergo surgical treatment until the irritable bowel has been resolved. Urgency of defecation, such as in patients after anterior rectal resection, must not be confused with anal incontinence.

In most patients, history-taking and a simple physical examination will give enough information to determine thè diagnosis, the severity of the problem and the decision as to what treatment should be instituted. There is an extensive list of physiologic tests for anal incontinence; although they may be of academic interest, they seldom change the decision about treatment or type of surgery. They include anorectal manometry, defecography, the 'enema challenge', electromyography, rectal compliance, and pudendal nerve terminal motor latency (PNTML). PNTML is used to assess the distal motor innervation of the pelvic floor muscle, and hence its degree of damage. This test may help to predict the outcome of surgery. It has been suggested that accompanying nerve damage to the pelvic floor muscle is a factor in the poor results of some sphincter repairs in patients with anal incontinence[19,20]. This pudendal nerve injury is often a result of childbirth but may not become manifest for many years.

Non-operative treatment

Medical treatment

Unless a patient has diarrhea, medications such as loperamide, diphenoxylate hydrochloride and codeine do not help, and the same is true of long-term use of anticholenergic agents. Certain foods that are known to firm the stool, such as bananas, rice, apple sauce and toast should be encouraged. Increasing bulk in diet may help the rectum to be better evacuated and to remain empty for the rest of the day. Similarly, a suppository helps to empty the rectum and diminish the chance of episodes of incontinence.

Biofeedback training

The aims of biofeedback are to improve anorectal sensation and to increase the strength of the external sphincter contraction. The basic training consists of a balloon inserted into the rectosigmoid area which is momentarily inflated (simulating the arrival of stool). The patient receives instantaneous feedback of sphincteric responses by viewing a polygraph. The instructor gives verbal reinforcement when correct responses are made, and tells the patient when the responses are wrong. The instructor periodically withholds the visual feedback to help the patient become independent of the apparatus. The advantages of biofeedback are the noninvasive nature of the procedure and the fact that it can be performed on an outpatient basis. The disadvantages are that it requires high motivation and the patient's full cooperation in responding to the cues and signals. It is time-consuming and may require up to 12 half-hour sessions[21]. Once the patient has learned the technique of contraction, he should continue to practice at home and whenever the sensation of intestinal distension and the urge to defecate is felt. A small portable anorectal biofeedback system and anorectal probe are available (Figure 5.5)

MacLeod[22] reported on 113 patients with anal incontinence in whom conventional sphincter exercises had been ineffective. They were treated by biofeedback: 89 in the office and 24 in the hospital rehabilitation department. They had an average of slightly over three one-hour sessions. They were followed up for six months or five years. 63% had either complete recovery of continence or at least a 90% decrease in the frequency of incontinence. When 13 cases of 'keyhole' deformity were excluded, the success rate rose to 71%. In this series, biofeedback was most effective in postobstetric and postoperative cases. It was less effective in those of neurologic origin and those caused by rectal prolapse. A success rate of 86% was obtained by Riboli and coworkers[21] in 21 cases (15 were secondary to surgical trauma and six were caused by old age). They also found that after successful biofeedback, the sensitivity of the rectum to endoluminal distension improved more than the external sphincter contraction. At the University of Minnesota, 44 patients completed treatment[23]; 30 of them, on self-assessment, felt that they had improved 100%. Forty of them experienced a 90% or greater reduction in the frequency of episodes of fecal incontinence. The improvement in continence appeared to be sustained. Relapse rates of 0–8% were reported, with follow-up periods of between six months and nine years.

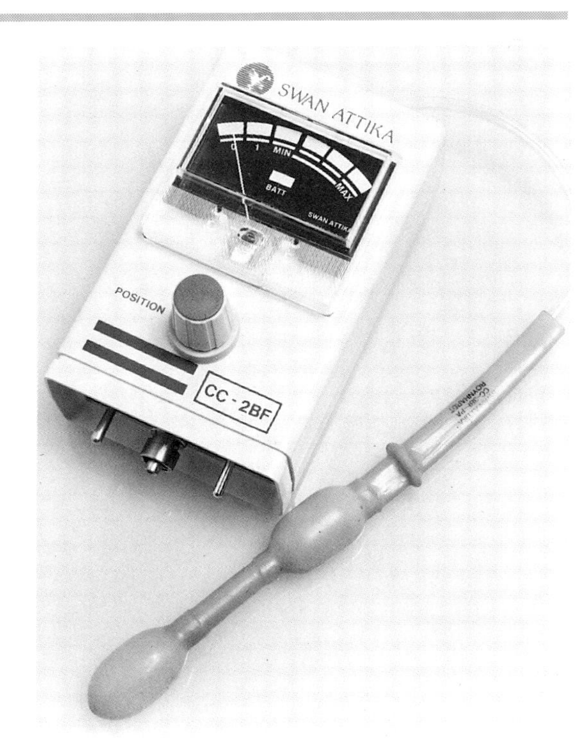

Figure 5.5: Swan Attika biofeedback system. (Courtesy of Biocare International, Wantagh, NY.)

Operative procedures

The patient should be prepared as for colon resection, ie with mechanical bowel preparation with oral or systemic antibiotics. In general, a diverting colostomy is not necessary. Immediately before the operation, a urinary catheter should be put in position and left there until wound pain has become minimal (usually in three or four days). Local wound care with irrigation and/or dressing is essential to minimize wound infection. Low-residue diet is instituted for four or five days to delay bowel movements. In some patients, antidiarrheal drugs such as loperamide or Lomotil (diphenoxylate, atropine) are helpful.

Overlapping sphincteroplasty

This technique is most suitable for patients with traumatic damage to the anal sphincter, such as obstetric tear, accidental injury to the sphincter muscle, and fistulectomy or fistulotomy.

*Technique** The patient is placed in the prone jackknife position under general or regional anesthesia. The perianal skin at the operative site is infiltrated with 0.25% bupivacaine containing 1 : 200,000 epinephrine to minimize bleeding (Figure 5.6**a**). A curved incision is placed around the anterior half of the anus and carried to at least a semicircle of the anus (Figure 5.6**b**). The anoderm,

*The technique described is for cases of injury at the anterior midline to the external sphincter muscle

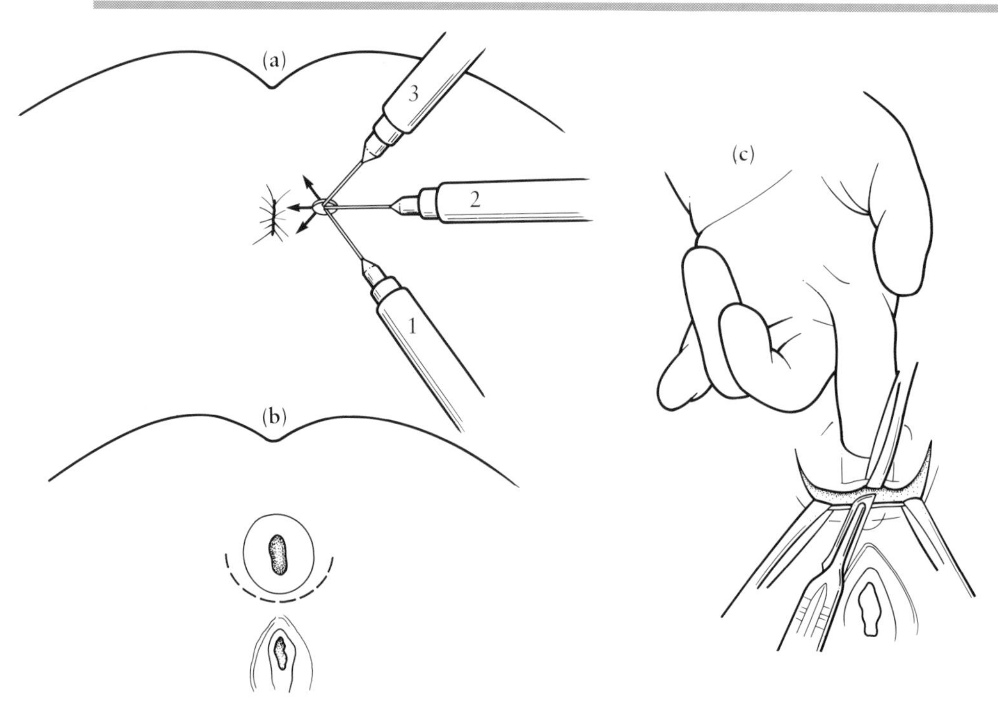

Figure 5.6: Overlapping sphincteroplasty. (**a**) Perianal skin is infiltrated with 0.25% bupivacaine containing 1 : 200,000 epinephrine. (**b**) A curved perianal incision is made. (**c**) Mobilization of anoderm.

along with the scar, is dissected from the surrounding tissues. Laterally, the internal sphincter muscle should be incorporated with this layer and separated from the external sphincter muscle (Figure 5.6**c**). The lateral edges of the retracted external sphincter muscle on each side are identified. The dissection is then carried proximally to the anorectal ring or the puborectalis muscle (Figure 5.6**d**) to where the scar tissue is transected. The lateral dissection should be adequate for wrapping the edges of the muscle together without tension (Figure 5.6**e**). The muscle ends are then overlapped around the anus (Figure 5.6**f**). It is important to excise the redundant muscle at each end that may not have an adequate blood supply. The muscle is wrapped around the anus and secured with mattress sutures of 3–0 Vicryl or Dexon (Figure 5.6**g**). At completion, the anal canal should admit one finger snugly (Figure 5.6**h**). The perineal body is resutured. The anoderm and the skin are tagged to the sphincter muscle (Figure 5.6**i**), and the wound is packed open with fine gauze (Figure 5.6**j**).

The results of overlapping external sphincteroplasty have been satisfactory. The improvement ranged from 85 to 97%, with an average follow-up of 13–67 months[24–27]. Most complications were minor, eg bleeding, infection, urinary retention and fecal impaction. The repair should not be performed before three months after the sphincter muscle injury, to allow the inflammation to subside with adequate scar formation.

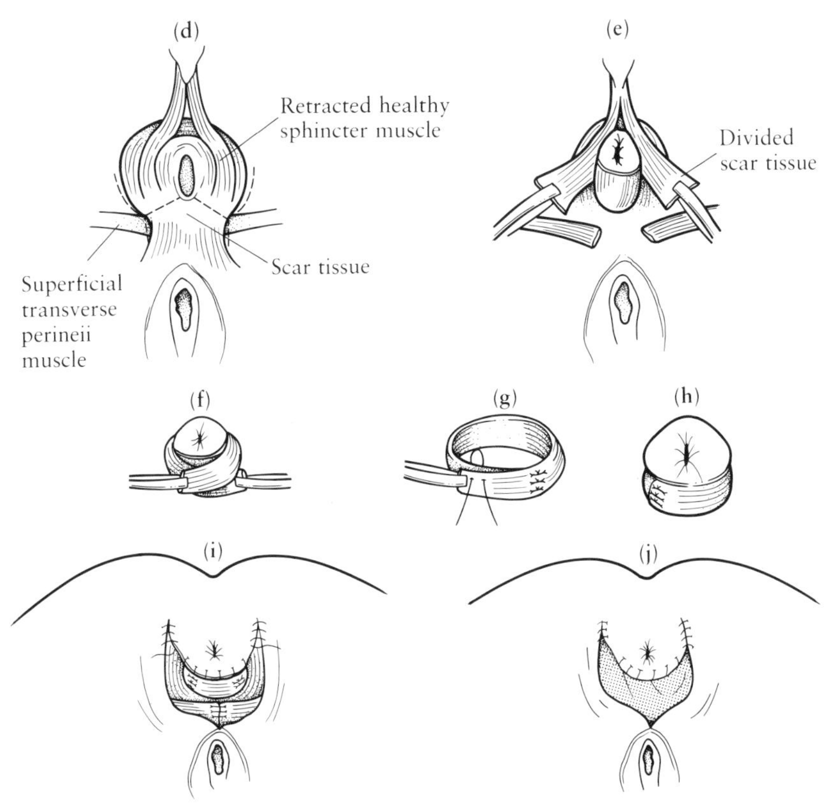

Figure 5.6: *continued* (**d**) Dissection of scar and external sphincter muscle, in the intersphincteric plane. (**e**) The severed muscle is adequately mobilized. (**f**) Muscle ends are overlapped over the anal canal. (**g**) Placement of mattress sutures. (**h**) At completion, the anal canal should admit one finger snugly. (**i**) Perineal body is reconstructed and anoderm is sutured to the sphincter muscle. (**j**) The wound is packed open. (Reproduced from Gordon 1992[47], by permission.)

Postanal repair

This technique is suitable for patients with incontinence without anatomic disruption of the external sphincter, such as in patients with rectal prolapse. The operation will tighten the sphincter muscle and lengthen the anal canal. Although originally thought to restore the anorectal angle, more recent studies have refuted this claim[28].

Technique The patient is placed in the prone-jackknife position. An angular or transverse incision is made between the anus and the coccyx (Figure 5.7**a**). The intersphincteric plane between the external and internal sphincter muscle is entered (Figure 5.7**b**). This plane is relatively avascular and can be easily dissected bluntly as one moves in a proximal direction up to the level of the puborectalis. At this point, the lipoareolar tissue is encountered and incised (Figure 5.7**c**) to enter the supralevator space. The levator ani muscle on each side is identified (Figure 5.7**d**). A suction drain is placed in the supralevator space and brought out through a separate stab wound. Sutures of 2–0 Vicryl or Dexon are placed on the ischiococcygeus (Figure 5.7**e**) and the pubococcygeus (Figure 5.7**f**). This muscle will not meet upon tying. The puborectalis (Figure 5.7**g**) and then the external sphincter muscle (Figure 5.7**h**) are then plicated. The subcutaneous tissue is closed (Figure 5.7**i**), after which the skin is approximated.

The results of postanal repair vary from series to series, because of the different methods of assessment, the degree of severity of incontinence, and the duration of follow-up. Browning and Parks[29] reported improvement of continence in 80% of 42 patients, with a mean follow-up of 13 months. They found that the operation effectively lengthened the anal canal and increased the anal pressure in patients with a successful clinical outcome. Yoshioka and Keighley[30] had similarly satisfactory results; in 116 patients who underwent this operation, with median follow-up of five years, the improvement was 81%. However, 60% of the patients still claimed urgency, 76% still leaked feces, and 52% continued to wear pads after the operation. In this series, the maximal resting anal pressure and the maximal squeeze pressure did not change significantly after the operation. The results indicated that the quality of continence after postanal repair was poor. Nevertheless, almost all the patients were grateful for the improvement that had been achieved. Orrom and coworkers[28] found satisfactory results in only 10 of 17 patients, after a follow-up of 15 months. There was significant improvement in sphincter pressure and mucosal electrosensitivity but there was no significant change in the anorectal angle.

Gracilis muscle transposition

This procedure is appropriate to repair the anorectum when bulk of the external sphincter muscle has been destroyed.

Technique The patient is positioned with both legs on stirrups. The perineum and both legs are prepared and draped so that both legs can be moved around from the stirrups. Three 3 cm incisions are made on the selected thigh over the gracilis muscle. It is mobilized and the tendon at its insertion at the knee is divided (Figure 5.8**a**). Care must be taken not to injure the neurovascular bundle at the proximal part of the muscle, an anatomical point that makes this muscle appealing for this indication. Two incisions are made at the anterior and posterior anus, and a circumferential tunnel is made to accommodate the gracilis muscle. The mobilized muscle is then passed through the subcutaneous passage (Figure 5.8**b**), encircling the anus from anterior to posterior (Figure 5.8**c**), and inserted to the contralateral ischial tuberosity (Figure 5.8**d**). Adduction of the thigh is needed to tighten the muscle around the anus to an index finger before sutures are placed and tied (Figure 5.8**e**). The wounds are then closed (Figure 5.8**f**).

The results of gracilis transposition for anal incontinence have been variable. Of the 22 patients operated by Corman[31], 14 were followed up for at least five years; the results were excellent in seven patients, fair in four, and poor in three. Christiansen and Colleagues[32] reported their experience with 13 patients with a median follow-up of 14 months; six patients were able to control solid and soft stool, four were continent only for solid stool, and two patients remained

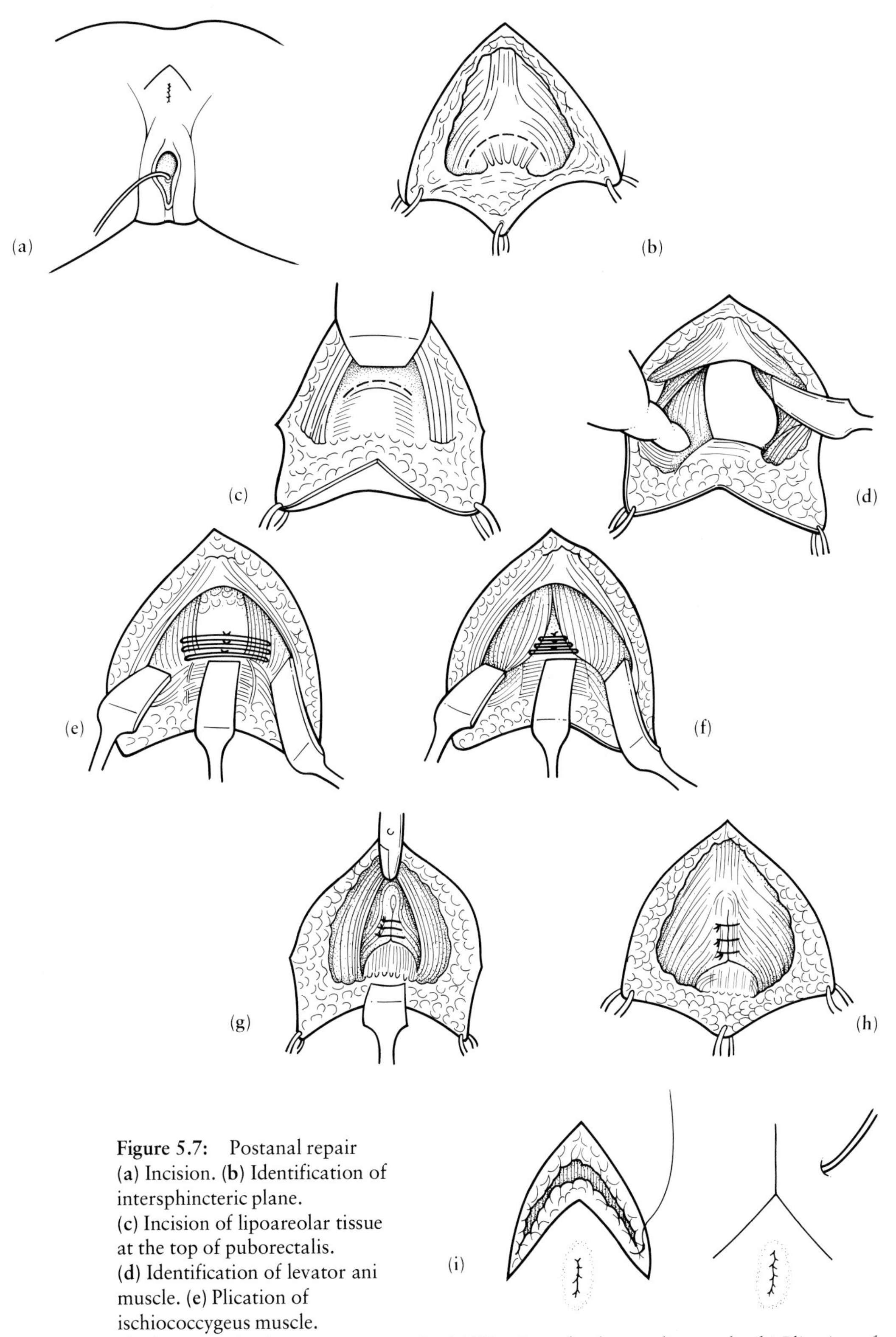

Figure 5.7: Postanal repair
(**a**) Incision. (**b**) Identification of intersphincteric plane.
(**c**) Incision of lipoareolar tissue at the top of puborectalis.
(**d**) Identification of levator ani muscle. (**e**) Plication of ischiococcygeus muscle.
(**f**) Plication of pubococcygeus muscle. (**g**) Plication of puborectalis muscle. (**h**) Plication of external sphincter. (**i**) Closure of subcutaneous tissue and skin. (Reproduced from Gordon 1992[47], by permission.)

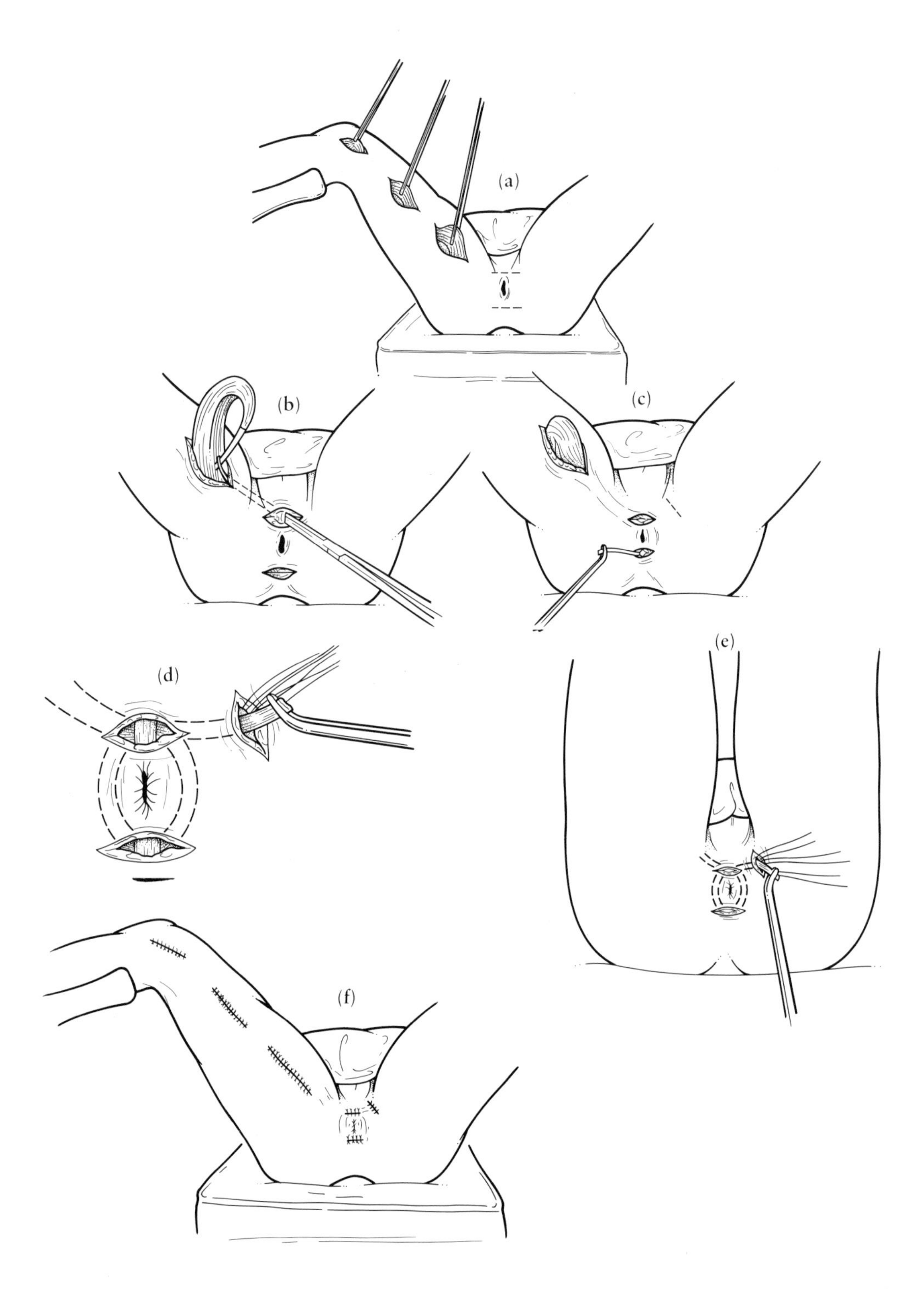

Figure 5.8: Gracilis muscle transposition. (**a**) Mobilization of gracilis muscle and division of tendon at its insertion. Dotted lines showed perianal incisions. (**b**) Passage of muscle through tunnel to anterior incision. (**c**) Passage of muscle through hemicircumference to posterior incision. (**d**) Passage of muscle through opposite hemicircumference of anus and placement of sutures to contralateral ischial tuberosity. (**e**) Adduction of thighs prior to tying sutures. (**f**) Completion.

incontinent as before the operation. Yoshioka and Keighley[33] reported failure in all six patients.

The unreliability of gracilis muscle transposition for anal incontinence is not surprising. George and Williams[34] cited its several drawbacks:

- Appropriate voluntary contraction of the transposed muscle is not reliably achieved.
- The nerve supply is such that reflex responses, ie sphincter contraction during episodes of raised abdominal pressure, do not occur.
- The gracilis muscle is predominantly a type 2 (fatiguable) muscle. This is inappropriate for sphincter function, which ideally requires a type 1 (fatigue-resistant) muscle.
- Transposition of the muscle involves a change in shape (from linear to loop), which may be mechanically disadvantageous.

George and Williams[34] used electrical stimulation to the transposed gracilis muscle, with the aim of altering the physiological characteristics of the gracilis muscle from type 2 to type 1 muscle. A stimulator and electric plate are implanted (Neuromed Inc., Miami, Florida) over the main nerve leading to the gracilis muscle and sutured to the relatively immobile adductor brevis. To reduce complications, especially muscular ischemia, the authors performed the procedure in three stages:

1 vascular delay ± defunctioning stoma. This consisted of dividing the minor distal vascular pedicles of the gracilis muscle (with preservation of its major proximal pedicle) and leaving the muscle in situ.
2 One month later, gracilis muscle transposition and implantation of stimulator and electrode were instituted. The low-frequency electrical stimulation was applied for 8–12 weeks.
3 The stoma were closed.

Physiological and histochemical analysis showed that the low-frequency electrical stimulation converts the type 2 muscle to type 1 in the majority of muscles. Of 20 patients who had previously had unsuccessful conventional procedures, there were 12 with functioning neosphincters, one who still had a colostomy, and one who had died seven months after the operation; in six patients the operation was still unsuccessful. Of 12 patients who had the gracilis transposition following sphincter excision (n = 9) or because of congenital absence of sphincter muscle (n = 3), eight had functioning neosphincters, three still had a colostomy, and one was a failure.

Bilateral gluteus maximus transposition

As with the gracilis, the gluteus maximus muscle can be used to reconstruct the external sphincter. Gluteus maximus muscle is a strong thigh extensor and lateral rotator of the hip. It originates from the upper part of the ileum, back of the sacrum, coccyx and sacrotuberous ligament, and inserts on the femur and iliotibial tract. It has a generous blood supply from the superior and inferior gluteal arteries supplemented by branches of the medial and lateral femoral circumflex arteries. Motor innervation is via the inferior gluteal nerve (L5, S1, S2). This factor must be considered as a cause of sphincter dysfunction secondary to spina bifida or myelomeningocele, which may warrant the use of a proximally innervated donor muscle, such as the gracilis (L2–4)[35].

Technique A slant incision is made on each side of the buttock, parallel to the caudal portion of the gluteus maximus muscle[35]. Similarly, a pair of curved incisions are made in the medial ischiorectal fossa. The lowest 4–5 cm of the origin of the gluteus maximus muscle (including a margin of periosteum) is detached from the lower part of the sacrum and coccyx. The muscle bundle is dissected from the main body of the gluteus maximus and the underlying sacrotuberous ligament, taking care not to injure its neurovascular supply (Figure 5.9). When the muscle flaps have been mobilized sufficiently to reach beyond the anus, they are bifurcated longitudinally, rotated inferiorly and tunneled subcutaneously to encircle the anus. The two ends of each transposed muscle bundle and its adjacent periosteum are joined to each other in an overlapping fashion using interrupted 2–0 Vicryl or Dexon, to form two opposing muscular slings (Figure 5.10). Suction drains are placed in the subcutaneous space and the incision is closed[35].

Pearl and colleagues[35] reported their experience of this operation in seven patients (five males and two females with ages ranging between 26 and 65 years); four patients had anal sphincter muscle destruction from multiple fistulotomies, two patients had bilateral pudendal nerve damage, and one had high imperforate anus. Six of the seven patients were continent to solid stool

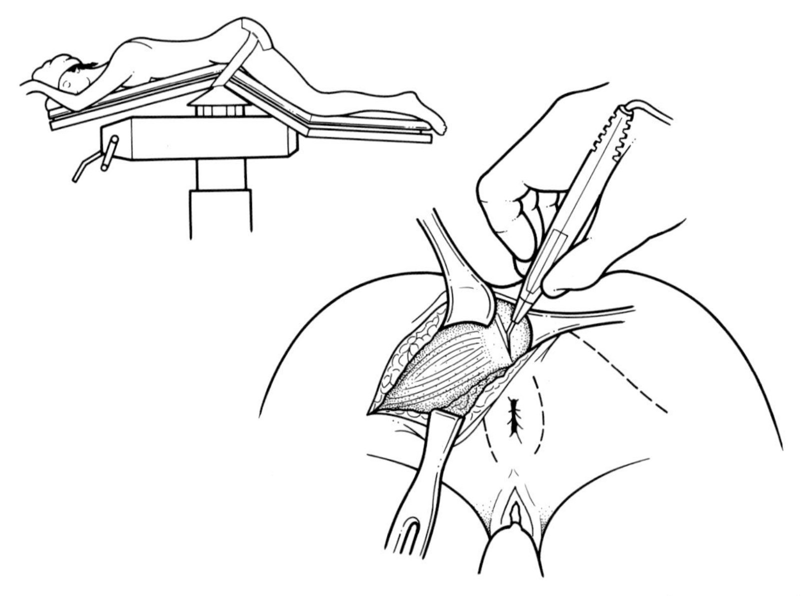

Figure 5.9: Bilateral gluteus maximus transposition. Patient is placed in prone jackknife position. Slant incisions are made. The lower 4–5 cm of the origin of gluteus maximus muscle including a margin of periosteum are detached from the sacrum and coccyx. (Reproduced from Pearl *et al.* 1991[35], by permission.)

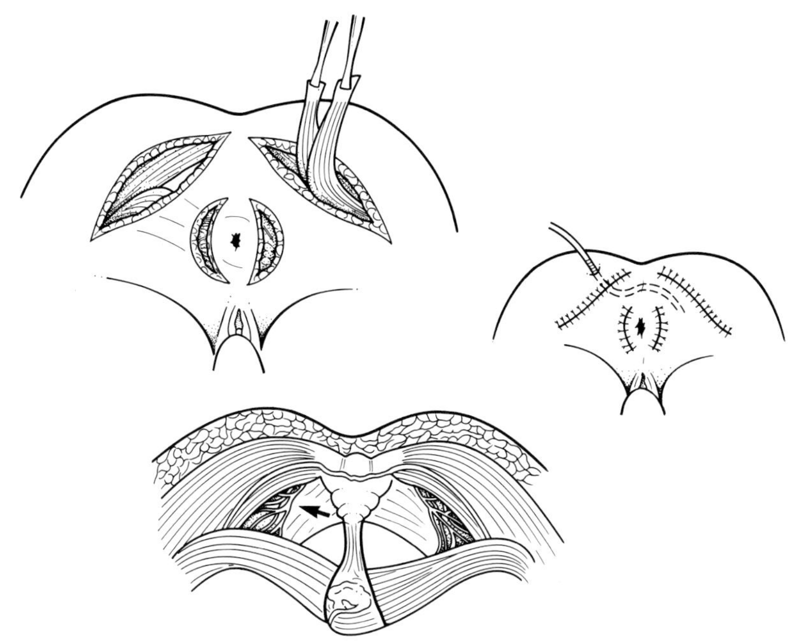

Figure 5.10: Bilateral gluteus maximus transposition. The detached gluteus maximus muscle is bifurcated, rotated inferiorly and tunneled subcutaneously to encircle the anal canal. Note the location of neurovascular bundles (arrow). Suction drain is placed subcutaneously and the skin closed. (Reproduced from Pearl *et al.* 1991[35], by permission.)

within three months after the operation. Of these, two were able to sense and control the passage of liquid stool, whereas only one was totally continent for gas.

Although this technique is not as well known as the gracilis repair, its advantages to the gracilis muscle are obvious: it is closer to the anus and the blood supply to the tip of the muscle is superior.

Artificial anal sphincter

As described earlier, each technique of sphincteroplasty is suitable for a certain type of anal sphincter injury. Anal incontinence due to neuromuscular disorders has not been within the range of surgical or other forms of treatment[36]. A new technique utilizing an artificial anal sphincter has now been used in humans, primarily in patients with anal incontinence due to neurological disorders and in patients who have failed other kinds of sphincteroplasty.

The artificial anal sphincter (American Medical System #800, St Paul, Minnesota) (Figure 5.11) consists of a cuff that is placed around the anal canal, a pressure-regulating balloon, and a pump placed in the scrotum or labia majora by which the patient can inflate and deflate the cuff. The inflated cuff will keep the anal canal closed and hence achieve continence. When the patient wishes to empty the rectum, the pump is squeezed four or five times, which (by means of a system of valves) empties the fluid from the cuff into the balloon, resulting in opening of the anal canal[36].

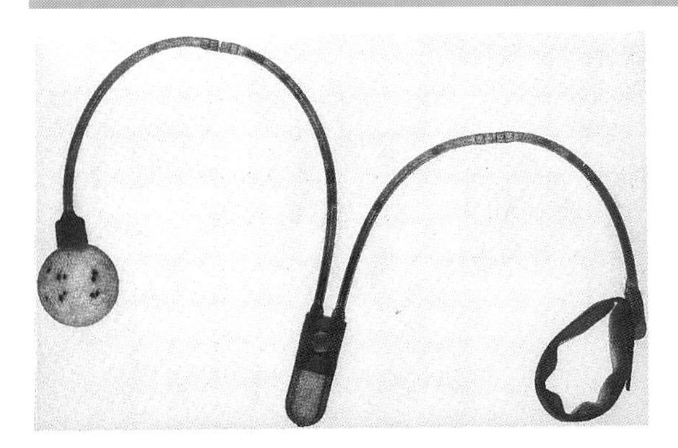

Figure 5.11: The artificial anal sphincter. Left, the pressure-regulating balloon; center, the pump (control assembly); right, the cuff. (Reproduced from Christiansen 1992[36], by permission.)

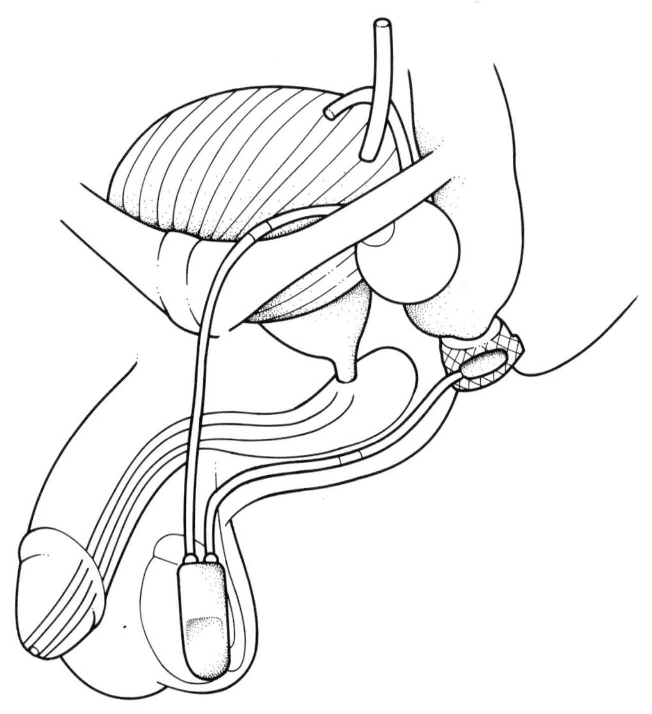

Figure 5.12: The artificial anal sphincter in position. The cuff is placed around the anal canal, the pressure-regulating balloon to the left of the bladder, and the pump in the scrotum. (Reproduced from Christiansen 1992[36], by permission.)

Technique The following technique was described by Christiansen[36]. The operation is performed with the patient in the lithotomy position. Two vertical incisions are made around the anus at 3 and 9 o'clock positions. Through these incisions, a tunnel is created around the anal canal. Pulleys are created posteriorly using the anococcygeal raphe and anteriorly using the raphe of the transverse perinei muscle. Through a subcutaneous tunnel, the pump is placed in the scrotum or labia majora. The pressure-regulating balloon is placed extraperitoneally on the left side of the urinary bladder. Finally, the three components are connected through subcutaneous tunnels with silastic tubing (Figure 5.12) (a defunctioning colostomy is not used). Christiansen[36] recommended prophylactic antibiotics, consisting of cefuroxime (750 mg), clindamycin (600 mg) and metronidazole (500 mg). These are given on induction of anesthesia and continued with three daily doses for eight days. The cuff is not inflated for three or four weeks, allowing the anal wound to heal.

Christiansen[36] reported his experience with this technique in 12 patients, (nine women and three men, with a median age of 49 years), all of whom had complete incontinence). Nine patients were incontinent due to the neurological disorders and three had traumatic damage to the sphincter that had been treated unsuccessfully by reconstructive procedures, including a gracilis transposition in one. In 10 patients, the system has subsequently functioned for more than six months. Five patients are almost completely continent, with only occasional leakage of gas. Three patients occasionally leak gas and liquid stool but none of them need to wear a pad. Two patients with irritable bowel syndrome require frequent use of laxatives and enemas. The anal canal pressures with the cuff deflated and inflated are 5–38 and 40–82 cm H_2O respectively. Severe complications from the operation have not been a problem. There was only one severe infection requiring removal of the system in one patient. There has been no erosion or extrusion of the system.

Wong and colleagues[37] reported artificial sphincter placement in 11 patients who had various causes of fecal incontinence including birth trauma (n = 3), major perineal trauma (n = 3), spinal cord disorder (n = 3), imperforate anus (n = 1), and neurogenic incontinence of unknown etiology (n = 1). The follow-up was 13 months (range 7–30 months). All patients achieved excellent continence, although one patient was intermittently incontinent of gas and another patient had occasional minimal soiling. Patient satisfaction was uniformly high.

At the time of writing this chapter, the artificial sphincter for anal incontinence has not been approved by the FDA for clinical use in the USA.

Encirclement of anus

The aim of this procedure is to narrow the patulous anus. It may help to control formed stool but offers little in the control of liquid feces or gas. Often the foreign body causes perianal abscess or fistula, or extrudes through the wound. The technique is the same as for rectal prolapse (see page 65).

Sigmoid colostomy

Not all patients are suitable for repair of anal incontinence. In these patients, and particularly in the elderly—if the patient cannot live with it—a well constructed sigmoid colostomy is an excellent option.

Management of rectocele

Rectocele is a herniation of the anterior wall of the anorectum to the posterior vaginal wall (Figures 5.13 and 5.14). Rectoceles can be divided into three anatomical types: low, high, and middle. Low rectocele presents with an abnormal anal sphincter and perineum and is often the result of major

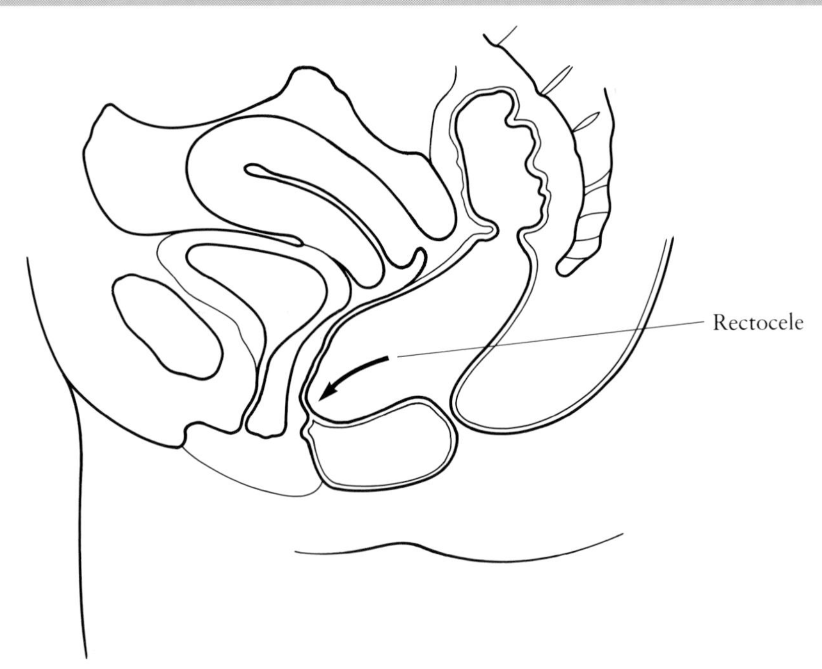

Figure 5.13: Rectocele. Sagittal view of the pelvis; herniation of anterior rectal wall to the vagina (arrow). (Reproduced form Capps 1975[42], by permission.)

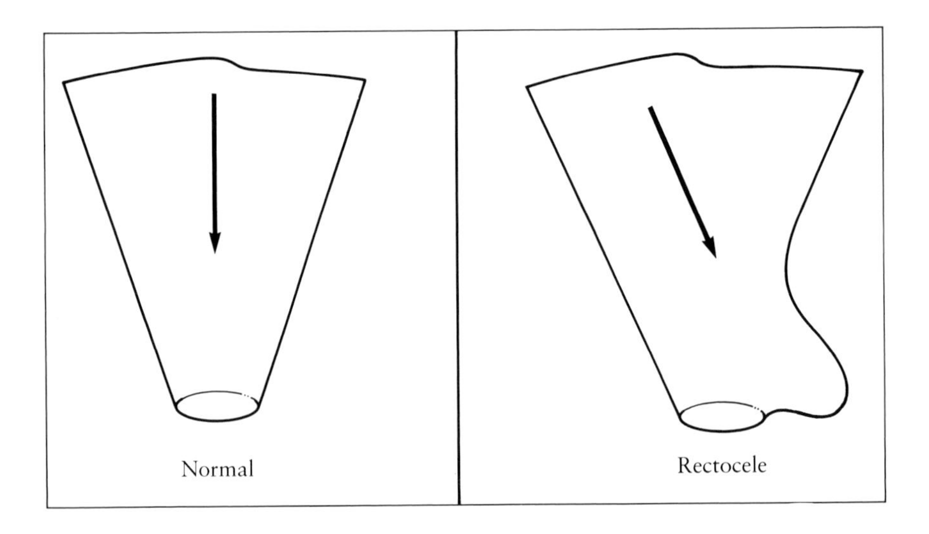

Figure 5.14: Rectocele. Diagrammatic illustration of the effect of defecation in normal and in rectocele. (Reproduced from Capps 1975[42], by permission.)

obstetrical trauma. High rectocele results from stretching of the upper third of the vagina and the cardinal and uterosacral ligaments. The defect begins 7–8 cm above the anal external sphincter and is often associated with complete genital prolapse and enterocele. Middle rectocele is by far the most common. The defect begins immediately above the anal external sphincter and proceeds cephalad for 3–7 cm[38]. The discussion here will include only the middle rectocele.

Common symptoms of rectocele are constipation, difficult evacuation, feeling of rectal or perineal fullness, anal pain and bleeding. Until recently, rectocele was seldom included in the differential diagnosis of chronic constipation.

The diagnosis of rectocele is best done by digital examination. With the index finger in the anorectum, the anterior rectal wall can be hooked into the vagina. One must keep in mind that not all rectoceles cause symptoms, and the severity of symptoms does not correlate with the size of the rectocele[39]. In the series reported by Johansson and colleagues[40], 71% of patients with rectocele had associated paradoxical sphincter reaction and 20% had rectal intussusception. In patients with rectocele, the investigation should include defecography to rule out these associated conditions and also to determine the degree of evacuation disturbance. A colonic transit time study should also be included in some cases. Surgical repair should be performed only if symptoms are thought to come from the rectocele. A transanorectal repair is simple and gives satisfactory results.

Technique

Mechanical bowel preparation is limited to tap-water enemas. Similar to hemorrhoidectomy, antibiotics are generally not given.

The patient is placed in the prone-jackknife position with the cheeks of the buttock taped apart. The anal canal and the perianal skin are infiltrated with 0.25% bupivacaine containing 1 : 200,000 epinephrine. The anterior anorectum is exposed using a Fansler anal speculum. An elliptical excision is made from the perianal skin and incorporates the external and internal hemorrhoids up to the level above the anorectal ring. The submucosal flaps are developed on each side to 1–1.5 cm laterally (Figure 5.15**a**). The muscle on each side of

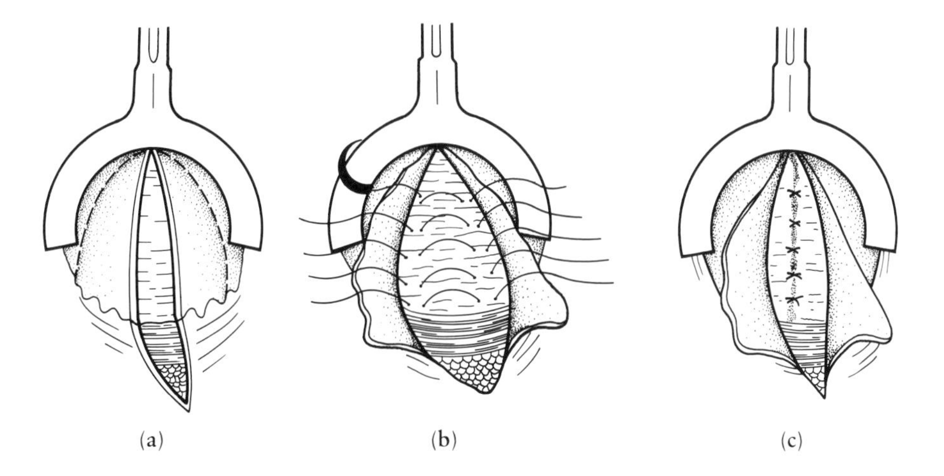

Figure 5.15: Rectocele repair. (**a**) An elliptical excision is made in the anterior anal canal, from perianal skin to apex of rectocele. Dissection is made under the submucosa on each side of the wound. (**b**) Placement of sutures. (**c**) With the sutures tied, the mucosa and submucosa are closed. (Reproduced from Cali *et al.* 1992[38], by permission.)

the wound is then approximated with 2–0 Vicryl or Dexon. It is important to place the index finger of the opposite hand in the vagina. The sutures have to incorporate the full thickness of the anorectal wall and a touch of the rectovaginal septum. Several such stitches are placed about 1 cm apart (Figure 5.15**b**). Once the sutures are tied, the redundant mucosa is trimmed and the mucosa is closed with running 3–0 chromic catgut (Figure 5.15**c**).

The results of transanorectal repair of rectocele have been good. Most series reported a success rate of 80–94%[41–45]. However, the follow-up in these patients was less than two years.

References

1 Auffret M (1882) Un cas de procidence du gros intestin d'une longueur de 90 centimetres. Operation par excision — Double rangu de suture — Mort. *J Med Chir Pharm.* **10**:650–2.

2 Miles WE (1933) Rectosigmoidectomy as a method of treatment for procidentia recti. *Proc R Soc Med.* **26**:1445.

3 Altemeier WA (1971) Nineteen years' experience with the one-stage perineal repair of rectal prolapse. *Ann Surg.* **173**:993–1001.

4 Williams JG (1991) Perineal approaches to repair of rectal prolapse. *Seminars Colon Surg.* **2**:198–204.

5 Prasad ML (1986) Perineal proctectomy, posterior rectopexy, and postanal levator repair for the treatment of rectal prolapse. *Dis Colon Rectum.* **29**:547–52.

6 Wassef R (1986) Rectal prolapse. *Curr Probl Surg.* **23**:402–51.

7 Delorme E (1900) Communication sur la tractement, des prolapsus du rectum to taux, par l'excision de la muqueuse rectale ou recto-colique. *Bull Mem Soc Chir Paris.* **26**:499–518.

8 Uhlig BE and Sullivan ES (1979) The modified Delorme operation: Its place in surgical treatment for massive rectal prolapse. *Dis Colon Rectum.* **22**:513–21.

9 Berman IR (1990) Delorme's transrectal excision for internal rectal prolapse: Patient selection, technique, and three-year follow-up. *Dis Colon Rectum.* **33**: 573–80.

10 Nivatvongs S (1991) Rectal prolapse: Techniques of transperineal repair. *Perspect Colon Rect Surg.* **4**:101–9.

11 Nay HR and Blair CR (1972) Perineal surgical repair of rectal prolapse. *Am J Surg.* **123**:577–9.

12 Moskalenko VW (1973) Modification of Delorme's resection of rectal mucosa for prolapse of the rectum. *Int Surg.* **58**:192–4.

13 Christiansen J and Kirkegaard P (1981) Delorme's operation for complete rectal prolapse. *Br J Surg.* **68**:537–8.

14 Gunderson AJ (1985) Reappraisal of Delorme's procedure for rectal prolapse. *Dis Colon Rectum.* **28**:721–4.

15 Corman ML (1988) Classic Articles in Colonic and Rectal Surgery: Carl Thiersch 1822–1895. *Dis Colon Rectum.* **31**:154–5.

16 Ambroze W L Jr (1992) Laparoscopic-assisted partial proctectomy with transanal anastomosis: A series of six cases. *Dis Colon Rectum.* **35**:21. (Abstract.)

17 Thorson AG (1992) Laparoscopic colectomy. *Dis Colon Rectum.* **35**:21–2. (Abstract.)

18 Berman IR (1992) Sutureless laparoscopic rectopexy for procidentia. Technique and implication. *Dis Colon Rectum.* **35**: 689–93.

19 Bartolo DC (1983) The role of partial denervation of the puborectalis in idiopathic fecal incontinence. *Br J Surg.* **76**:664–7.

20 Laurberg S (1988) Delayed external sphincter repair for obstetric repair. *Br J Surg.* **75**:786–8.

21 Riboli EB (1988) biofeedback conditioning of fecal incontinence. *Arch Phys Med Rehab.* **69**:29–31.

22 MacLeod JH (1987) Management of anal incontinence by biofeedback. *Gastroenterol.* **93**:291–4.

23 Lowry AC (1992) Biofeedback for fecal incontinence. *Seminars Colon Rect Surg.* **3**:110–14.

24 Fang DT (1984) Overlapping sphincteroplasty for acquired anal incontinence. *Dis Colon Rectum.* **27**:270–272.

25 Pezim ME (1987) Sphincter repair of fecal incontinence after obstetrical or iatrogenic injury. *Dis Colon Rectum.* **30**:521–5.

26 Arnaud A (1991) Sphincter repair without overlapping for fecal incontinence. *Dis Colon Rectum.* **34**:744–7.

27 Fleshman JW (1991) Anal sphincter repair for obstetric injury: Manometric evaluation of functional results. *Dis Colon Rectum.* **34**:1061–7.

28 Orrom WJ (1991) Comparison of anterior sphincteroplasty and postanal repair in the treatment of idiopathic fecal incontinence. *Dis Colon Rectum.* **34**: 305–10.

29 Browning GGP and Parks AG (1983) Postanal repair for neuropathic fecal incontinence: Correlation of clinical result and anal canal pressures. *Br J Surg.* **70**:101–4.

30 Yoshioka K and Keighley MRB (1989) Critical assessment of the quality of continence after postanal repair for fecal incontinence. *Br J Surg.* **76**: 1054–7.

31 Corman ML (1985) Gracilis muscle transposition for anal incontinence: Late results. *Br J Surg.* **72** (Suppl):S21–2.

32 Christiansen J (1990) Gracilis muscle transposition for fecal incontinence. *Br J Surg.* **77**:1039–40.

33 Yoshioka K and Keighley MRB (1988) Clinical and manometric assessment of gracilis muscle transplant for fecal incontinence. *Dis Colon Rectum.* **31**:767–9.

34 George BD and Williams NS (1992) Electrically stimulated gracilis neoanal sphincter. *Seminars Colon Rect Surg.* **3**:104–9.

35 Pearl RK (1991) Bilateral gluteus maximus transposition for anal incontinence. *Dis Colon Rectum.* **34**: 478–81.

36 Christiansen J (1992) The artificial anal sphincter. *Seminars Colon Rect Surg.* **3**:98–100.

37 Wong WD (1992) An artificial sphincter for anal incontinence. *Dis Colon Rectum.* **35**:P4. (Abstract.)

38 Cali RL, Christensen MA, Blatchford G J *et al.* (1992) Rectoceles. *Seminars Colon Rect Surg.* **3**:132–7.

39 Yoshioka K (1991) Physiologic and anatomic assessment of patients with rectocele. *Dis Colon Rectum.* **34**:704–8.

40 Johansson C (1992) Association between rectocele and paradoxical sphincter response. *Dis Colon Rectum.* **35**:503–9.

41 Sullivan ES (1968) Transrectal perineal repair: An adjunct to improve function after anorectal surgery. *Dis Colon Rectum.* **11**:106–14.

42 Capps WF (1975) Rectoplasty and perineoplasty for the symptomatic rectocele. A report of fifty cases. *Dis Colon Rectum.* **18**:237–43.

43 Kubchandani IT (1983) Endorectal repair of rectocele. *Dis Colon Rectum* **26**: 792–6.

44 Sehapayak S (1985) Transrectal repair of rectocele. An extended armamentarium of colorectal surgeons. A report of 355 cases. *Dis Colon Rectum*. **28**: 422–33.

45 Sarles JC (1989) Endorectal repair of rectocele. *Int J Colorectal Dis*. **4**:167–71.

46 Labow S *et al.* (1980) Perineal repair of rectal procidentia with an elastic fabric sling. *Dis Colon Rectum*. **23**:467–9.

47 Gordon PH (1992) Anal incontinence. In: Principles and practice of surgery for the colon, rectum and anus. 346–7. Quality Medical Publishing, Inc, St Louis.

6

Transanal Endoscopic Microsurgery

LEE SMITH

Introduction

Minimal access surgery for tumors of the rectum has become possible in the past 10 years because of new instruments specifically designed for the purpose. The instruments are the creation of Gerhard Buess of Tubingen, Germany[1–5]. Exposure is the problem that the surgeon faces in dealing with upper rectal lesions. Long operating proctoscopes, long instruments, magnification with a binocular operating microscope, and insufflation of carbon dioxide to keep the rectal side walls from collapsing make this technique possible.

Indications

This minimal access surgical procedure may be applied to both benign and malignant lesions. Any benign lesion which is within reach of the scope may be treated by transanal endoscopic microsurgery (TEM). The critical factor is for the proximal edge to be visualized and excised with a margin. Malignant lesions may also be removed with these tools. Even those cancers that are beyond help, ie metastases to distant organs, may be palliated by 'coring out' an opening through the blocked lumen or excising the primary with the expectation that the metastases will subsequently take the patient's life. Small carcinomas may be selected for excision by this technique. More radical surgery is advisable if the cancer is completely invading the wall.

Rectal prolapse is a condition that may be treated by a modification of rectal excision. In this instance, the rectum is opened posteriorly and the rectal wall is attached to the sacral fascia. In this fashion a rectopexy is achieved. The posterior wall of the rectum is then closed. Clearly there is a risk of infection in the space that is created posteriorly.

Alternatives to endoluminal microscopic surgery

First, any benign tumor that can be removed by standard snaring techniques via an endoscope should be removed in this way. Those that cannot be snared lend themselves to excision. We prefer excision so that pathologic examination can be performed effectively. Cryosurgery, electrosurgery and laser surgery do not provide an opportunity for pathologic examination or proper histologic staging. The approach to a rectal lesion may be accomplished by dilating the anus for direct visualization and excision, making parasacral incisions and approaching via the posterior wall of the rectum (Kraske approach)[6], or splitting the sphincter for wider visualization (York-Mason approach)[7]. The problem with the transanal approach in former times was exposure. The problem with the parasacral incision is the frequent presence of fistualization. The problem with the York-Mason approach is the sphincter incision which must be reapproximated and is then expected to function normally. The abdominal approach allows the upper half of the rectum to be accessed, especially in thin patients. In obese patients access may be difficult: a low pelvic anastomosis is needed, but this is more likely to leak than other gastrointestinal anastomoses. Leakage or a tenuous anastomosis may require a temporary ostomy proximally. At the same time, the ureters are in jeopardy during dissection. The pelvic nerves (both autonomic and somatic) may be bruised or incised, resulting in a neuropathy. Nerves to the genitals, bladder and sphincter mechanism of the anus may be compromised with resultant bladder weakness, impotence and/or anal sphincter dysfunction.

Preoperative staging

In 1932 Cuthbert Dukes described a classification for rectal cancer[8]. The unfortunate factor is that this staging is performed on a postoperative specimen or at postmortem examination; thus this information is obtained after surgery. Recently attempts have been made to stage a cancer prior to the operation. This effort requires clinical and imaging studies to decide the depth of spread of a cancer.

The tumor/node/metastasis (TNM) system has become a standard classification. For purposes of local excision, the T portion of this classification is the most important. In order to understand subsequent comments in this discussion, I will define the T1–T4 local staging of the tumor (Figure 6.1). A T1 tumor is one which is invasive to the level of the submucosa, sparing the muscularis propria. A T2 carcinoma invades into the muscularis propria but not through it. The T3 lesion invades through the entire bowel wall to the adjacent fat. A T4 carcinoma is one that has spread through the wall and to an adjacent organ or side wall of the pelvis.

Before embarking upon a local excision, the surgeon must decide whether the cancer is of full thickness (T3) or not. The first step is a clinical appraisal. The digital examination is extremely important in staging the rectal cancer if it is within reach of the finger. The size can be estimated, the mobility

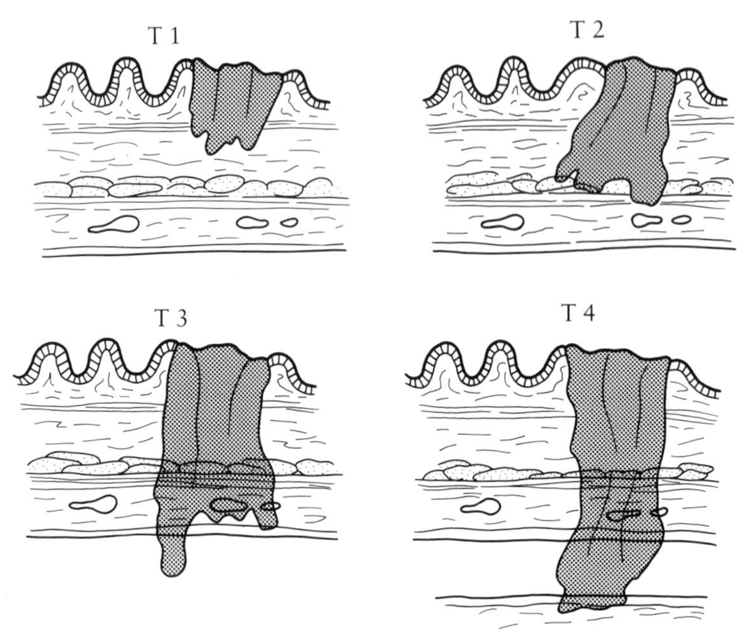

Figure 6.1: Classification of depth of carcinoma penetration. The stages are divided into four levels. T_1 is into the submucosa. T_2 extends into the muscularis propria. T_3 is full thickness and breaks into the surrounding tissues. T_4 carcinoma extends into an adjacent structure or the pelvic sidewalls.

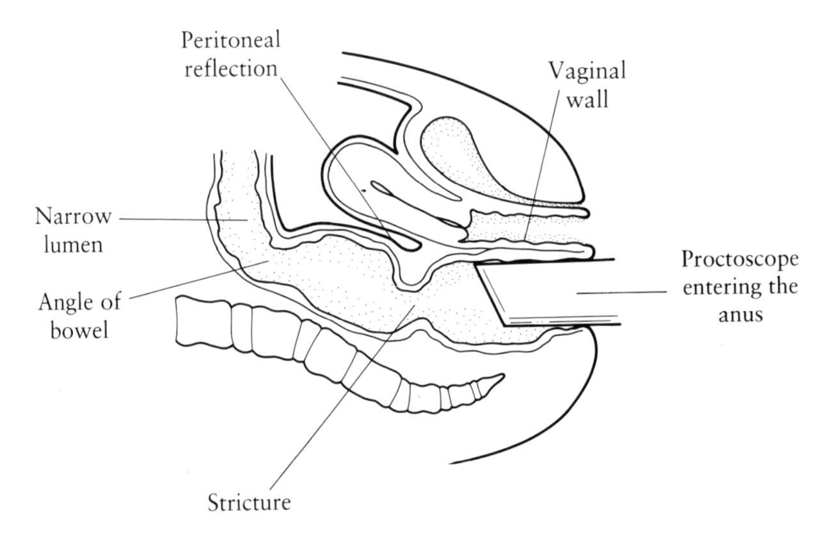

Figure 6.2: Difficulties and dangers. Narrow points, stenoses and angulation may prevent introduction of the 4 cm diameter operating proctoscope to the proximal margin of the tumor.

determined, and satellite nodules may be appreciated. A large tumor which feels tethered has probably grown through the bowel wall. Another critical estimate is whether the peritoneal cavity may be immediately beneath the tumor or, in the female, whether the vagina is adjacent (Figure 6.2).

Rigid sigmoidoscopy

Rigid sigmoidoscopy is also an essential part of the investigation. The distance markings on the rigid scope allow more exact determination of the level within the rectum that the tumor is situated. Proximal and distal margins may be measured. Another important determination is the circumferential orientation of the tumor. This knowledge is important for positioning the patient subsequently at surgery. Hence it must be stated whether the tumor is anterior, posterior, right lateral or left lateral. The proximal margin of the tumor must be visible and it must be decided whether a scope which is 4 cm in diameter might be introduced to the proximal extent of the tumor. Factors that prohibit complete entry of the scope are strictures (either from previous surgery or from pathology), folds or angulation (Figure 6.2).

Rectal ultrasound

Rectal ultrasound has become a standard tool for evaluating the extent of bowel wall penetration by carcinoma[9,10]. This relatively inexpensive technique is superior to both the CT scan and the MRI scan for examination of the layers of the bowel wall. This technology has allowed us to visualize lymph nodes or satellite deposits that are otherwise hidden before surgery. Lymph nodes that are enlarged are highly suspicious for metastatic carcinoma. However, the presence of lymph nodes in the area of the carcinoma elicits concern regarding possible local spread of the carcinoma.

Computed tomography is of value when trying to determine whether there are additional lesions hidden within the abdomen and pelvis. The CT scan is particularly useful for evaluating the liver.

Colonoscopy or barium enema evaluation is best performed prior to surgery. Other proximal adenomas or carcinomatous lesions might dictate a different therapeutic approach.

Preoperative care

Informed consent is necessary to ensure that the patient understands the procedure, its alternatives and the potential complications (see p. 59).

Bowel preparation is a vital requirement, and the importance of colorectal cleanliness must be emphasized to the patient. My preference is to use a four litre oral saline lavage solution. Some patients object to the volumes, but when it is finally taken, the colon is the cleanest that it can be for surgery. After completing the prep, the patient is told to avoid any sort of solid food until after surgery.

Generally speaking, prophylactic antibiotics are used to minimize the chance of infection and should cover both aerobes and anaerobes. I use oral neomycin and metronidazole in three doses on the afternoon and evening before surgery.

In addition, a broad-spectrum cephalosporin is employed parenterally at the time of the procedure and continued for 24 hours. This combination of preoperative oral and intraoperative parenteral antibiotics reduces both the anaerobic and aerobic flora, minimizing the chance of sepsis.

The operation

Equipment

The operating proctoscopes are 4 cm in diameter and either 15 or 20 cm in length (Figure 6.3). There is an obturator with each scope, which creates a tapered tip for easier introduction into the rectum, and two face plates that fit on the proctoscope (Figure 6.4, 6.5). The first one is a glass 'window' so that

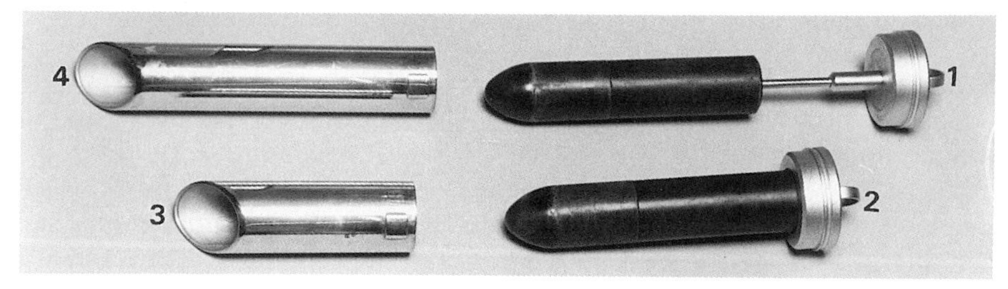

Figure 6.3: The operating proctoscopes and obturators. **1** and **2**, the obturators for their respective 15 cm (3) and 20 cm (4) operating scopes.

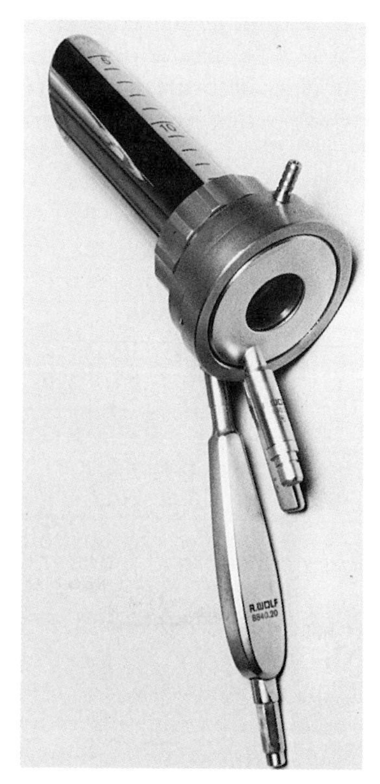

Figure 6.4: Operating proctoscope with window face plate. This nonmagnified window is used to center the beveled tip of the scope over the tumor.

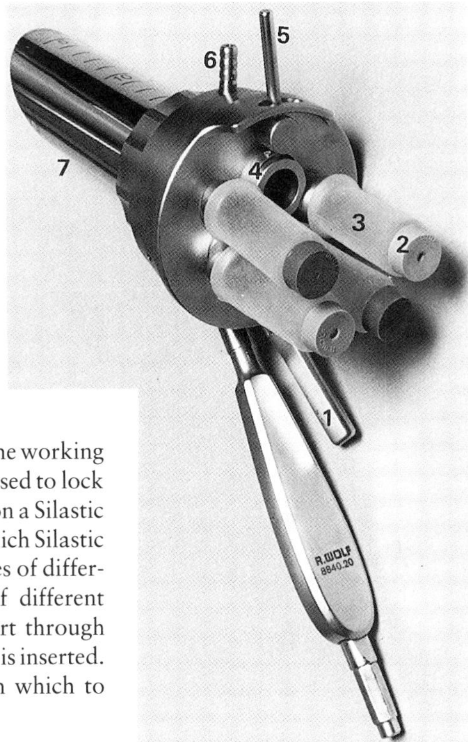

Figure 6.5: Operating proctoscope with the working face plate locked onto the scope. **1**, handle used to lock the face plate onto the scope. **2**, rubber cap on a Silastic sleeve (**3**). Note there are four ports onto which Silastic sleeves are applied. The caps may have holes of different sizes to accommodate instruments of different diameters and yet prevent gas leak. **4**, port through which the shaft of the binocular microscope is inserted. **6**, port which is connected to a tube with which to monitor CO_2 pressure. **7**, scope barrel.

the tumor can be directly visualized and the scope tip can be placed over it (Figure 6.4). The second face plate is designed for use during the operation (Figure 6.5) and has five ports. The center port is for the binocular operating microscope (Figure 6.6). The microscope has a long optical shaft which is placed through the operating proctoscope. Within the shaft of the binocular scope there is a narrow channel through which a monocular scope shaft may be inserted. This gives the assistant a view of the operating field so that he can properly coordinate suction and irrigation. The same monocular scope can be attached to a video camera so that the view can be displayed on a television monitor (Figure 6.6). (3).

The working face plate has four other ports to which silastic sleeves are attached. On the tips of the sleeves are rubber caps (Figures 6.5, 6.6), with small holes to permit the introduction of long narrow instruments while still maintaining a gas-tight system (Figure 6.5).

The insufflation machine is built for use with these gas-tight scopes (Figure 6.7). It has the ability to insufflate at a rate of 6 L min^{-1}. The recommended pressure during procedures is 15 mmHg. The vacuum pump creates suction pressure which is less than the carbon dioxide insufflation pressure, so that one does not lose exposure due to collapse of the rectum.

The long instruments that reach through these scopes are reuseable. Their tips are like miniaturized, standard operating instruments (Figure 6.8). There is a needle holder, right and left angled scissors, a clip applier, an electric knife, right and left angled forceps, and a suction-irrigation probe (Figure 6.9).

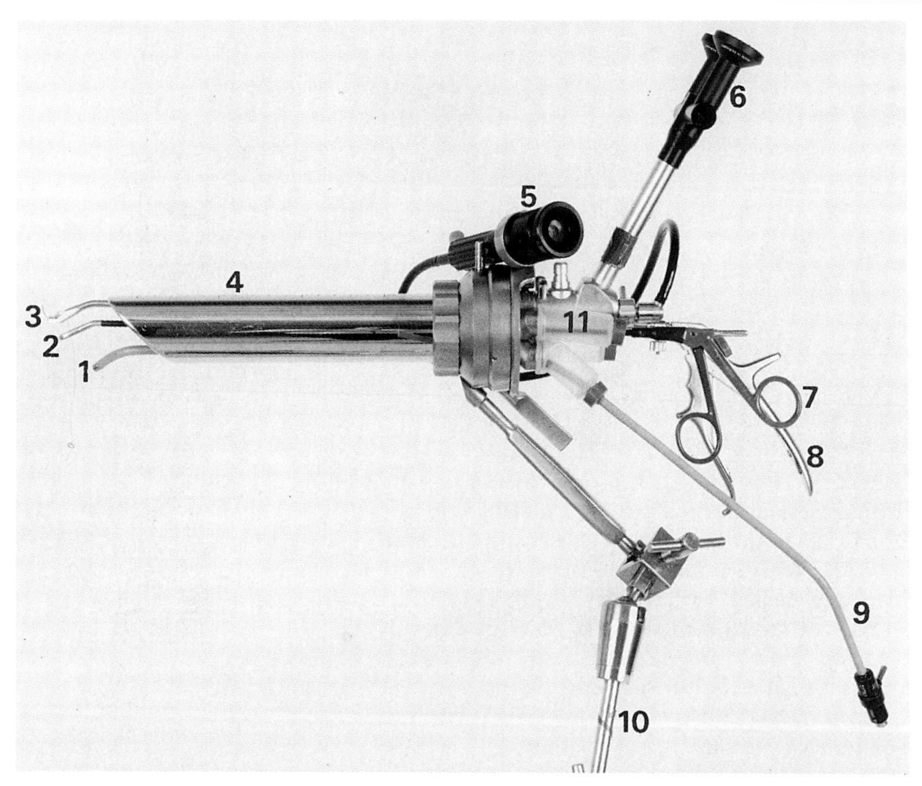

Figure 6.6: The scope assembled. The connecting tubes are not connected. **1**, suction probe. **2**, forceps. **3**, needle holder. **4**, scope barrel. **5**, assistant's monocular microscope which views through a channel in the shaft of the binocular microscope. **6**, binocular microscope. **7–9**, handles of the needle holder, forceps, and the suction probe respectively. **10**, Martin arm which fixes the scope to the operating table. **11**, Silastic sleeves through which the instruments are inserted.

An electrocautery machine is essential for cutting tissue and coagulating vessels. The forceps, knife and suction irrigation probe may be connected to an electrocautery unit (Figure 6.10).

Whenever setting up the operating room, the circulating nurse should be sure that an instrument set for laparotomy is available. Snares should be available in case portions of the tumor prove to be removed more easily in this fashion.

Anesthesia

One may operate using general anesthesia, spinal injection or epidural injection. So far patients have tolerated anesthesia well.

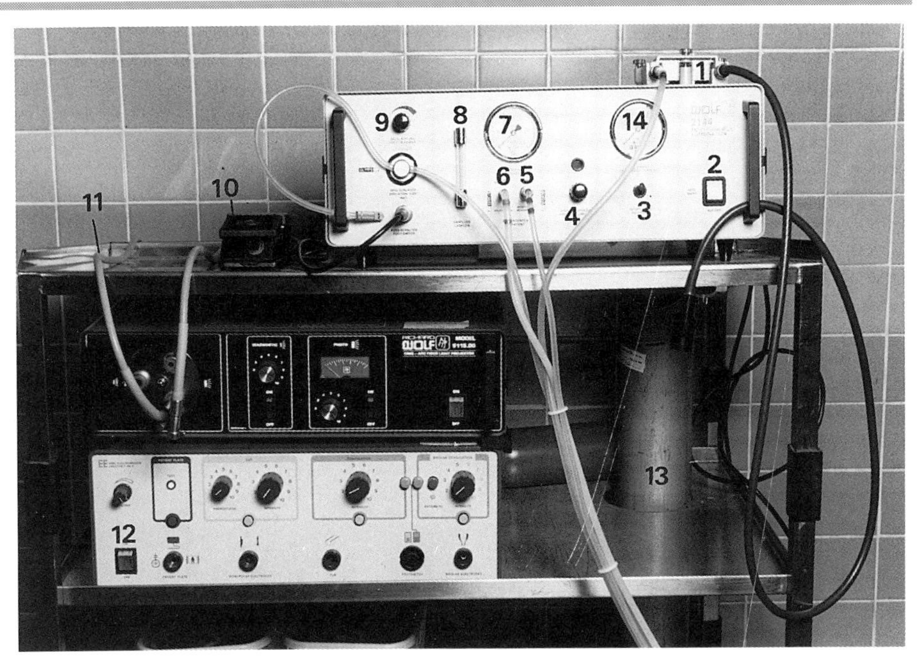

Figure 6.7: The insufflation machine, light source, and electrocautery machine. **1**, suction pump. **2**, power switch. **3**, CO_2 flow switch. **4**, flow rate regulator. **5**, CO_2 outflow port. **6**, port for monitoring pressure in the rectum. **7**, gas pressure gauge. **8**, CO_2 flow indicator. **9**, regulator for suction pressure. **10**, foot pedal which turns on the irrigation. **11**, cable to the light source. **12**, power switch to the electrocautery. **13**, the CO_2 tank. **14**, gauge for the CO_2 tank volume.

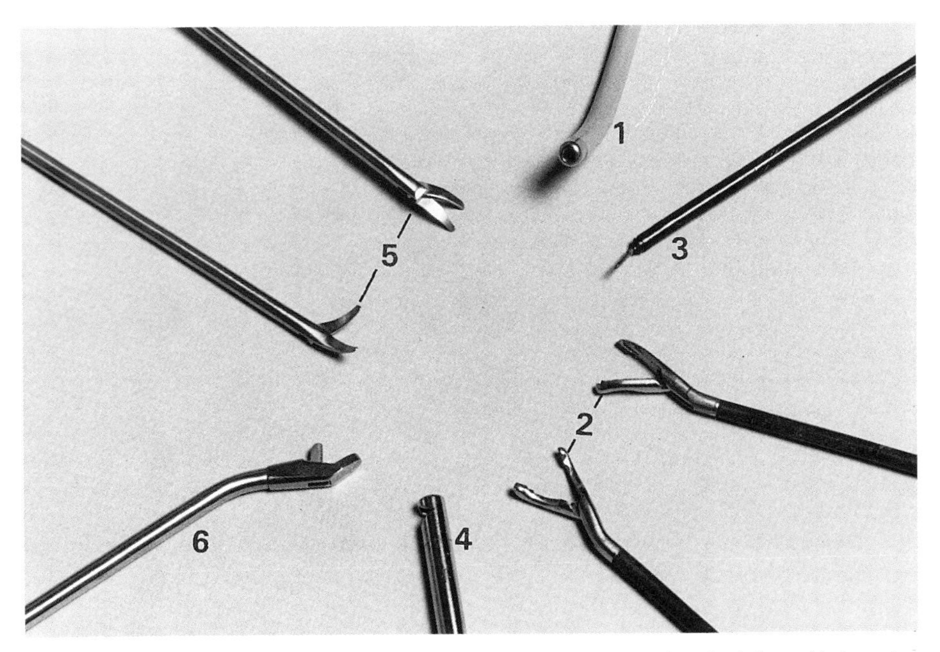

Figure 6.8: Tips of the long TEM instruments. **1**, irrigation–suction. **2**, right and left angled forceps. **3**, electric knife. **4**, clip applier. **5**, right and left angled scissors. **6**, needle holder.

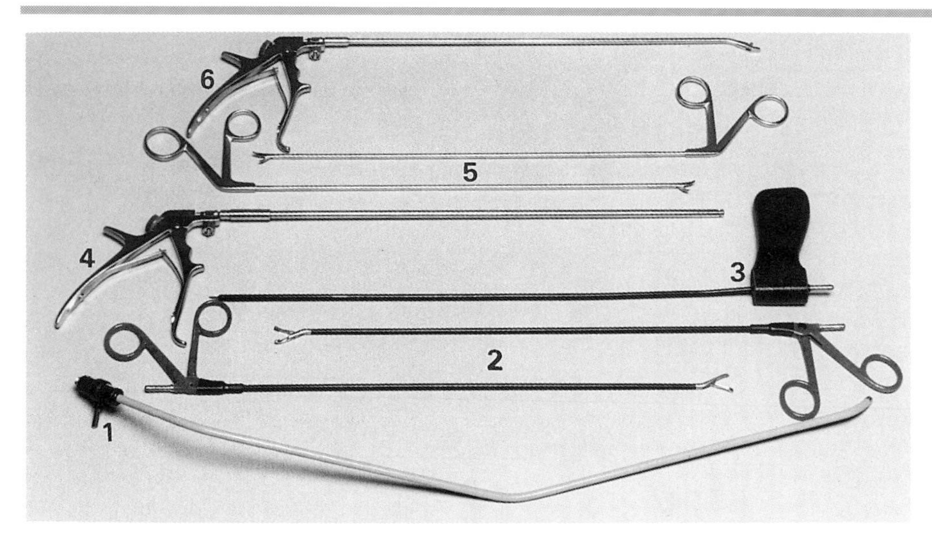

Figure 6.9: The long TEM instruments. **1**, suction–irrigation probe. **2**, left and right angled forceps. **3**, electric knife. **4**, clip applier. **5**, right and left angled scissors. **6**, needle holder.

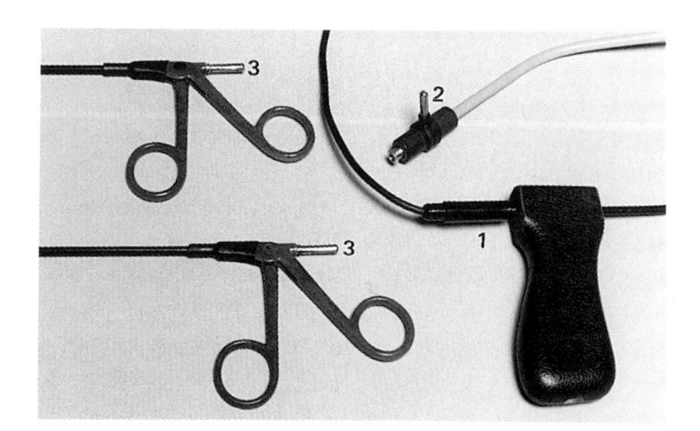

Figure 6.10: Electrified instruments. **1**, electric knife. **2**, suction–irrigation. **3**, right and left angled forceps.

Position

The patient is positioned on the table so that the center of the tumor is directly down toward the operating table and the scope tip opening is straight over the tumor. The patient may be in the right lateral, left lateral, supine (in candy-cane type stirrups) or prone jackknife positions. Making the patient comfortable in the prone jackknife position is the most difficult preoperative activity because of the flexed lower legs.

Technique[10,11]

A Foley catheter is inserted to keep the bladder decompressed. A vaginal prep is necessary in case the vagina is entered. A rectal prep is also necessary to minimize the risk of contamination of the operative site. The multiple lines to the operating scope may be passed across the patient's body to keep them out of the way of the surgeon. (There are lines for suction–irrigation, electrocautery, carbon dioxide pressure insufflation, light, and carbon dioxide monitoring.)

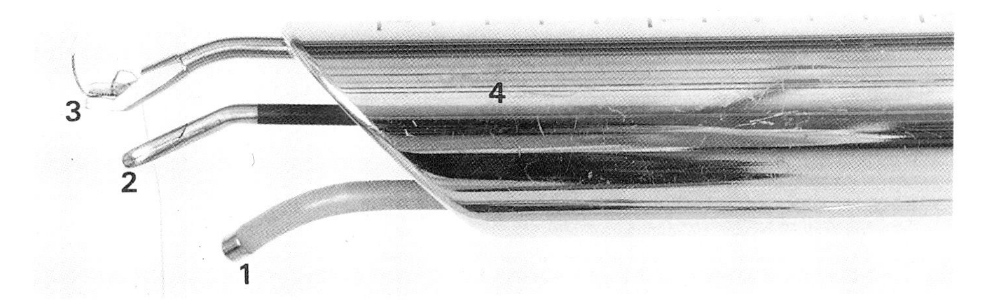

Figure 6.11: Instruments projecting through the operating proctoscope. **1**, suction–irrigation probe. **2**, forceps. **3**, needle holder. **4**, scope barrel. Note the 3–0 PDS suture held by the needle holder. It is 6 cm in length with a silver clip clamped onto the tip of the suture. This clip will be the first 'knot'.

The equipment must be checked to see that it is working appropriately and that there are no carbon dioxide leaks. After the scope has been introduced, the obturator is removed and the window face plate is used to cover the open proctoscope and make the rectum gas-tight so that it will retain the insufflated carbon dioxide gas (Figure 6.4). When the face plate on the operating proctoscope is locked in position, the Martin arm is affixed to the table so that the operating proctoscope can be clamped onto it (Figure 6.6). Carbon dioxide is run at 6 L min^{-1} until a pressure of 15 mmHg is achieved. The operating proctoscope should be placed over the right portion of the tumor first. The electrocautery knife is used to outline the lesion at a distance of 1 cm from the edge of the tumor (Figure 6.12). With a cancer this margin might be wider. I generally create a small tab of additional normal tissue to the right with my initial outline so that I can use it to lift the specimen while maintaining traction; therefore my forceps will not crush or touch the tumor itself (Figure 6.13). A special long syringe may be used to inject a dilute epinephrine solution around the margins to help minimize blood loss.

On the burn outlining the tumor, the knife is used to cut down to the chosen level (Figure 6.14). If one is certain that the tumor is benign, the dissection is performed at the submucosal level. However, most of the time a full-thickness cut-down to fat is employed. The electrocautery device has high-frequency and electrocoagulation settings. The high-frequency setting cuts very readily but also produces large amount of smoke which must be evacuated. A general principle is to work from the right side of the tumor toward the left in transverse fashion (Figure 6.13). In order to keep the work site in the center of the field, shifting the scope is frequently necessary. The operating table may be turned to the right or left to change positions, the scope may be pulled back and reinserted or turned, and the surgeon may tilt his head sideways to see through the scope. The instruments are kept parallel within the scope and are not allowed to cross. If they cross, tip mobility is restricted considerably.

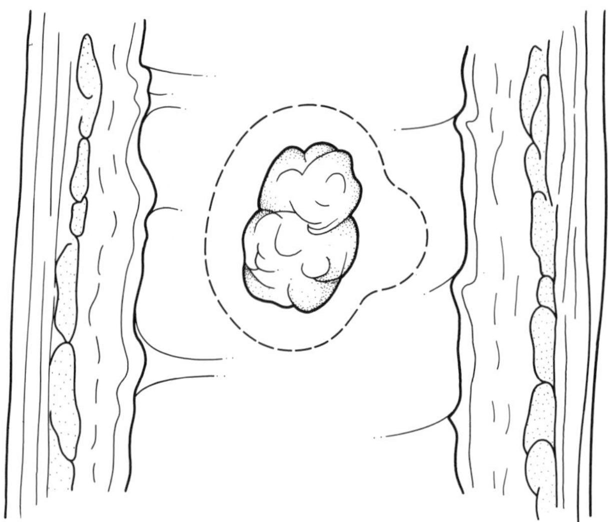

Figure 6.12: The tumor outlined. The dots represent points of eschar created by the electric knife. These dots are at least 1 cm away from a carcinoma. A tab is created to the right so that tissue can be grasped without touching the tumor.

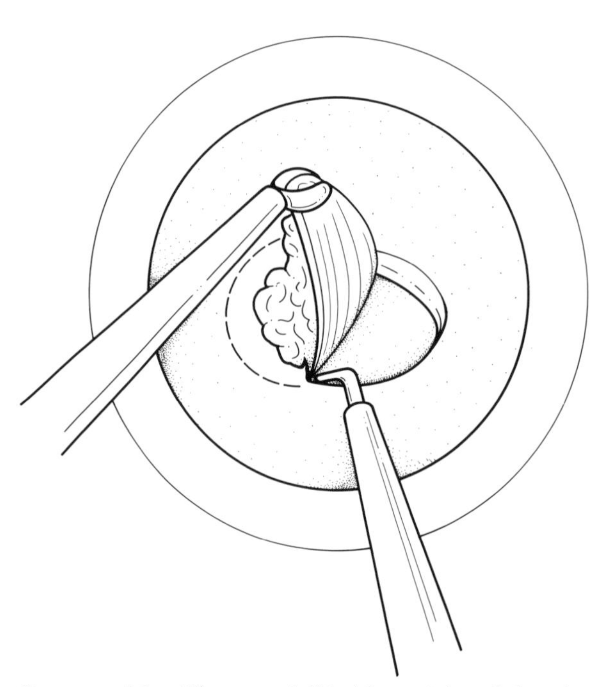

Figure 6.13: Tumor excision. The tumor is lifted from right to left as the tumor is undercut.

Whenever bleeding vessels are encountered, electrocoagulation should be instituted immediately. Once vision is lost it is very difficult to recover. As the dissection proceeds, the tumor is lifted and undercut. The wound may be closed when the tumor has been removed.

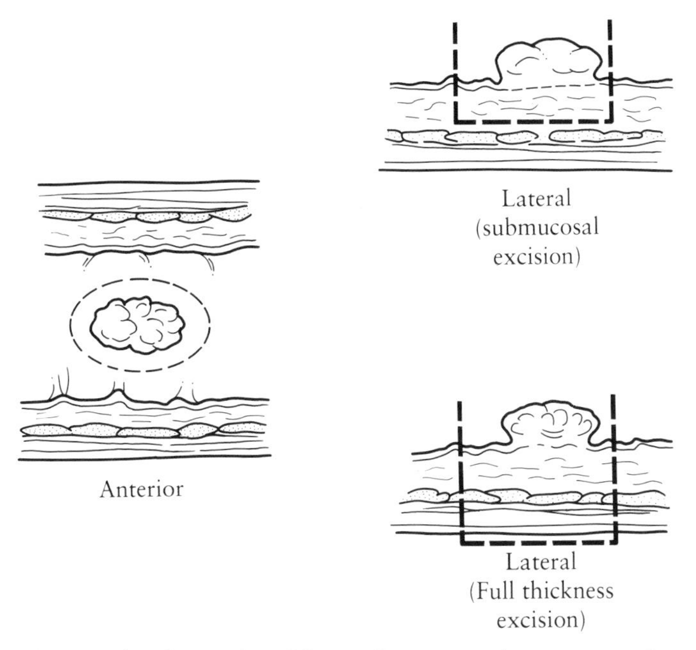

Figure 6.14: Depth of resection. The outline is cut down upon. Then the depth is determined based upon whether the tumor is benign or malignant. Benign tumors may be resected in the submucosal plane. A carcinoma must be resected full thickness.

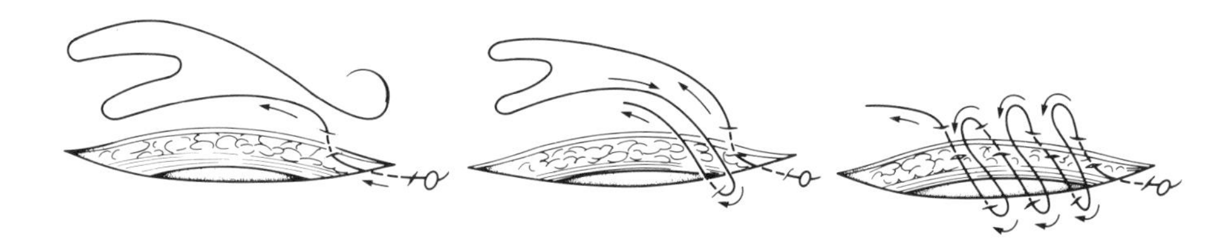

Figure 6.15: Closure of the wound. The 3–0 PDS suture, which is cut in 6 cm lengths, has a silver clip which will bind as it is pulled through tissue: hence tying a knot is avoided. The sewing progresses from right to left. Several pieces of PDS may be used if the incision is long.

Ordinarily 3–0 PDS is used for closure. Spilt clips are first applied to the suture, and another clip at the end of the suture line is used in place of a knot. (Figure 6.11). Sewing is performed, beginning at the right end of the excision site. The closure is carried toward the left from the right; hence it is a transverse closure, minimizing the chance for stenosis (Figure 6.15).

The most difficult procedures are those for large benign adenomas. When such an adenoma is circumferential or almost circumferential the margins are difficult to recognize, especially as the excision progresses and the specimen is in the way of direct vision. Therefore identifying-stay sutures are applied as the excision takes place. By keeping the proximal cut margin in relationship to the distal cut edge, the lumen will be maintained and more easily closed later. The stay sutures may be removed subsequently after the running PDS suture has been applied. For closure, the patient and/or scope will often be moved in order to center the work field and keep control of the proximal margin.

Postoperative care

The patient is restricted from oral intake for a day. Clear liquids may be offered on the second day, and if these are tolerated a solid diet is then allowed. Some patients with small lesions, however, may be discharged home at once, and can take clear liquids immediately.

If cancer is found to extend full thickness through the bowel wall, then more radical surgery should be offered. Signs such as poor differentiation, venous or lymphatic invasion or growth into the fat surrounding the rectum should prompt the surgeon to recommend radical surgery because this group is at high risk for recurrence. If the tumor did not enter the muscularis propria in its growth, the operation is usually curative. If the tumor has grown into the muscularis propria (T2 extension), radiation therapy may be added if radical surgery is declined. This latter choice may be adequate in most cases. On discharge, patients require pain medication, stool softeners and additional oral fluid intake to keep the stool soft.

Complications

Early complications include rectovaginal fistula, perforation into the free peritoneal space, infection and hemorrhage. If a perforation to the vagina or the peritoneum is discovered, it should be repaired immediately; hence a well prepped bowel and vagina may be closed primarily and healing may be expected. Laparoscopy or laparotomy may be necessary to close an intraperitoneal perforation. Fever suggests infection, and antibiotics should be administered specifically to attack those flora of colonic origin.

Sphincter injury and incontinence manifested by soiling may be recognized as a late complication. If a benign tumor recurs, it may be reexcised or destroyed locally. If a malignant tumor recurs in the margin of the resection, local resection may be tried again if it is tiny. However, if the carcinoma is large or distant from the original site, a low anterior resection or abdominoperineal resection should be employed.

Only one death has been reported in the literature using these techniques, and it was due to a pulmonary embolus. Other nonspecific complications include pneumonia and urinary tract infection.

Results

Recurrence of properly selected cancers is unusual. Buess and colleagues[5] reported the recurrence of only one of 51 T_1-N_0-M_0 carcinomas. Of four T_2-N_0-M_0 carcinomas treated at the George Washington University Medical Center, two have recurred. They were converted to abdominoperineal resections and both patients are alive and free of disease. Anterior resection was recommended for another patient who had invasion of lymphatics. This patient is alive three years after TEM excision plus radiation, without evidence of disease.

For adenomas, careful follow-up has been necessary because small sites of villous tumors have recurred adjacent to suture lines. These have been easily treated in the office by electrocoagulation. Buess *et al.*[5] reported a 4% recurrence rate after excision of villous adenomas.

References

1 Buess G, Thiess R, Gunther M *et al.* (1984) Endoscopic operative procedure for the removal of rectal polyps. *Coloproctol.* **6**:254–60.

2 Buess G, Thiess, R, Gunther M *et al.* (1985) Endoscopic surgery in the rectum. *Endoscopy.* **17**:31–5.

3 Buess G, Kipfmuller K, Hack D *et al.* (1988) Technique of transanal endoscopic microsurgery. *Surg Endosc.* **2**:71–5.

4 Buess G, Kipfmuller K, Hack D *et al.* (1988) Clinical results of transanal endoscopic microsurgery. *Surg Endosc.* **2**:245–50.

5 Buess G, Mentges B, Manncke K *et al.* (1991) Minimal invasive surgery in the local treatment of rectal cancer. *Int J Colorect Dis.* **6**:77–81

6 Kraske KP (1885) Zur Extirpation hochsitzender Mastdarm Krebs. *Verh Deutsch Ges Chi.* **14**:464–74.

7 York-Mason A (1970) Surgical access to the rectum – a transsphincteric exposure. **63**:91–4.

8 Dukes CE (1932) The classification of cancer of the rectum. *J Pathol N Bacteriol.* **35**:323–32.

9 Beynon J, Foy DMA, Roe AM *et al.* (1986) Endoluminal ultrasound in the assessment of local invasion in rectal cancer. *Br J Surg.* **73**:474–7.

10 Hildebrandt V, Fiefel G, Schwarz HP *et al.* (1986) Endorectal ultrasounds instrumentation and clinical aspects. *Int J Colorectal Dis.* **1**: 304–8.

11 Saclarides TJ, Smith L, Ko ST *et al.* (1992) Transanal endoscopic microsurgery. *Dis Colon Rectum* **35**:1183–91.

12 Smith L (1993) Transanal endoscopic microsurgery for rectal neoplasms. *Gastrointest Endosc Clin N Am.* **3**:329–41.

7

Laparoscopic Approach to Suspected Appendicitis

MARGRET ODDSDOTTIR AND JOHN G HUNTER

Historical introduction

The early anatomical drawing which Leonardo da Vinci did in 1492 can be said to represent the earliest appearance of the appendix in the literature. The first reported appendectomy was done in 1735 by Claudius Amyand, Serjeant-Surgeon to George II. He removed a perforated appendix with a fecal fistula through a right inguinal hernia using a scrotal incision[1]. The first appendectomy with the correct preoperative diagnosis was done was Lawson Tait in 1880[2]. In 1886 Reginald H Fits, at the Association of American Physicians, awakened the medical profession to the significance of the appendix vermiformis undergoing inflammation (acute appendicitis) and the need for its early removal to prevent the complications previously reported[2]. A few years later Charles McBurney described point tenderness in the right lower abdominal quadrant, indicative of appendicitis, and popularized the 'muscle-splitting' incision[3]. Little in the diagnosis and treatment of appendicitis has changed since then.

More than 80 years have elapsed since laparoscopy was introduced. Only recently, however, have advances in optics, video transmission and high-resolution video monitoring opened the door to its use for many surgical procedures, diagnostic and therapeutic. Today one can inspect the peritoneal cavity and pelvis much more thoroughly with the laparoscope than with a small laparotomy or muscle-splitting incision. Laparoscopic appendectomy for the uninflamed appendix was first reported in Germany in 1983 by Semm, a gynecologist and the true father of operative laparoscopy[4]. In 1985 Flemming, from New South Wales, reported a laparoscopic assisted appendectomy for the treatment of acute appendicitis[5]. In 1987 Schreiber, from Germany, reported laparoscopic appendectomy for the treatment of acute appendicitis[6]. Since then many reports have been published indicating that laparoscopic appendectomy is safe and feasible in most settings[7–14]. However, the specific indications, benefits and possible drawbacks of laparoscopic appendectomy have yet to be established.

Diagnosis

Acute appendicitis is very common, affecting one out of every 14 individuals in the USA over an average lifetime[15]. Acute appendicitis is the commonest cause for an operation in patients with acute abdominal pain. In the USA alone about 500,000 appendectomies are performed each year, more than half of these for acute appendicitis[16].

The clinical presentation of acute appendicitis is often confusing. Appendicitis can be mistaken for diseases of any organ within the abdomen. When the presentation is classic, the diagnosis proves to be wrong at surgery in 5–30% of cases[15,17]. In women of child-bearing age, the incidence of false-positive diagnosis is even higher; up to 45% of patients operated on for acute appendicitis have a normal appendix[17–19]. Despite these high false-positive rates, the overall rate of perforation is 21%[15]. In children less than five years of age, and patients aged 65 years or more, the perforation rate is up to 50% and is associated with significant morbidity and mortality[15,17]. When other medical conditions are present, or the patient has received antibiotics or steroids, the diagnosis of appendicitis becomes even more difficult.

The inherent error rate of 5–30% in the diagnosis of appendicitis is accepted by most clinicians. A negative appendectomy rate of less than 10% for a surgeon is generally felt to be too low, indicating that he is operating too infrequently, increasing the risk of rupture in those he chooses not to explore. Therefore exploration is advised on the assumption that the danger when appendicitis is missed is greater than that of an unnecessary abdominal exploration. However, removal of the normal appendix is not entirely inconsequential. Apart from the inconvenience and cost of the hospital stay, there is a measurable incidence of wound infection and long-term sequelae[17,19,20]. In a review of 1000 appendectomies, the rate of normal appendices removed was 20%[17]. The wound infection rate was 4% and the total morbidity was 15% for patients undergoing removal of the normal appendix.

Is it estimated that from laparotomy alone, about 50% of patients will have significant adhesions[22–24]. If appendectomy is added, up to 70% will have adhesions in the lower abdomen[4,19–21]. These adhesions have been associated with infertility, chronic lower abdominal pain and bowel obstruction. In a series of 2465 patients undergoing laparoscopy for various pelvic problems, 68.1% had previous open appendectomy adhesions. In 55% of patients who were infertile after appendectomy, periovarian and peritubal adhesions were felt to be responsible.

There has been little progress in the diagnosis of appendicitis in the past several decades. A thorough history and physical examination remain the most accurate preoperative investigation. The use of plain films of the abdomen, looking for abnormal gas pattern, appendicolith, soft tissue density in the right lower quadrant and levoscoliosis, was evaluated in 154 patients with suspected appendicitis who had undergone appendectomy[40]. Of the abnormal findings, only the presence of abnormal gas pattern was associated with appendicitis. The abnormal gas pattern was related to the degree of inflammation and was found in 62% of patients with acute appendicitis and 97% of patients with gangrenous appendices.

The value of visualizing the appendix with contrast medium to rule out the diagnosis of appendicitis has been much debated[37,38,41,42]. By looking for persistent non-visualization or partial visualization, pressure defects on the cecum and irritability or spasms of the ileocecal region, Ferzli and colleagues found that barium enema had an accuracy of up to 91.5%, with 96% specificity and 83% sensitivity[41]. Other authors have not been able to show such high diagnostic value for barium enema[37,38,42]. Fedyshin and coworkers found barium enema to be of limited use, except when the entire appendiceal lumen filled with contrast, in which case acute appendicitis could be virtually ruled out[42]. Selective use of barium enema in children does not appear to reduce the number of negative explorations[37].

Ultrasonography has also been used to aid the diagnosis of appendicitis. Ultrasonography is very operator-dependent, requiring skilled and dedicated personnel. In a recent study ultrasonography had 76% accuracy, 78% sensitivity and 73% specificity, as compared to 89, 95 and 84% respectively for the clinical assessment[25]. In another report, 111 patients were evaluated for possible appendicitis with ultrasonography. Ultrasonography resulted in changes in the proposed management in 26% of patients[43]. Prompt surgical therapy was performed as a result of ultrasonography in 47 of the 111 patients and the negative laparotomy rate was 8.5%.

Finally, CT scans can be of value, especially in the evaluation of advanced appendicitis. In a study of 40 patients with suspected periappendiceal abscess (pain, fever, palpable mass), CT scan reliably differentiated between an abscess and a phlegmon in all, but there were three errors in diagnosis, including a ruptured cecal lymphoma, a ruptured cecal diverticulum and a ruptured corpus luteum cyst[44].

Diagnostic laparoscopy can reliably identify those patients who have appendicitis and also (less reliably) those who do not[18,30,33]. Nowzaradan and colleagues found that, with diagnostic laparoscopy in patients with suspected appendicitis, the correct diagnosis was made 98% of the time[30]. Leape and Ramenofsky reduced their negative appendectomy rate from 10 to 1% by using laparoscopy in patients with suspected appendicitis but equivocal or insufficient clinical findings[26]. With diagnostic laparoscopy, the patient can be spared many noninvasive tests, long observation time and unnecessary laparotomies. During diagnostic laparotomy for suspected appendicitis, the entire abdomen can be explored and coexisting pathologic conditions identified. The viewing capabilities through the laparoscope far exceed that of exploration through a right lower quadrant incision. Diagnostic laparoscopy causes minimal adhesions, if any, and is associated with very low morbidity[4,23]. Adding an appendectomy extends the role of the laparoscope in the management of suspected appendicitis, and causes little additional morbidity[8,26]. In their updated review of 1253 laparoscopic appendectomies, Pier *et al.* reported a complication rate of 1%[13]. For open appendectomies, Lewis *et al.* reported a complication rate of 18.5% and mortality of 0.8%[17].

The absolute contraindications for laparoscopic appendectomy are the same as those for diagnostic laparoscopy. These are the inability to tolerate general anesthesia, uncorrected coagulopathy, advanced bowel obstruction and extensive adhesions.

Laparoscopic appendectomy: technique

Preoperative preparation

The preoperative care for laparoscopic appendectomy is similar to that for a standard open approach. The minimum laboratory investigations needed include a complete blood count and urine analysis. If perforation is suspected, broad-spectrum intravenous antibiotics are administered, otherwise only prophylactic antibiotics are indicated. There is generally no need for preoperative radiologic procedures.

Procedure

Laparoscopic appendectomy is a two-person procedure, requiring only a surgeon and an assistant (scrub nurse, resident or physician assistant). Both stand at the patient's left side, facing the video monitor across the table (Figure 7.1).

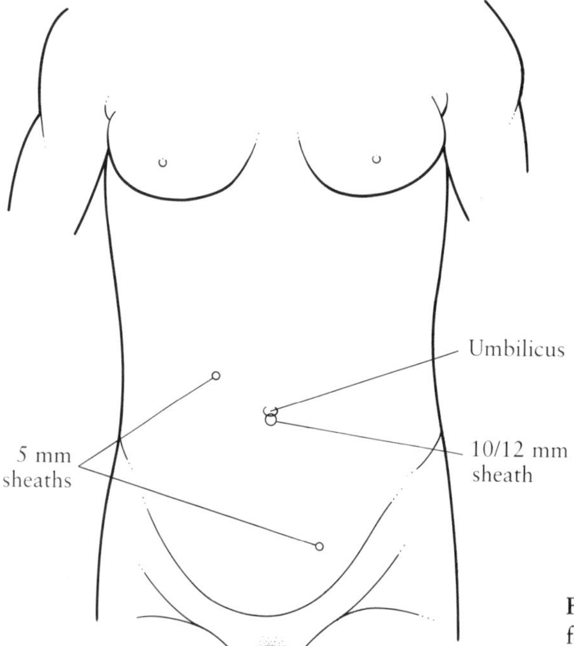

Figure 7.1: Port placement for laparoscopic appendectomy. The location and size of the ports are changed as necessary.

The patient is placed supine on the operating table. If pelvic pathology is suspected in the female patient, she is placed in the lithotomy position and a uterine manipulator inserted. Due to increased intra-abdominal pressure generated during laparoscopy, sequential compression stockings are suggested. A Foley catheter and naso-gastric tube are placed after the patient is asleep. It is important to decompress the stomach and the bladder to minimize the risk of injuring them during cannula insertion and to provide adequate exposure of the operative field. The patient should be in the Trendelenburg position to allow gravity-assisted retraction of the transverse colon and omentum. The patient is draped widely to allow access to the entire abdomen, and a laparotomy instrument set is kept within the operating room.

Pneumoperitoneum

Pneumoperitoneum is established using either the Verres needle or the open technique through the umbilicus. The procedure is initiated as a three-puncture technique, adding a fourth port if necessary. First a 10/12 mm trocar is placed in the umbilical area and subsequently the laparoscope is put in place. A 30° forward oblique viewing telescope aids in the diagnostic evaluation. The abdomen is explored visually. A 5 mm trocar is placed either suprapubically or in the left lower quadrant. A probe or a grasping instrument through this port will facilitate exposure during the exploration. If the diagnosis of appendicitis is correct and an appendectomy is to be performed, the third trocar (5 mm) is placed in the right upper quadrant. A fourth port (5 mm) in the right lower quadrant may be necessary for traction on the appendix, but often a catgut loop inserted through a trocar, alongside an instrument, will serve to expose the appendix adequately.

Mobilizing the appendix and cecum

To facilitate exposure, the appendix and cecum are mobilized as needed by sharply incising the lateral peritoneal attachments along the line of Toldt. It is important to see the entire appendix for the diagnosis of acute appendicitis, since early in the course of the disease only the tip of the organ may be inflamed[33]. With the appendix mobilized, it is elevated and stretched toward the pelvis by a grasper placed through the left lower abdominal port. Alternatively a loop ligature is placed over the distal portion of the appendix to be used as a handle for retraction.

Mesoappendix

Various techniques described for the dissection and division of the mesoappendix include the use of loop ligatures, clips, bipolar electrocoagulation and linear intestinal stapling devices. If loop ligatures and clips are to be used, windows are created as necessary around the vessels in the mesoappendix with a blunt dissecting instrument. The vessels are either clipped or tied with a loop ligature and divided (Figure 7.2). When a stapling device is used to secure the mesoappendix, the umbilical 10/12 mm port is used for the device. Visualization of the procedure occurs with a 5 mm telescope placed through the left lower quadrant trocar. A vascular cartridge is loaded into the stapler, placed across

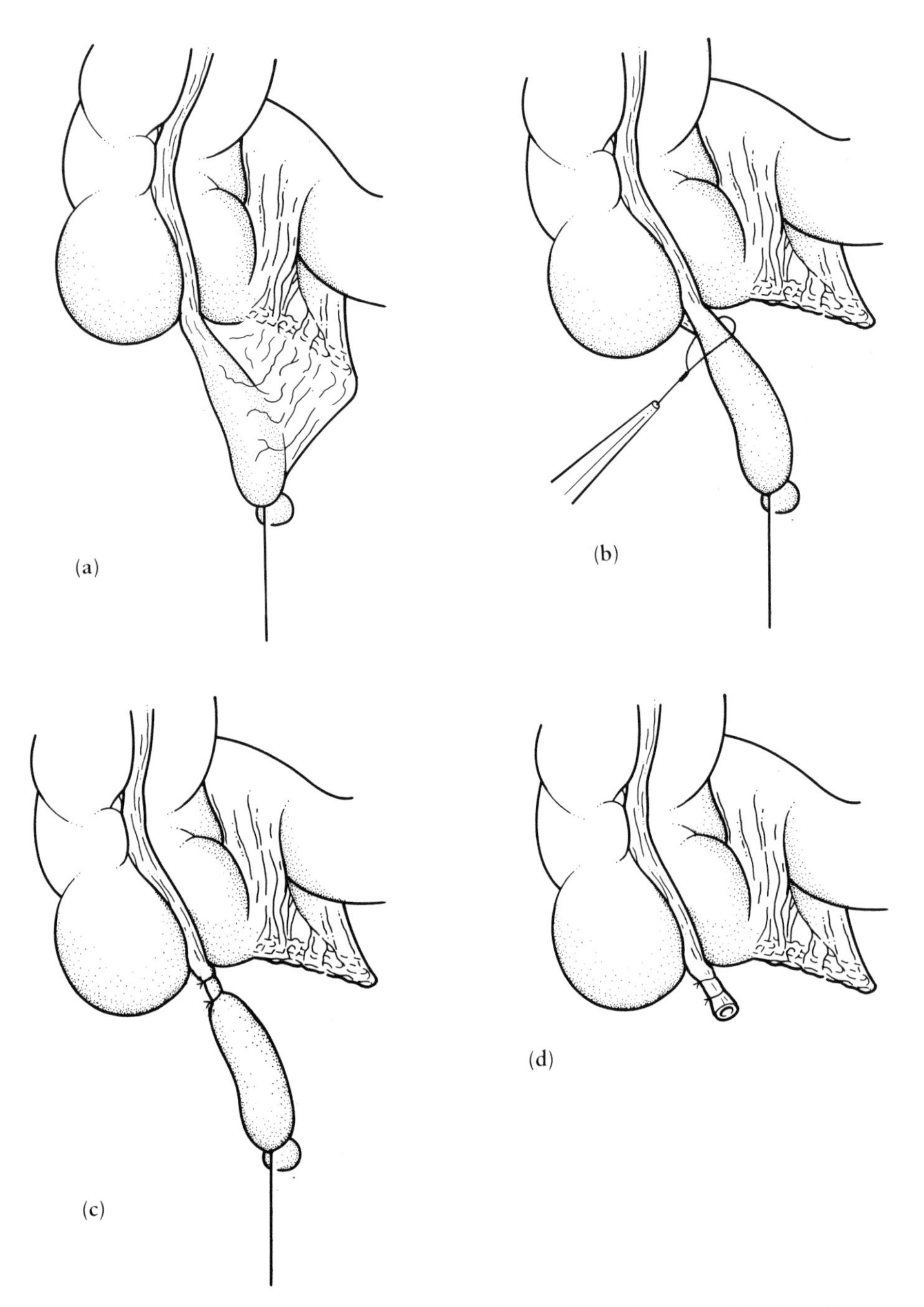

Figure 7.2: Laparoscopic appendectomy using clips and loop ligatures. (**a**) A loop ligature has been placed on the tip of the appendix for retraction. Division of the mesoappendix is begun using clips for hemostasis. (**b**) Mesoappendix completely divided. Pretied loop ligatures are passed towards the base of the appendix. (**c**) Three ligatures are tied at the base of the appendix. The first two ligatures are 5 mm apart, the third is 1 cm distal to the proximal two. (**d**) Appendectomy completed. The appendix is divided, leaving two ligatures on the stump.

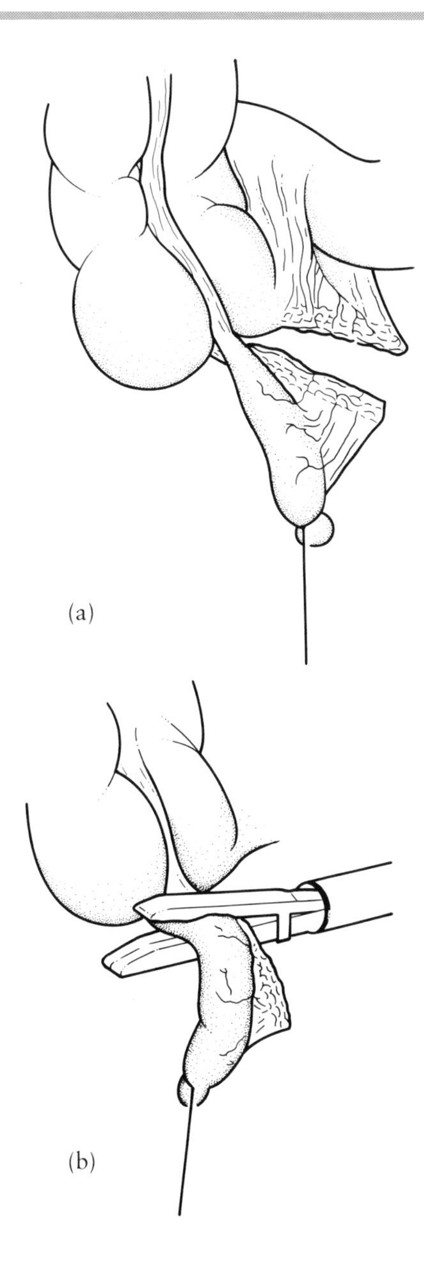

Figure 7.3: Laparoscopic appendectomy using stapling device. (**a**) The mesoappendix is divided using a vascular cartridge in the stapler. (**b**) The stapler is reloaded with a gastrointestinal cartridge and the appendix is transected at its base.

the mesoappendix and fired (Figure 7.3). Any residual bleeding can be controlled with a clip placed across the staple line. Finally the appendix can be skeletonized from tip to base by coagulating the mesoappendix with bipolar coagulation forceps and subsequently dividing it with scissors in the coagulated area[13].

Resection of the appendix

With the mesoappendix divided, the base of the appendix is exposed. The appendix can be resected using either pretied loop ligatures or the stapling device. With the first technique, three chromic catgut loops are passed over the tip of the appendix and secured at the base of the appendix. Two ligatures are placed 5 mm apart, close to the cecum, and the third tie is placed 1 cm distal to the first two. The appendix is transected between the ties, leaving two loops on the cecal end. The appendix can be transected using scissors, electrocautery or laser energy. If monopolar electrocautery is used to cauterize the appendiceal stump, there is a risk of thermal injury of the appendiceal base. This can result in necrosis and a subsequent stump leak. Sterilization of the stump with either electrocautery or iodine swab is advocated by some authors, but has never been proven necessary. Invagination of the stump is also unnecessary[35], but if one wants to invert the tip of the amputated appendix, this can be done using a needle and suture and either external or internal knotting techniques. If a stapling device is used, it is loaded with a gastrointestinal staple cartridge, placed across the base of the appendix and fired.

Removal of the appendix

Removal of the appendix is done in one of two ways. If the appendix is small enough, it is grasped and pulled through the 10/12 mm trocar to prevent direct wound contact. Larger trocars can replace the 10/12 mm trocar if the appendix is large and edematous. Alternatively, a sterile specimen retrieval bag is placed into the abdomen and the appendix placed inside. The same procedure used in removing the gallbladder during cholecystectomy is used to extract the bag and appendix. When the appendix is removed in this manner, it is helpful to release the pneumoperitoneum to allow the fascia to stretch and accommodate the passage of the bag and its contents. This is the preferred method for the extraction of necrotic or perforated appendices. The fascia is closed at the umbilicus and where any 10/12 mm ports were placed. The skin incisions are closed with a subcuticular suture, staples or sterile adhesive tapes.

Complicated appendicitis

The laparoscopic approach to complicated appendicitis may be superior to open appendectomy. The visibility for dissection of inflamed tissue and irrigation of the entire abdomen can be accomplished without extension of the incision. Drainage can be performed and the wound is less exposed to the infected tissue.

Retrocecal appendix

If the appendix is not identified during the initial exploration, the cecum is mobilized sharply with scissors or electrocautery along the peritoneal reflection. Atraumatic bowel graspers are used for retraction of the cecum. Reflecting the cecal pole up and to the left will often expose the appendix, which then can be removed as described above. In this location, however, the appendix (especially the tip) may be covered by adhesions, making the operation difficult. If that is the case, retrograde dissection should be performed. For retrograde resection of the appendix, the trocar placement is the same as for the usual antegrade resection. Once the cecum and the base of the appendix have been identified, a window is created in the mesoappendix, near the base. The appendix can be transected with a stapler or between ligatures as described above. The ligatures are placed in continuity, using external or internal knot tying, before dividing the appendix. The cut end of the appendix is retracted to expose the mesoappendix. The mesoappendix is transected in a reversed manner, using the same techniques as for antegrade transection.

Gangrenous appendix

When the appendix is necrotic or gangrenous, the anatomy is often obscure. An exudate can usually be seen in the area of the cecal pole or in the pelvis. With careful blunt dissection the large phlegmonous appendix can usually be identified and shelled out from its inflamed bed. Once mobilized, the appendix is resected in the same manner as described above. When the appendix is gangrenous or perforated, it should be extracted in a sterile bag to minimize contamination. When the appendix is removed in this manner, the umbilical cannula is removed, pneumoperitoneum evacuated and the bag and its contents extracted. The cannula is replaced to inspect the operative area and to irrigate as necessary.

Perforated appendix

For the perforated appendix, similar steps are followed as for the necrotic appendix. If the perforation is close to the tip of the appendix, an attempt to close it off with a loop ligature is sometimes possible. If the perforation is close to the base, ligation or stapling of the stump close to the perforated or necrotic areas is risky and can be impossible. The cecum should instead by mobilized adequately and the appendix removed by applying the gastrointestinal stapler across the base of the cecum. The appendix is extracted using a sterile bag as described above.

Appendiceal abscess

If an appendiceal abscess is suspected, the Trendelenburg position is avoided to prevent contamination of the upper abdomen. When the diagnosis is known prior to surgery, the abscess is identified by bluntly dissecting the adherent bowel loops away. The abscess cavity is aspirated dry and irrigated. Then the appendectomy is performed as described above. A drain should be left in the abscess cavity. The drain can be pulled in through the umbilical trocar and out one of the 5 mm trocar sites or if necessary through a separate stab wound incision in the right lower quadrant.

Conversion to open procedure

The only absolute contraindication for laparoscopic appendectomy is the inability to safely obtain a pneumoperitoneum under general anesthesia. Early in the experience with laparoscopic appendectomy, advanced and complicated appendicitis were considered indications for conversion to an open procedure. However, with improved technique and increased experience, most appendiceal conditions can be managed laparoscopically. Moreover, most skilled laparoscopic surgeons find that the complicated appendicitis can often be better managed through the laparoscope than through a small muscle-splitting incision. The view is better, abscesses are easier identified and treated, and the entire abdomen may be explored and lavaged.

Nevertheless, a prudent surgeon will occasionally have to convert a laparoscopic appendectomy to an open procedure. The various reasons that may lead to conversion include:

- time restrictions
- inability to gain exposure
- fear of intestinal injury
- extensive phlegmon
- inability to recognize the base of the appendix
- extensive adhesions
- uncontrolled bleeding.

Postoperative care

The Foley catheter, naso–gastric tube and the sequential compression stockings are discontinued in the recovery room. Oral fluid may be started immediately postoperatively if the appendicitis and appendectomy have been uncomplicated. An unrestricted diet is resumed if the patient tolerates liquids. Antibiotics are continued if clinically indicated (phlegmon, gangrene and perforation). Discharge from the hospital occurs as soon as the patient feels fit, within 24 hours. Return to normal activity is unrestricted.

Results

Many reviews of laparoscopic appendectomy have been published in the past five years. These reviews indicate that laparoscopic appendectomy has some advantages over the open technique in exposure, diagnostic capabilities and cosmetic results. In some studies hospital stay, morbidity and rehabilitation are decreased when laparoscopic appendectomy is performed. Open appendectomy does not require specially trained operating room personnel or special operating room equipment, and it is less expensive.

Recent reports

Saye and colleagues reported three years' experience with laparoscopic appendectomy beginning in 1988[10]. Of their 109 procedures, the appendectomy was performed in addition to other primary pelvic procedures in 85% of cases, principally enterolysis and ablation of endometriosis. Laparoscopic appendectomy was performed for acute appendicitis in only 10 patients, including one with perforated appendix. Patients who had appendectomies as secondary procedure were discharged at a mean interval of 23 hours following surgery, but those with acute appendicitis were discharged 36 hours following appendectomy. The appendectomy required no increase in operating time over standard open appendectomy, and the average time for appendectomy was 20 minutes after laparoscopic access was achieved. The patients usually returned to normal activity after three or four days.

The largest reported series of laparoscopic appendectomies comes from Germany[9,13,34]. Between May 1987 and September 1991, laparoscopic appendectomy was attempted in 933 patients (Table 7.1). The procedure was converted to an open procedure in 18 cases (2%), most of which occurred during

Operative time	15–20 minutes
Conversion rate	18 (2%)
Normal pathology	112 (12%)
Wound infection	14 (1.7%)
Stump leak	1 (0.1%)
Abscess formation	2 (0.2%)

Table 7.1: Experience of laparoscopic appendectomy in 933 patients[13].

the initial phase of the study period. These conversions to open technique were required because of extensive adhesions, extreme obesity, bleeding, abnormal vermix position, abscess or perforation. With improved equipment and experience, none of these were a problem later on in the study. Pathologic examination showed that 12% had no evidence of acute appendiceal inflammation.

Nonrandomized prospective data comparing the results of open versus laparoscopic appendectomy in the USA have recently been published; perforated appendices were excluded[14]. The results indicate a trend towards increased use of laparoscopy in females for diagnosis, with a high percentage of normal appendices removed (Table 7.2). The laparoscopic procedures took longer than the open ones, a mean of 88 minutes versus 59 minutes respectively (Table 7.2). The hospital stay and return to normal activity were similar in both groups, but the hospital cost was significantly higher in the laparoscopic group (a mean of $ 6838 versus $ 5439). The wound infection rate was lower in the laparoscopic group. They concluded that their data did not show clear superiority of one approach over the other; however, the laparoscopic technique was advantageous in cases of diagnostic uncertainty and the obese patients.

In the pediatric population, Gilchrist and colleagues compared their nonrandomized prospective data and found that the patients who had laparoscopic appendectomy spent significantly fewer days in hospital and returned earlier to unrestricted activity than those who had had an open procedure[11]. The operations took similar lengths of time if the appendicitis was uncomplicated;

	Open	Laparoscopic
Number	39	34
Gender M/F	24/15	11/23
Mean operative time (minutes)*	59 ± 20	88 ± 32
Mean hospital stay (days)	2.8	2.9
Normal pathology	6 (15.4%)	12 (35%)
Mean hospital cost	$5430	$6838
Wound infection	1 (2.6%)	0
Mean return to activity (days)	17.6	16.6

Table 7.2: Laparoscopic appendectomy versus open appendectomy[14].
*$p < 0.05$.

	Open	Laparoscopic
Number	32	30
Mean operative time (minutes)	51 (range 15–100)	61 (range 20–130)
Mean hospital stay (days)*	2.8 (range 1–7)	2.5 (range 1–7)
Normal appendix	7 (23%)	0
Complications	4 (12%)	0

Table 7.3: Prospective randomized trial, open versus laparoscopic appendectomy[12].
*$p < 0.05$.

otherwise the laparoscopic approach took significantly longer. The laparoscopic procedure was approximately $1000 more expensive, but because of shorter hospital stays for the laparoscopic group the total hospital cost was comparable.

Retrospective analysis of laparoscopic appendectomy in 465 children by Valla and coworkers also indicated more rapid recovery and return to normal activities[8]. They used two operative techniques, laparoscopically assisted and laparoscopic appendectomy, and found no difference in results. A total of 14 (3%) postoperative complications were identified, including incisional effusion, incisional hernia, abscesses and early small bowel obstruction.

The only prospective randomized trial of open versus laparoscopic appendectomy was published by Attwood and colleagues[12]. Thirty patients were randomized to laparoscopy and 32 to open appendectomy. Of the 30 patients who underwent laparoscopy, 27 appeared to have an inflamed appendix (which was successfully removed at laparoscopy in 25), but the three normal appendices were left in situ. The median operating time for the open procedure was 51 minutes, versus 61 minutes for the laparoscopic approach (Table 7.3). The authors noted that the time taken to perform laparoscopic appendectomy steadily declined during the study period. The mean lengths of hospital stay were two and three days for laparoscopic and open exploration respectively. The four complications that occurred were all in the open group. The laparoscopic group spent fewer days in bed, had less pain, returned earlier to work and were more satisfied with their scars.

The preliminary results from our multicenter randomized prospective study, comparing open appendectomy with laparoscopic stapled or laparoscopic loop ligature appendectomy, are equivocal (Table 7.4). Of the first hundred patients, the laparoscopic appendectomies took slightly longer and had the same complication rate. There were only three conversions to open procedures. There were no differences in length of hospital stay or return to regular activities.

		Laparoscopic	
	Open	Stapled	Ligature
Number	32	23	39
Mean operative time (minutes)	67	81	75
Conversion	NA	2	1
Mean hospital stay (days)	2.5	2.65	3.41
Complications	3	1	3
Mean return to full activity (days)	11.2	11.3	11.9

Table 7.4: Multicenter randomized prospective trial of appendectomy.

Complications

Most reports of laparoscopic appendectomy show a very low incidence of intraoperative and postoperative complications (in the range of 1–2%)[9,12,13,30]. For diagnostic laparoscopy alone, the incidence of complications is even lower. Lewis *et al.*, in their review of 1000 open appendectomies, reported a complication rate of 18.5%, about half of which were wound infections[17].

The most commonly reported complications of laparoscopic appendectomy are wound infection, bleeding, abscess, stump leak and pain. The wound infection rate is much lower than with open appendectomy[9,12,17,20]. Pier *et al.* reported a few cases of omphalitis during the initial phase of their study, but this problem was subsequently eliminated by careful preoperative cleansing of the umbilicus[9]. Other reports have reported few or no wound infections[12,14]. During the laparoscopic procedure the appendix never comes in contact with the skin, decreasing the risk of infection.

Bleeding is usually overestimated during laparoscopic procedures, because of the magnification of the camera. During the early phase of most laparoscopic surgeons, conversion to open technique will occur for bleeding[9]. However, with experience most bleeding can be handled laparoscopically by the use of clips, ligatures or coagulation.

Postoperative abscesses are uncommon with the laparoscopic technique[12,30]. The reported incidence of abscesses during conventional appendectomy is 4.3%[17]. With the improved view through the scope, better lavage and cleaning of the operative field is accomplished. There are rare reports of subhepatic and subphrenic abscesses, possibly due to spreading of infected fluid while the patient is in the Trendelenburg position[34]. This is an unproven theory and the incidence of abscesses has never been compared between the two methods.

Stump leak is another rare complication[6,13]. It may be related to excessive coagulation of the stump causing tissue necrosis. If electrocoagulation of the stump is performed, or the stump is handled in any other harmful way, it should be invaginated.

Pain after laparoscopic procedures is generally perceived as being less than for open procedures, requiring fewer analgesics. However, subphrenic and subscapular pain does occur, mostly on the operative day and the day after. Careful evacuation of all insufflated carbon dioxide and blood will minimize the incidence of this pain.

Discussion

Laparoscopic appendectomy is a minimal access technique. Advantages of the laparoscopic approach over open surgery include better exposure and visualization of the appendix and abdominal viscera, better diagnostic capability and improved cosmetic results. Laparoscopic appendectomy is probably associated with less postoperative morbidity, and probably results in fewer adhesions than a standard appendectomy, although this is still to be proven by long-term follow-up[23,30,36]. Some of the published reports do not show significant benefits of the laparoscopic approach for the otherwise healthy patient with a near certain diagnosis of appendicitis. However, with up to 30% of patients undergoing negative appendectomy and the overall perforation rate in the range of 20%, there is a place for improvement in both diagnosis and treatment. This large group of patients is exposed to significant morbidity, whether of the unnecessary procedure or their disease. When used judiciously, laparoscopy is both diagnostic and therapeutic, saving time and the need for radiologic attempts at diagnosis.

When the diagnosis of appendicitis is firm, the arguments against the use of laparoscopy are as follows:

- the same length of hospitalization is required for open and laparoscopic appendectomy
- laparoscopic appendectomy requires surgical and nursing expertise
- the standard appendectomy incision is not substantially longer than the combined incisions for laparoscopic appendectomy
- laparoscopic appendectomy is more expensive and will probably take longer to complete.

The risk of spillage or contamination may be greater when using laparoscopic methods to remove gangrenous or perforated appendices than during conventional open appendectomy[27].

There is some controversy about what to do if the diagnostic laparoscopy for possible appendicitis reveals a normal appendix[9,12,28,29]. Most surgeons agree that appendectomy should be considered. Early appendicitis can be difficult to diagnose; with its focus of luminal inflammation on histologic examination, it can look normal externally and therefore be missed on diagnostic laparoscopy[30]. Appendectomy not only eliminates the chance of missing early stage appendicitis, but also removes future diagnostic dilemmas associated with abdominal pain, especially in female patients of child-bearing age. The laparoscopic removal of a normal appendix seems to be associated with very low morbidity[23].

It is well established that an uninflamed appendix can be safely removed during laparotomy[31]. The incidence of complications of appendectomy performed in association with cholecystectomy, hysterectomy and cesarean section is no greater than when these procedures are performed alone. Laparoscopic appendectomy was initially practiced only as incidental appendectomy during pelviscopic surgery, without any reported complications[4]. Ferzli and colleagues reported on three incidental appendectomies during laparoscopic cholecystectomy, using the same ports[32]. They concluded that appendectomy is safe as long as the cholecystectomy is uncomplicated. Incidental laparoscopic appendectomy is surgically simple and probably safe, using the same criteria as for the open case[23,31].

Who benefits from laparoscopic appendectomy?

The subset of patients who could particularly benefit from the laparoscopic approach to suspected appendicitis are as follows.

Females child-bearing age

The negative appendectomy rate for this group of patients is as high as 45%[15,17,20]. The possibility of gynecological disease, in particular pelvic inflammatory disease, makes the diagnosis of appendicitis difficult. The difficulty of diagnosis and the hazard of missing an acute appendicitis explain the high rate of normal appendiceal pathology. Conventional appendectomy with or without normal pathology has significant long-term sequelae in this group of patients, related to adhesions, chronic pelvic pain and infertility[19,21].

The elderly with lower abdominal pain

Appendicitis is not a benign disease in the patient over 60 years of age. The perforation rate is more than 50% and is associated with significant morbidity and mortality. Other serious diseases (diverticulitis, perforated cecal/sigmoid carcinoma, cholecystitis etc) frequently found in this age group can mimic the presentation of appendicitis. It is of particular importance to make the diagnosis as soon as possible in the elderly.

Children

Like the elderly, children have a high incidence of perforated appendicitis, in particular those under the age of five[15,17]. Laparoscopy is safe in children, and should be strongly considered when the diagnosis is unclear. The laparoscopic approach could prevent undue delay while waiting for noninvasive diagnostic procedures.

The mentally or physically impaired

A good history and/or physical examination can be impossible to obtain from the mentally or physically impaired patient. These patients commonly present late, the diagnosis is difficult and the outcome often poor.

The obese

The physical examination can be difficult in the morbidly obese patient. Large incisions are needed to gain access to the abdomen, they offer poor visualization of the abdomen and are subsequently fraught with wound complications. Obesity does not interfere with laparoscopy as long as the trocars and instruments are long enough.

Summary

The use of the laparoscope in the management of suspected appendicitis was initially limited to diagnostic laparoscopy[18,33]. Its use was advocated to decrease the high number of unnecessary appendectomies and the associated morbidity. The development of laparoscopic appendectomy during the past decade has further extended the use of the laparoscope in the management of appendicitis. It is of some concern, however, that the number of normal appendices being removed has not decreased. As the availability of the laparoscope and the number of skilled laparoscopic surgeons increase; the question of overuse may become an issue. Laparoscopy should probably be used sooner rather than later when the surgeon is worried enough to admit and submit the patient to multiple noninvasive tests. It must be kept in mind, however, that laparoscopy requires general anesthesia and does carry some risk. It is costly, and requires an operating room and skilled personnel. Therefore laparoscopy should be used judiciously, and should not replace clinical evaluation and repeat observation of the minimally ill outpatient who has atypical right iliac fossa pain.

References

1 Creese PG (1953) The first appendectomy. *Surg Gynecol Obstet.* **97**:643.

2 Herrington JL (1991) The vermiform appendix: its surgical history. *Contemp Surg.* **39**:36–44.

3 McBurney C (1889) Experience with early operative interference in cases of disease of the vermiform appendix. *NY State Med J.* **50**:676.

4 Semm K (1983) Endoscopic appendectomy. *Endoscopy.* **15**:59–64.

5 Flemming JS (1985) Laparoscopically directed appendectomy. *Aust NZ Obstet Gynaecol.* **25**:238–40.

6 Schreiber JH (1987) Early experience with laparoscopic appendectomy in women. *Surg Endosc.* **1**:211–16.

7 Gangal H T and Gangal MH (1987) Laparoscopic appendectomy. *Endoscopy.* **19**:127–9.

8 Valla JS, Limonne, B, Valla V *et al.* (1991) Laparoscopic appendectomy in children: report of 465 cases. *Surg Laparosc Endosc.* **1**:16–172.

9 Pier A, Gotz F and Bacher C (1991) Laparoscopic appendectomy in 625 cases: from innovation to routine. *Surg Laparosc Endosc.* **1**:8–13.

10 Saye WB, Rives DA and Cochran EB (1991) Laparoscopic appendectomy: three years' experience. *Laparosc Endosc.* **1**:109–15.

11 Gilchrist BF, Lobe TE, Schropp KP *et al.* (1992) Is there a role for laparoscopic appendectomy in pediatric surgery? *J Ped Surg.* **27**:209–14.

12 Attwood SEA, Hill ADK, Murphy P G *et al.* (1992) A prospective randomized trial of laparoscopic versus open appendectomy. *Surgery.* **112**:497–501.

13 Pier A, Gotz F, Bacher C *et al.* (1993) Laparoscopic appendectomy. *World J Surg.* **17**:29–33.

14 Molnar RG, Apelgren KN and Kisala JM (1993) Open versus laparoscopic appendectomy: an update. *Surg Endosc.* **7**:121.

15 Adiss DG, Shaffer N, Fowler B *et al.* (1990) The epidemiology of appendicitis and appendectomy in the United States. *Am J Epidemiol.* **132**: 910–25.

16 National Inpatient Profile (1989) Healthcare Knowledge Systems.

17 Lewis FR, Holcroft JW, Boey J *et al.* (1975) Appendicitis. *Arch Surg.* **110**:677–84.

18 Whitwoth CM, Whitworth PW, Sanfillipo J *et al.* (1988) Value of diagnostic laparoscopy in young women with possible appendicitis. *Surg Gynecol Obstet.* **167**:187–90.

19 Lehmann-Willenbrock E, Mecke H and Riedel HH (1990) Sequelae of appendectomy, with special reference to intra-abdominal adhesions, chronic abdominal pain, and infertility. *Gynecol Obstet Invest.* **29**:241–5.

20 Chang FC, Hogle HH and Welling DR (1973) The fate of the negative appendix. *Am J Surg.* **126**:752–4.

21 Riedel HH and Haag G-M Spatfolgen nach Appendektomie unter besonderer Berucksichtigung von Unterbauchverwachsungen, chronischen Unterbeschwerden und Sterilitat. *Zentbl Gynakol.*

22 Lowe RJ, Boyd DR, Folk FA *et al.* (1989) The negative laparotomy for abdominal trauma. *J Trauma.* **111**:1101–12.

23 Semm K (1988) Die pelviskopische appendektomie. *Dtcsh Med Wochenschr.* **113**:3–5.

24 Bindel E and Ortmann G (1978) Der Dunndarmileus als fruhkomplikation nach appendektomie. *Artzl Fortbild.* **72**:757.

25 John H, Neff U and Kelemen M (1993) Appendicitis diagnosis today: Clinical and ultrasonic deductions. *World J Surg.* **17**:243–9.

26 Leape LL and Ramenofsky ML (1980) Laparoscopy for questionable appendicitis. *Ann Surg.* **191**:410–13.

27 Easter DW (1993) The diagnosis and treatment of acute appendicitis with laparoscopic methods. In: Hunter J G and Sackier JM (Eds) *Minimally invasive surgery.* McGraw-Hill. New York. pp. 171–7.

28 MacFadyen BV, Wolfe BM and McKernan JB (1992) Laparoscopic management of the acute abdomen, appendix, and small and large bowel. In: MacFadyen BV and Ponsky JL (Eds). *The surgical clinics of North America: laparoscopy for the general surgeon.* WB Saunders, Philadelphia. pp. 1169–83.

29 Geis WP, Miller CE, Kokoszka JS *et al.* (1992) Laparoscopic appendectomy for acute appendicitis: Rationale and technical aspects. *Contemp Surg.* **40**:13–19.

30 Nowzaradan Y, Westmoreland J, McCarver CT *et al.* (1991) Laparoscopic appendectomy for acute appendicitis: indications and current use. *J Laparoendosc Surg.* **1**:247–57.

31 Storm PR, Turkelson ML and Stone HH (1983) Safety of incidental appendectomy. *Am J Surg.* **145**:819–22.

32 Ferzli G, Ozuner G and Castellano MR (1992) Incidental appendectomy during laparoscopic cholecystectomy. *J Laparoendosc Surg.* **2**:165–6.

33 Deutsch AA, Zelikovsky A and Reiss R (1982) Laparoscopy in the prevention of unnecessary appendicectomies; a prospective study. *Br J Surg.* **69**:336–7.

34 Pier A and Gotz F (1992) Laparoscopic appendectomy. In: Cuschieri A, Buess G and Perissat J (Eds) *Operative manual of endoscopic surgery*. Springer, Berlin. pp. 194–208.

35 Engstrom L and Fenyo G (1985) Appendicectomy: assessment of stump invagination versus simple ligation: a prospective, randomized trial. *Br J Surg*. **72**: 971–2.

36 O'Reilly MJ, Reddick EJ, Miller WD *et al.* (1993) Laparoscopic appendectomy. In: Zucker KA (Ed.) *Surgical laparoscopy update*. Quality Medical Publishing, St Louis. pp. 301–26.

37 Gilbert SR, Emmens R W, Putnam TC *et al.* (1985) Appendicitis in children. *Surg Gynecol Obstet.* **161**:261–5.

38 Rajagopalan AE, Manson JH, Kennedy M *et al.* (1977) The value of the barium enema in the diagnosis of acute appendicitis. *Arch Surg.* **112**:531.

39 Ceres L, Alonso I, Lopez P *et al.* (1990) Ultrasound study of acute appendicitis in children with emphasis upon the diagnosis of retrocecal appendicitis. *Pediatr Radiol.* **20**:258–61.

40 Janus C (1986) Diagnosis of acute appendicitis: How useful is the abdominal X-ray? *Digestive Surg.* **3**:27–31.

41 Ferzli GE, Ozuner G, Davidson PG *et al.* (1990) Barium enema in the diagnosis of acute appendicitis. *Surg Gynecol Obstet.* **171**:40–2.

42 Fedyshin P, Kelvin FM and Rice RP (1984) Nonspecificity of barium enema findings in acute appendicitis. *AJR*. **143**:99–102.

43 Puylaert JBCM, Rutgers PH, Lalisang RI *et al.* (1987) A prospective study of ultrasonography in the diagnosis of appendicitis. *N Engl J Med.* **317**:666–9.

44 Barakos JA, Jeffrey RB, Federle MP *et al.* (1986) CT in the management of periappendiceal abscess. *AJR*. **146**:1161–4.

8

Minimal Access Approach to Volvulus

RICARDO GOES AND ROBERT W BEART JR

Introduction

In the last few years there has been a rapid increase in the use of laparoscopic surgery in a wide variety of gastrointestinal disease, both on an elective[1–8] and emergency basis[7,9–11]. Unfortunately for the treatment of colonic volvulus the experience is still small[10,11]. In addition to the capability to resect bowel, the laparoscopic techniques of visceral fixation of areas of the gastrointestinal tract and the creation of stomas have also been described[1,2,4,10–12]. The value of these techniques in elderly and high-risk patients has been demonstrated[7].

The treatment of colonic volvulus is based initially on endoscopic decompression. However, surgical treatment is always indicated. Emergency derotation of the bowel, or resection followed by creation of a stoma or primary anastomosis, can be used when endoscopic decompression fails. The best technical option will be guided by the patient's general clinical conditions, the type and severity of associated diseases, and the viability of the affected bowel segment. This chapter discusses some important features related to colonic volvulus, and the use of laparoscopic procedures as diagnostic and therapeutic alternatives for colonic volvulus. Theoretically, laparoscopy can be useful for diagnostic confirmation and assessment of the viability of the bowel loop.

General considerations

Colonic volvulus has been described since ancient time[13,14] and occurs all over the world, with great variations in its frequency and etiological factors. While it is a rare condition in the developed countries, it is a very common cause of intestinal obstruction in Africa, India, Iran, Pakistan, South America and Eastern Europe[13,14]. In 31 international series reviewed by Ballantyne[13], the sigmoid colon was the most affected segment (76%) followed by the cecum

(21.8%), transverse colon (1.9%) and the splenic flexure (0.2%). The average age of those with the condition was 40 years, but it can be diagnosed in anyone, neonates and in the elderly[13,14].

Colonic volvulus is 10 times more frequent in males than females. Current data on sigmoid volvulus related to Chagas' megacolon, however, do not show any predominance of sex or race[13,15].

Etiology

The etiology of colonic volvulus includes congenital or acquired factors (e.g. high-fiber diets or destruction of the colonic myoenteric plexus in the Chagas' megacolon)[13,15]. However, many cases are idiopathic. Another important cause of colonic volvulus is the association between chronic constipation and neurological and psychiatric disorders, particularly in patients who are institutionalized[13,14,16–18].

Pathophysiology

Torsion of the bowel loop may occur in different ways and will depend on etiology and location. In the sigmoid, it is associated with a redundant loop and a very narrow mesentery (Figure 8.1). For the cecum, the torsion is related to incomplete parietal fixation and can be either an axial bowel rotation or an anterior folding of the cecum[14] (Figure 8.2).

Torsion may be followed by gangrene as a result of the progressively impeded arterial blood supply and venous thrombosis. Necrosis can occur in less than 24 hours.

Clinical features

The onset of symptoms can be acute or subacute, and gangrene is not related to the duration of the symptoms. Symptoms may not be very typical during the initial phase, and subsequently there may be some delay before a correct diagnosis can be made[14].

The main symptoms are abdominal pain, asymmetric distension and constipation, and about 40–60% of patients have a history of previous attacks. If the twisted colon maintains a normal blood supply, even under severe distension, the patient may remain stable[15]. On the other hand, if the pain becomes more severe and the clinical condition of the patient worsens, it may be an indication that bowel necrosis has occurred. The patient should be taken to the operating room promptly, as delay may lead to perforation with a high morbidity and mortality.

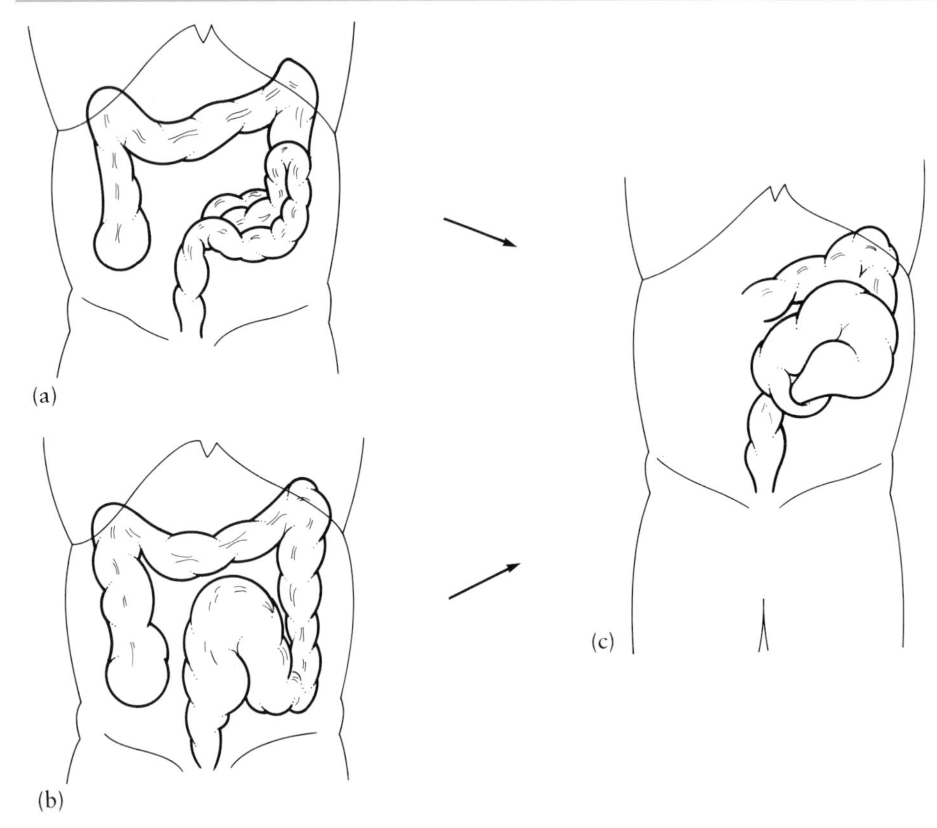

Figure 8.1: Pathophysiology of sigmoid volvulus. (**a**) Redundant loop. (**b**) Narrow mesentery. (**c**) Axial rotation of the sigmoid colon.

The overall mortality from colonic volvulus is about 10% but can reach 80% when the bowel segment is perforated[13]. Mortality is also related to the location of the volvulus and is higher in the sigmoid colon (7–40%) than the cecum (0–17%) in a series reviewed by Brothers and colleagues[18].

Radiology of the abdomen can be used to diagnose colonic volvulus, which appears as a distended loop, sometimes in the very characteristic shape as seen in sigmoid volvulus (figure 8.3). If the radiological findings are not typical, a barium enema may show the area of the torsion as having a 'bird-beak' appearance.

Non-operative treatment

The treatment of colonic volvulus depends on the location of the torsion, the clinical condition of the patient and the presence or absence of necrosis. Successful outcome depends partly on the appropriate choice of procedure and partly on minimal delay between diagnosis and operation. The main purpose

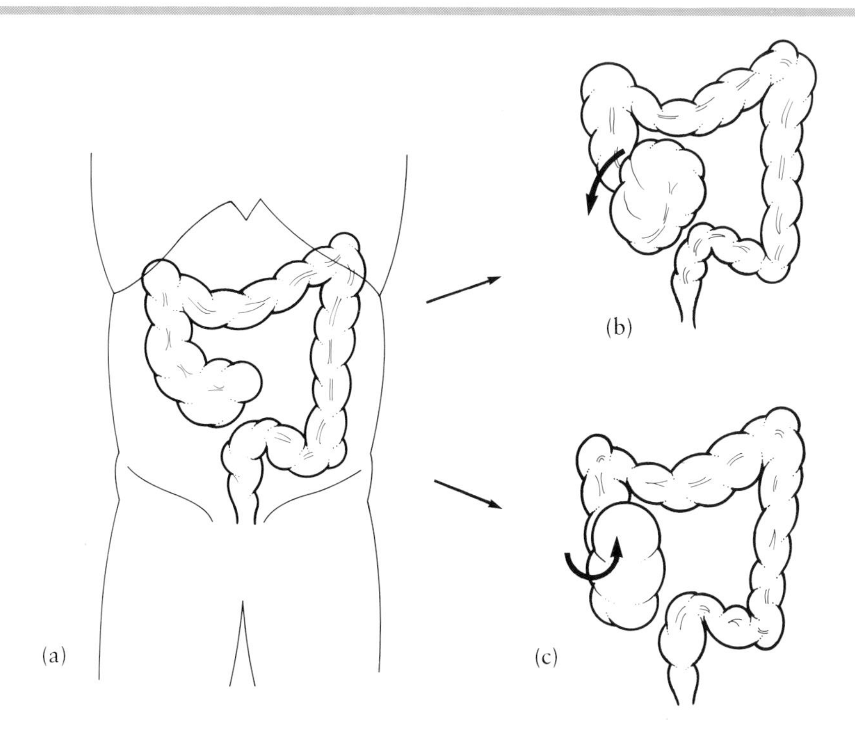

Figure 8.2: Pathophysiology of cecal volvulus. (**a**) Incomplete fixation of the cecum. (**b**) Axial torsion. (**c**) Anterior folding.

of treatment in the acute phase is to relieve the obstruction. If the bowel is viable, endoscopic decompression is the procedure of choice.

After the report of Bruusgaard in 1947[19], deflation of the distended bowel by sigmoidoscopy and tube placement became the preferred treatment for sigmoid volvulus. To perform such a procedure, the tube must be lubricated very well and then inserted gently through the area of the torsion. As soon as the sigmoidoscope has reached the distended loop, spontaneous deflation begins (which can be helped using a suction device). Successful deflation will allow detorsion of the volvulus. This procedure is effective in about 80% of cases[14].

With the development of the colonoscope, it became possible to decompress more proximal segments[20–22]. One great advantage of the flexible scope is that it allows the viability of the bowel segment to be assessed by examination of the mucosa. After deflation, one can also place a large-bore tube in the distended loop, allowing recovery of the bowel and preparation for elective operative treatment[23,24].

Some factors, however, may render the endoscopic procedure more difficult or even impossible, and make operative treatment mandatory. Excessive fecal material preventing the endoscopist from reaching the site of obstruction or clinical deterioration may make endoscopy undesirable or impossible[14].

After endoscopic decompression there is a high frequency of recurrence of volvulus[25]. The effectiveness of the colonoscope in decompressing more proximal segments, such as the cecum, has not been proved. Some authors even

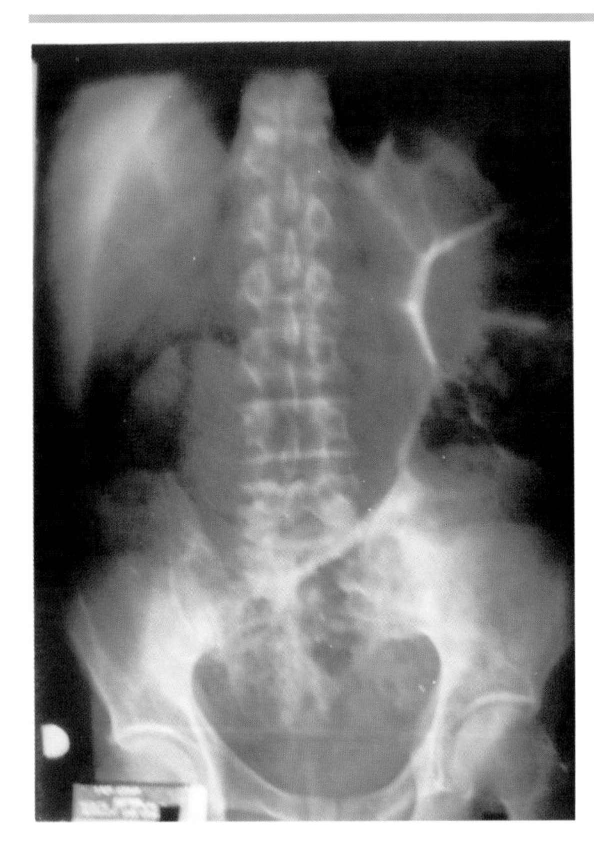

Figure 8.3: Volvulus of sigmoid colon.

report a worsening in the prognosis related to the delay in definitive surgical treatment and to the higher risk of perforation of a necrotic bowel[18]. As soon as cecal volvulus is diagnosed, therefore, the patient should be admitted to surgical treatment.

Operative treatment

Surgical treatment of colonic volvulus at diagnosis was recommended by Moynihan[26] at the beginning of this century, and it was accepted as the treatment of choice until the introduction of endoscopic decompression, mainly for sigmoid volvulus. Surgery is necessary even if deflation has been successful, since the recurrence rate is high. If there is clinical suspicion of peritonitis secondary to gangrene or perforation, surgical treatment should be initiated as soon as possible[13,20,27,28].

Numerous techniques are possible, depending on the viability of the bowel loop. If the operative finding is a volvulus, with bowel in good condition, then the following alternatives are acceptable:

- detorsion of the bowel loop alone, although this procedure is associated with very high rates of recurrence (80%) and mortality (25%)[14]

- detorsion and fixation of the loop to the parietal peritoneum, though this technique also has a very high rate of recurrence (40%)[29]
- colonic mucous fistula[30,31], which has much better results[14]
- segmental resection of the affected bowel and creation of a stoma or a primary anastomosis.

In the management of cecal volvulus, surgical intervention is required; however, it is debatable whether the procedure of choice is resection, cecostomy, detorsion alone or detorsion plus cecopexy.

For the sigmoid colon, primary resection and anastomosis are acceptable if the colon is clean and the patient is in a satisfactory clinical condition[32]. This option is controversial in an emergency situation, and may require on-table colonic lavage[33,34]; as a rule, however, patients with necrotic bowel must always have a resection, and a safer option is the construction of a proximal enterostomy (Hartmann) or a double-loop enterostomy (Paul Mikulicz).

Videolaparoscopy

Despite the rapidly increasing experience with laparoscopic surgery in a wide variety of gastroenterologic diseases, both on an elective[1–8] and an emergency basis[7,9–11], there is limited experience with its use in the treatment of colonic volvulus. At present, endoscopic decompression and laparotomy remains the standard procedure for the treatment of this disease.

Techniques

Patients are prepared and draped in the usual fashion and the equipment is placed so that the television screen can be seen adequately from both sides of the field. A recommended operating room configuration is shown in Figure 8.4. The umbilicus is not an appropriate place to put a video camera, because it does not allow adequate visualization of all areas of the colon. For this reason, we routinely place the endoscope in the upper abdomen. Although we have attempted to place it in the midline and right upper quadrant, the falciform ligament is usually encountered, and therefore we prefer to place the endoscope in the left upper quadrant, to the left of the midline, using the Hasson technique. Once the abdomen has been entered, and the intraabdominal cavity is visualized, additional ports can be placed as shown in Figure 8.5. 10–12 mm ports are placed at the site of camera placement and in the suprapubic area. The upper portal allows for visualization of the lower two-thirds of the abdomen. When it is necessary to visualize either the flexures or the transverse colon, the camera can be moved to the supraumbilical port. 5 mm ports are placed in the right and left lower quadrants at the lateral third of the rectus sheath. This approximates the site of colostomy placement. The operating surgeon then uses

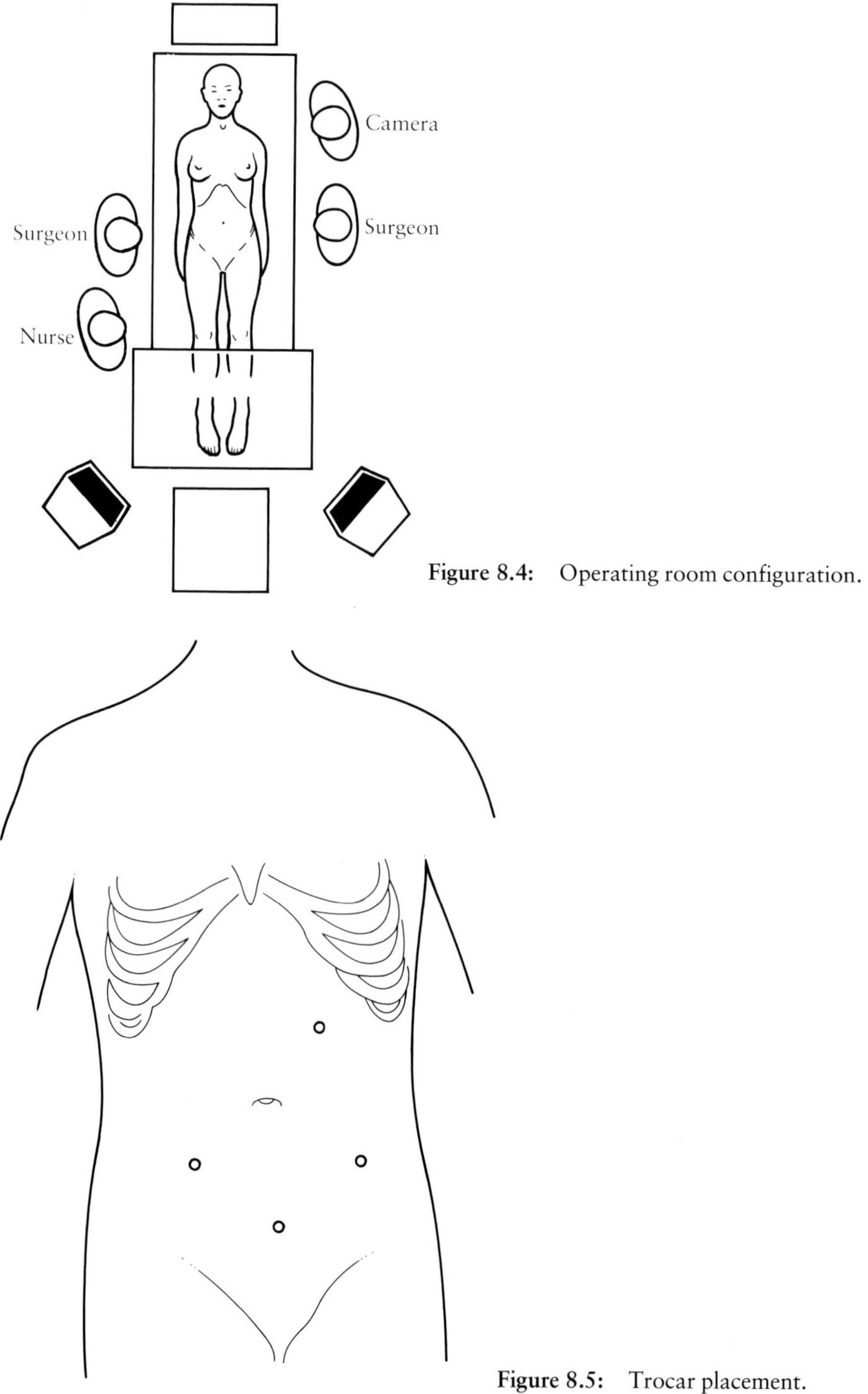

Figure 8.4: Operating room configuration.

Figure 8.5: Trocar placement.

the suprapubic port and the 5 mm port which is on the opposite side of the abdomen, from the segment of colon being handled. The assistant uses the operative port on the site of the colon being handled, and an additional operative port can be placed for the assistant if he is capable of using the two-hand technique. The patient is then placed in a steep Trendelenburg position and rotated away from the side of the colon being handled. The small bowel can be pushed out of the way of the operative field, and the operation can be initiated.

After confirming the diagnosis, and having established the viability of the affected bowel segment, the next task is to attempt laparoscopic detorsion of the volvulus, allowing free transit of intestinal contents. Evacuation may be helped by using colonoscopy intraoperatively to aspirate contents, or by placing a large-bore tube inside the distended loop via the anus. Fixation of the bowel loop after detorsion is an optional technique, but the patient should be prepared promptly for elective surgery as detorsion and colonic plication is associated with a high rate of recurrence, and would be considered definitive only in very ill patients and those having an absolute contraindication for colonic resection.

An alternative laparoscopic procedure is to make a colonic mucous fistula (Figure 8.6). After the confirmation of a viable colon, the intestinal contents can be aspirated through the colonoscope (or by needle aspiration of the colonic

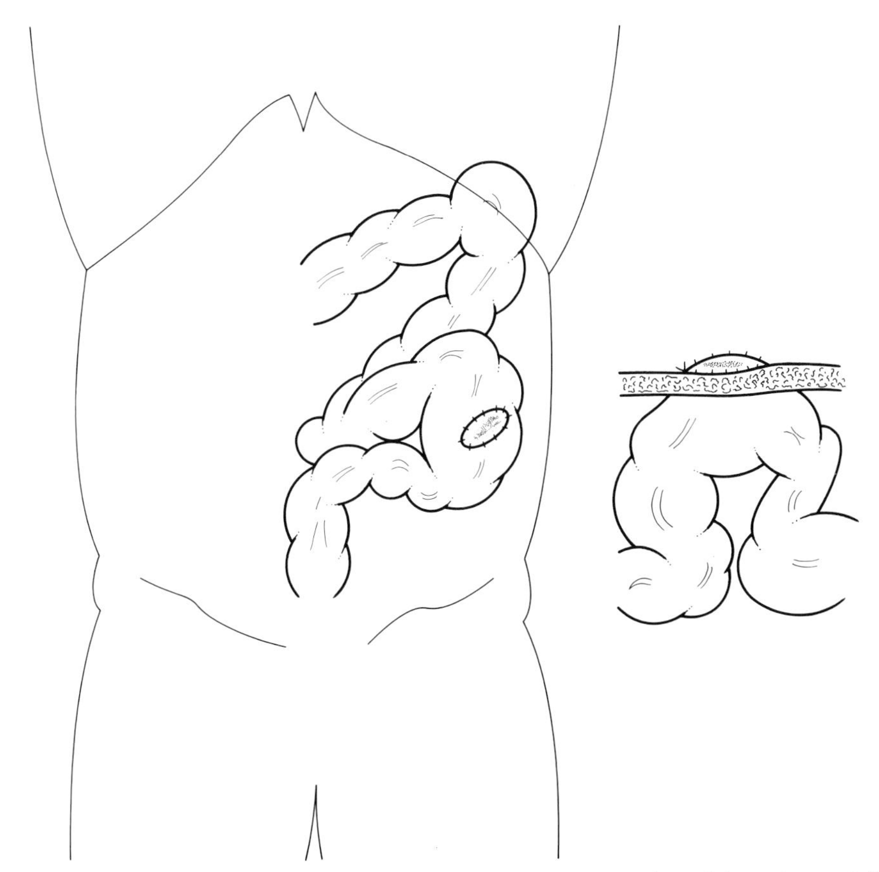

Figure 8.6: Sigmoid colon mucous fistula. After derotation, bowel loop is partially delivered outside and fixed to the abdominal wall as a mucous fitula.

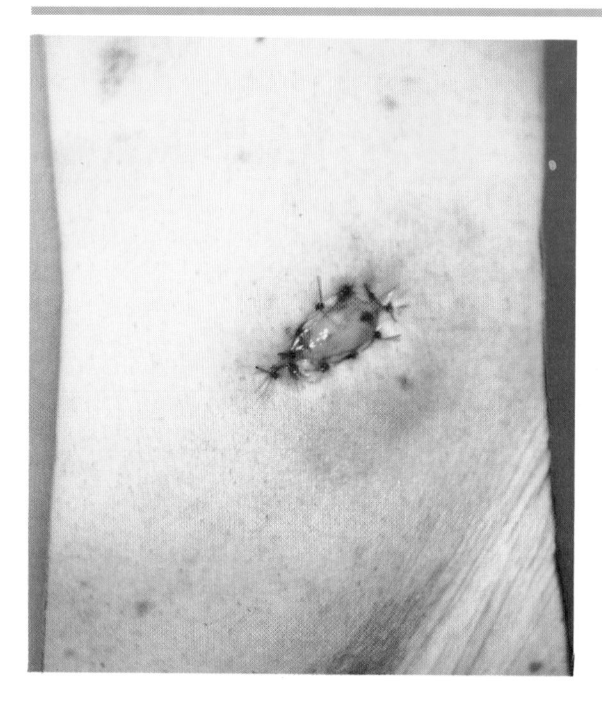

Figure 8.7: Bowel loop delivered and fixed to border of the incision.

wall). The antimesenteric border of the affected bowel loop is identified, grasped and delivered through a small incision of about 3 cm placed adjacent to the left lateral port. After complementary needle aspiration of intestinal gas, the colonic wall may be fixed to the border of the incision, using separate stitches of chromic catgut (2.0). In order to avoid fecal spillage into the abdominal cavity, opening the bowel may be delayed until the fifth postoperative day (Figure 8.7).

If a resection is to be performed, dissection is initiated by retracting the segment of colon towards the midline and dividing the lateral peritoneal reflections. This should be carried out widely. Particular care should be taken to free the entire peritoneum, which binds both the terminal ileum and the distal sigmoid. Only when these are free can the retroperitoneum be fully exposed and the bowel mobilized. We prefer electrocautery for this technique, and use a paddle electrocoagulation device as opposed to the hook which tends to become entangled with mesenteric vessels and fat.

The bowel is bluntly reflected toward the midline until the ureter is identified; the ureter is then freed over the length of the involved segment of bowel. Once the bowel is fully mobilized and the ureter identified, the bowel is retracted laterally and the medical aspect of the mesentery is incised with electrocautery using blunt dissection. The mesentery is then placed on traction, thereby placing the primary feeding vessel on traction as well. Using the paddle dissector, and alternating blunt dissection with electrocautery, the primary vessel can then be identified and ligated. Using double hemoclips we ligate the artery and vein separately, on the proximal and distal ends, and then divide the vessels. The divided vessels are ligated with the pretied Roeder loops, and the adjacent avascular segments of mesentery are carefully dissected and divided.

It is usually unnecessary to complete the mesenteric dissection of the segment to be resected, as this can be carried out extracorporeally. If an intracorporeal anastomosis is to be performed, then the mesentery must be dissected completely. However, there are currently no satisfactory techniques for intracorporeal anastomosis which do not leave the bowel open, risking fecal contamination. For this reason, and because of the need to remove an intact specimen, we generally favor a small incision which removes the specimen and allows completion of the anastomosis extracorporeally.

Once the mobilization is completed, the bowel is grasped through the nearest operative port. For the right colon, this usually means a port in the right lower quadrant; while for the left and sigmoid colon, this usually means the left lower quandrant or suprapubic midline ports. A small incision is made adjacent to this incision, and the bowel is visualized. The bowel is then grasped with a Babcock clamp and drawn into the wound. A 5 cm incision is generally large enough, unless the pathology dictates a larger incision. A finger is inserted through this incision and the window in the dissected mesentery is identified. With traction on this window, the mobilized bowel can be drawn completely into the incision and the undissected mesentery identified. This mesentery can then be divided and ligated between clamps. Once the mesenteric dissection is completed, non-crushing bowel clamps are placed on the bowel, crushing clamps are placed on the segment to be removed, and the bowel is divided. For sigmoid volvulus, primary anastomosis may be inappropriate in the emergency setting, and alternative strategies would include creation of a stoma, the Hartmann procedure or the Paul Mikulicz procedure. For proximal volvulus, primary anastomosis may be performed more frequently, and this can be done with the surgeon's preferred technique. The re-anastomosed bowel is then returned to the abdomen. The incision is closed in two layers, with running suture, and the abdomen is re-insufflated. The previously placed ports are all left in situ, except the port through which the bowel was removed, that defect having been closed. The abdomen is then carefully inspected for adequate hemostasis, irrigated with saline and all blood clots removed. The ports are removed under direct visualization and the port sites closed. This completes the surgical dissection. Drains can be placed as indicated through the port sites.

Therapeutic possibilities of laparoscopy

The advantage of laparoscopic treatment of colonic volvulus may be in confirming the diagnosis and assessing the viability of the bowel. Laparoscopy may also be indicated in older patients, who have associated pathological conditions, or those with psychiatric and neurological disorders. The indications for laparoscopic colectomy are essentially the same as for traditional colectomies. The use of this technology in no way alters traditional surgical judgements or compromises the traditional value of surgical techniques. Initial experience with this technology suggests that it may be more difficult in abdomens that have undergone multiple previous procedures, resulting in significant intraabdominal adhesions. Although theoretically any adhesion can be taken down with laparoscopic techniques, the procedure may be so prolonged as to increase the risks for the patient inappropriately. When utilizing this technology, it is important that the surgeon adopts an appropriate philosophy. This technology provides an alternative to traditional surgical techniques, but not an *exclusive* alternative. The patient should not be subjected to a procedure which compromises the effectiveness of the surgical procedure or unnecessarily subjects the patient to increased risks of a prolonged procedure. If, in the middle of a procedure, the surgeon feels that the efficacy or safety of the procedure is being affected, then it is appropriate to abandon laparoscopic surgery and return to traditional surgical techniques. There is nothing about laparoscopic surgery which should compromise one's ability to continue with an open procedure, and conversion to an open technique should not be viewed by the physician as a failure. Therefore the entire procedure should not be unduly prolonged, nor should an adequate resection be compromised.

As in traditional open surgery, the optimum laparoscopic procedure in the management of cecal volvulus has yet to be established. Laparoscopic cecopexy has been suggested as a satisfactory option; in the single reported case, however, the volvulus recurred less than two years later, and was managed by right hemicolectomy[11]. Another option which may be applicable to the laparoscopic management of cecal volvulus would be colonic resection, which is now well accepted[35–37]. Further data on results of laparoscopic procedures for this condition are required to establish their role.

The development of laparoscopic-assisted colectomy requires increased skill in bowel mobilization, resection, creation of enterostomies and mechanical anastomosis[6–8,35,36]. A very important point is that in the elderly, those in poor clinical condition or with grave associated diseases, urgent treatment is necessary. This must have two basic objectives: (1) to relieve the obstruction, and (2) to minimize the recurrence of the volvulus, either by the use of detorsion plus mucous fistula or by segmental bowel resection, both possible by laparoscopy.

References

1 Edelman DS *et al.* (1991) Laparoscopic gastrostomy. *Surg Laparosc Endosc.* **1**:251–3.

2 Lange V *et al.* (1991) Laparoscopic creation of a loop colostomy. *J Laparoendosc Surg.* **1**:307–12.

3 Sharpe DR and Redwine DB (1992) Laparoscopic segmental resection of the sigmoid and recto sigmoid colon for endometriosis. *Surg Laparosc Endosc.* **2**:120–4.

4 Umehara Y *et al.* (1992) Laparoscopic gastropexy in a patient with chronic gastric volvulus. *Surg Laparosc Endosc.* **2**:261–4.

5 Roby R *et al.* (1993) Laparoscopic-assisted excision of a solitary cecal ulcer. *J Laparoendosc Surg.* **3**:405–9.

6 Sackier J (1993) Laparoscopic colon and rectal surgery. In: Hunter JG, Sackier JM (eds) *Minimally Invasive Surgery*, 1st Edn. McGraw-Hill, New York.

7 Schirmer BD *et al.* (1993) Laparoscopic colon surgery in the high-risk patient population. SAGES, Phoenix, Arizona. (Abstract.)

8 Zucker KA *et al.* (1994) Laparoscopic-assisted colon resection. *Surg Endosc.* **8**:12–18.

9 Bastug D F *et al* (1991) Laparoscopic adhesiolysis for small bowel obstruction. *Surg Laparosc Endosc.* **1**: 259–62.

10 Miller R *et al.* (1992) Laparoscopic fixation of sigmoid volvulus. *Br J Surg.* **79**:435.

11 Shoop SA and Sackier JM (1993) Laparoscopic cecopexy for cecal volvulus. *Surg Endosc.* **7**:450–4.

12 Reiner DS *et al.* (1991) Laparoscopic Stamm gastrostomy with gastropexy. *Surg Laparosc Endosc.* **1**:189–92.

13 Ballantyne GH (1982) Review of sigmoid volvulus. Clinical patterns and pathogenesis. *Dis Colon Rectum.* **25**:823–30.

14 Gibney EJ (1991) Volvulus of the sigmoid colon. *Surg Gyn Obstet.* **173**:243–55.

15 Habr-Gama A (1993) Chagasic megacolon In: Boucher IAD, Allan RN, Hodgson HJF and Keighley MRB (eds) *Gastroenterology*, 2nd edn. WB Saunders, Philadelphia.

16 Shepherd JJ (1969) The epidemiology and clinical presentation of sigmoid volvulus. *Br J Surg.* **56**:353–9.

17 Lane RH and Todd IP (1977) Idiopathic megacolon: a review of 42 cases. *Br J Surg.* **64**:305–10.

18 Brothers TE *et al.* (1987) Endoscopy in colonic volvulus. *Ann Surg.* **206**:1–4.

19 Bruusgaard C (1947) Volvulus of the sigmoid colon and its treatment. *Surgery.* **22**:466–78.

20 String ST and DeCosse JJ (1971) Sigmoid volvulus. An examination of the mortality. *Am J Surg.* **121**:293–7.

21 Ghazi A *et al.* (1976) Treatment of volvulus of the colon by colonoscopy. *Ann Surg.* **183**:263–5.

22 Anderson MJ *et al.* (1978) The colonoscope in cecal volvulus: report of three cases. *Dis Colon Rectum.* **21**:71–4.

23 Procaccino J and Labow SB (1989) Transcolonoscopic decompression of sigmoid volvulus. *Dis Colon Rectum.* **32**:349–50.

24 Wyman A and Zeiderman MR (1989) Maintaining decompression of sigmoid volvulus. *Surg Gyn Obstet.* **169**:265–6.

25 Drapanas T and Stewart JD (1961) Acute sigmoid volvulus: concepts in surgical treatment. *Am J Surg.* **101**:70–7.

26 Moynihan BG (1905) *Abdominal Operations.* WB Saunders, Philadelphia.

27 Berenyl MR and Schwarz GS (1967) Megasigmoid syndrome in diabetes and neurological disease, review of 13 cases. *Am J Gastroenterol.* **47**:310–20.

28 Arnold GJ and Nance FC (1973) Volvulus of the sigmoid colon. *Ann Surg.* **177**:527–37.

29 Shepherd JJ (1968) Treatment of the volvulus of the sigmoid colon: a review of 425 cases. *Br Med J.* **1**:280–3.

30 Tanga MR (1974) Sigmoid volvulus: a new concept in treatment. *Am J Surg.* **128**:119–21.

31 Moreira H (1979) Tratamento cirurgico do volvulo do sigmoide no megacolon chagasico: nova tecnica cirurgica. *Rev Goiana Med.* **25**:73.

32 Armstong DN and Ballantyne GH (1993) Colonic surgery for acute conditions: volvulus of the colon. In: Fielding LP and Goldberg SM (eds) *Operative Surgery: Surgery of the Colon, Rectum and Anus*, 5th edn. Butterworth-Heinemann, Oxford.

33 Bolt DE (1956) The management of the volvulus of the sigmoid colon. *Br J Surg.* **44**:172–5.

34 Kourtesis GJ and Motson RW (1988) Primary anastomosis in emergency distal colonic surgery after on-table colonic lavage. *Aust NZ Surg.* **58**:961–4.

35 Beart RW (1993) Laparoscopic assisted right hemicolectomy. In: Fielding LP and Goldberg SM (eds) *Operative Surgery: Surgery of the Colon, Rectum and Anus*, 5th edn. Butterworth-Heinemann, Oxford.

36 Quattlebaum JK Jr *et al.* (1993) Laparoscopically assisted colectomy. *Surg Laparosc Endosc.* **3**:81–7.

37 Beart RW (1994) Laparoscopic colectomy: status of the art. *Dis Colon Rectum.* **37** (Suppl.):S47–9.

9

Laparoscopic Diagnosis, Staging and Follow-up of Colorectal Malignancies

FREDERICK L GREENE AND DOUGLAS A DORSAY

Introduction

Until the late 1980s, laparoscopy was used primarily as a diagnostic modality except in the field of gynecology, where it was successfully applied to tubal ligation. More complex procedures were hindered by the need to manipulate the laparoscope with one hand and the inability of assistants to visualize the intra-abdominal proceedings. The development of videolaparoscopy freed more hands and enabled increasingly complex manipulations. The first laparoscopic cholecystectomy was performed in 1987[1], and since then this approach has been widely adopted. The arguments for the laparoscopic approach are strong. Bowel function returns faster and postoperative pain is much less than with a formal laparotomy. Hospital stay is usually shorter and return to baseline functional level is faster. For these reasons, minimal access techniques are being adapted for all areas of abdominal and thoracic surgery.

This chapter considers their potential application in the diagnosis, staging and follow-up of colorectal malignancies. This is an area that has been little explored; by necessity much of what follows is speculative or extrapolated from the traditional approach to these problems as well as other applications of laparoscopy. Much will depend on the development of appropriate new techniques and the instrumentation to realize them, tempered by their judicious application.

Diagnosis

As always, the foundation of diagnosis rests on a thorough history and physical examination. Other than testing a stool sample for the presence of heme, laboratory studies play little part in the diagnosis of colorectal malignancy, although anemia, hypokalemia or elevated hepatic enzymes may prompt further evaluation. Carcinoembryonic antigen is generally felt to be a poor screening test for colorectal cancer due to frequent false-negative results (particularly when a tumor is potentially curable)[2] and the high cost of frequent false-positive results[3]. Its usefulness in the follow-up of colon cancer continues to be debated. Currently the definitive diagnosis depends on radiology and/or endoscopy. These should be considered complementary, and every effort should be made to evaluate thoroughly the entire colon and rectum.

Sigmoidoscopy, either rigid or flexible, engenders little morbidity and only moderate discomfort, and is easily performed without anesthesia. As such, it is usually the first invasive step in the evaluation of complaints attributable to the large bowel. Rigid sigmoidoscopy permits evaluation of the distal 20 cm of the rectosigmoid colon and has been estimated to detect one third of intraluminal tumors[4]. A flexible sigmoidoscope may consistently reach 55 cm and permit visualization of an additional 30% of lesions.

Even if sigmoidoscopy is positive, further evaluation of the colon is warranted by the finding of synchronous malignancies in 1.5–7.6% of known colorectal cancers, and synchronous polyps in another 25–40%[5]. Colonoscopy and/or air-contrast barium enema may be used to complete this evaluation. Once again, this choice is controversial in that each study has unique advantages and disadvantages. Generally, air-contrast barium enema is the next step and, if of adequate quality, will discern most significant lesions and localize them anatomically. If this study is equivocal, inadequate or negative in the face of signs or symptoms of colonic malignancy, then colonoscopy should be performed. This will permit

- small polyps to be detected
- samples to be taken for biopsy
- extraluminal masses to be distinguished from intraluminal ones.

Further information may be obtained from magnetic resonance imaging or computed tomography with or without biopsy. These scans are particularly useful in staging or in identifying the origin of mural or extrinsic masses.

These steps will provide a diagnosis in the great majority of cases; however, occasionally events may conspire to prevent diagnosis without open exploration. Examples include:

- an extraluminal mass that cannot be biopsied by CT or ultrasound guidance
- stricture preventing adequate colonoscopy or barium enema, with non-diagnostic biopsies
- inadequate visualization of the colon due to redundancy or other anatomic factors
- obstruction or perforation requiring urgent or emergent exploration.

If there is reason to suspect malignancy, this should be followed by celiotomy, exploration, biopsy and extirpation with curative or palliative intent. It is at this point that laparoscopy becomes a diagnostic option.

In the past, laparoscopic diagnosis would have offered no advantage over an open procedure because, even when colorectal malignancies are unresectable, palliative procedures may provide significant benefits in terms of survival and quality of life. Furthermore, a negative laparoscopic examination would not have completely ruled out disease. Recently, however, 'laparoscopically assisted' colectomies[6,8] and bypass and diverting procedures[9] have been developed which offer significant palliation with greatly shortened recovery times. Therefore, in the narrowly defined group which might avoid laparotomy based on discovery of distant metastases or local spread not amenable to en bloc resection, laparoscopy may be indicated as a diagnostic tool to be followed by palliative laparoscopic colectomy, bypass procedures or ablative procedures. Laparoscopic colectomy may fail to achieve adequate nodal clearance which is the key factor in both staging and achieving curability. Until there are studies which indicate that nodal (mesenteric) dissection with laparoscopic techniques is comparable with open methods, laparoscopic colectomy for malignancy must be approached with caution.

Laparoscopic diagnosis, especially in the identification of hepatic metastases, is based on gross appearance and the histologic examination of tissue obtained by fine-needle aspiration, or core-needle, forceps or excisional biopsy. Two new techniques may prevent the loss of tactile feedback during laparoscopic exploration. The first is the laparoscopic two-dimensional ultrasound probe which can be used to identify and delineate primary tumors as well as hepatic or nodal metastases. The second is the application of radioimmunolocalization techniques to laparoscopic examination of the abdomen. An example is the development of second-generation monoclonal antibodies directed against the tumor-associated glycoprotein 72 antigen (TAG-72)[10]. Utilizing these highly sensitive and specific markers, laparoscopic localization and staging could be followed by celiotomy for curative resection, or resection of 'occult' metastases identified by these techniques.

Staging

Current staging of colorectal cancer requires preoperative, intraoperative and histopathologic findings. Each contributes to subsequent decision-making, and the methods and information derived from them overlap. For example, tissue may be obtained for histologic examination during colonoscopy or CT-guided biopsy during intraoperative excisional biopsy or examination of the resected specimen. Evidence of distant metastasis may materialize during preoperative evaluation or intraoperatively. The result is an algorithm leading to a limited number of therapeutic options. These options include:

- doing nothing
- adopting a palliative approach

- minimizing tumor load in anticipation of adjuvant therapy
- resecting for cure, with or without adjuvant therapy.

The goal of tumor-staging is to determine the optimal therapy while inflicting minimal morbidity at the lowest cost. To stage colorectal carcinoma adequately, one must:

1. resect the primary tumor and assess the extent of local invasion
2. harvest tissue from epicolic, paracolic, intermediate and mesenteric or iliac lymph nodes
3. inspect the peritoneal surface for metastases
4. search for evidence of hepatic metastases.

All of these are achievable with laparoscopic techniques, and this ability will probably improve along with advances in instrumentation and technology.

The real advantage of preoperative staging may be seen in the management of rectal carcinoma, especially in patients at greater risk for major abdominal exploration and conventional resection. If laparoscopy uncovers hepatic or advanced local regional disease palliative modalities such as laser ablation, local transanal resection or intracavity radiation therapy may be viable options.

Techniques

Although diagnostic laparoscopic procedures may be performed with local anesthesia and intravenous sedation, we prefer to use general anesthesia. Careful preoperative assessment and optimization of cardiopulmonary function are mandatory. A carbon dioxide pneumoperitoneum creates severe stresses which may lead to hemodynamic compromise or hypercapnia in the patient with marginal functional reserve. Aggressive mechanical and antibiotic bowel preparation is essential if therapeutic measures are being considered. In addition, we normally administer a second- or third-generation cephalosporin as prophylaxis.

Surgeon position and trocar placement

Surgeon position and trocar placement depend upon the suspected location of the primary tumor as well as the location of any previous abdominal incisions. In general, trocar placement should allow access to the area of interest from multiple angles, and close inspection of the liver, peritoneum and lymph node bearing regions. Additional trocars may be placed as needed for retroperitoneal nodal or liver biopsies. Although we usually place an infraumbilical 10 mm trocar for the camera following insufflation via a Verres needle, this may be modified in the presence of previous abdominal incisions. In this instance a Hasson trocar may be inserted using an open technique or, if there is a midline scar, the trocar may be inserted in the left iliac fossa lateral to the rectus abdominus muscle. This decision may be aided by preoperative CT or ultrasound which may suggest focal adhesions to the anterior abdominal wall. Initially, two additional trocars (usually 12 mm, to permit application of stapling devices if needed) are inserted parallel to the region of interest under laparoscopic vision. If the lesion involves the ascending or descending colon or cecum, the additional ports are placed cephalad and caudad to the camera port in the linea alba (Figure 9.1). If we are approaching the transverse colon or rectosigmoid, the trocars are oriented transversely, just above or below the umbilicus at the linea semilunaris (Figure 9.2).

It is not uncommon to encounter adhesions in the previously operated abdomen. These are taken down with scissors using unipolar electrocautery. Extensive adhesions may warrant conversion to an open procedure. Generally the patient is in the supine position; however, for procedures such as a laparoscopic abdominoperineal resection, stapled end-to-end anastomosis, pull-through procedure or intraoperative colonoscopy, then the patient should be placed in the dorsal lithotomy position. A fully adjustable operating table is essential and should be used freely to enlist gravity as an ally in obtaining exposure. The surgeon is usually positioned opposite the focus of attention. During diagnostic procedures this focus may change, and the surgeon should reposition him or herself accordingly.

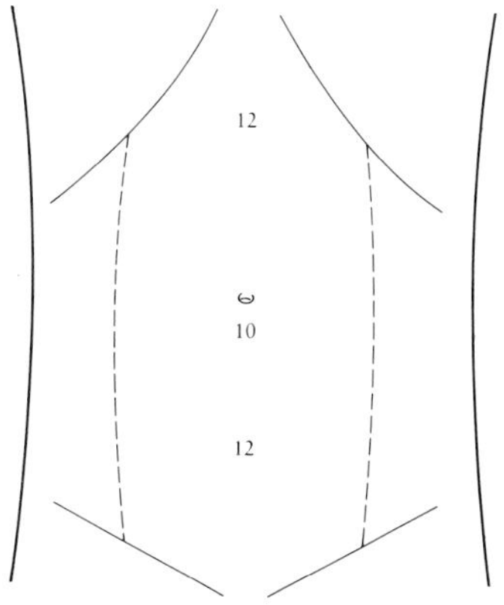

Figure 9.1: Primary trocar placement for approaching the ascending or descending colon or cecum.

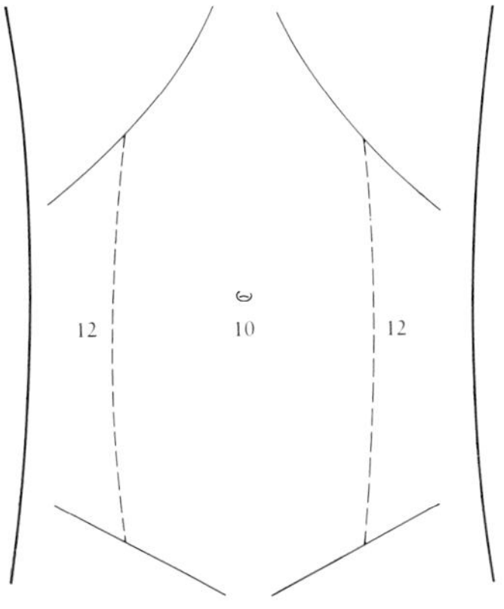

Figure 9.2: Primary trocar placement for approaching the transverse colon or rectosigmoid.

Lesion identification and examination

Upon entering the peritoneal cavity, the primary lesion should first be identified unequivocally. Copies of the barium enema and CT scans should be available for review. If colonoscopy is performed preoperatively and the lesion is small, it should be tattooed at that time. If doubt exists, the tumor can be definitively identified with intraoperative colonoscopy. Once identified, the serosa is inspected for signs of penetration. If bulky, the region is examined for invasion of adjacent viscera or the abdominal wall. The omentum, peritoneal surfaces, and, in women, the ovaries are then examined for metastatic implants. Biopsies are taken from suspicious lesions and sent for frozen and permanent section. Examination of the liver is performed in conjunction with information derived from preoperative ultrasound or CT scans. Visualization of the diaphragmatic and inferior surfaces is aided by use of a wide retractor and a 30° or 45° laparoscope. The recent introduction of flexible laparoscopes should facilitate the examination. Metastatic lesions may appear as whitish superficial plaques or surface dimpling. Identification of metastatic lesions is aided by remotely palpating the hepatic surface with a blunt-tipped probe. Surface lesions are biopsied with cup forceps and deep lesions with a percutaneous, laparoscopic-guided core-needle biopsy.

Laparoscopic ultrasound with a linear array 7.5 MHz probe was introduced in 1984 and used to identify an intra-hepatic lesion and guide a needle biopsy[11]. Another group[12] used a 3.5 and 5 MHz probe on the tip of a flexible laparoscope to visualize pancreatic and hepatic malignancies in 20 patients with disease previously diagnosed by CT scanning or extracorporeal ultrasound. This technique is only now being reintroduced, using phased array technology, and it should greatly enhance the sensitivity of laparoscopic detection of hepatic metastases.

Staging of rectal carcinoma

Staging of rectal carcinoma may require the laparoscopic evaluation of pelvic lymph nodes. This is performed with the same (transverse) trocar arrangement and the patient in Trendelenburg position. An additional 5 mm trocar may be placed in the midline, halfway between the umbilicus and pubic symphysis to facilitate exposure. The inguinal ligament, pubic tubercle and internal inguinal ring are identified, and beginning ventral to the inguinal ligament and just lateral to the medial umbilical ligament, the peritoneum is incised with scissors and unipolar cautery. This incision is then carried dorsally to a point just proximal to the bifurcation of the iliac vessels. The peritoneal edges are grasped medially and laterally, and freed up using a blunt dissector using care to avoid injury to the obturator vessels and nerve. The ureter is carefully identified while the nodal tissue surrounding the hypogastric vessels is grasped and dissected free. Hemostasis is maintained with judicious use of multiple clips and electrocautery. If no further dissection is to be carried out in the pelvis, then the peritoneal defect is closed with a running absorbable suture using a 'ski' needle. This is then repeated on the opposite side. If resection of the lesion is planned, then the lymph node dissection can be carried out in continuity with the specimen.

Occasionally a patient with known colorectal cancer may have CT evidence of para-aortic lymphadenopathy but no other known metastatic disease. In such cases, positive tissue will profoundly affect therapy. In general, laparoscopic access to this region is extremely awkward due to the presence of the small bowel. Despite this, Salky and colleagues[13] obtained a biopsy diagnosis in 16 of 19 patients with retroperitoneal pathology approached laparoscopically and, in 1992, Childers and Surwit reported a laparoscopic para-aortic lymph node biopsy resulting in a diagnosis of non-Hodgkin's lymphoma[14]. Herd and colleagues[15] recently described the development of an elegant technique using a porcine model which may ease this procedure. With the animal in steep Trendelenburg, the retroperitoneum was opened beginning lateral to the right common iliac vessels. After extending the incision cephalad, a pretied 0 chromic gut ligature is passed through one of the trocars lateral to the umbilicus and secured on the peritoneal edge (Figure 9.2). The end of the

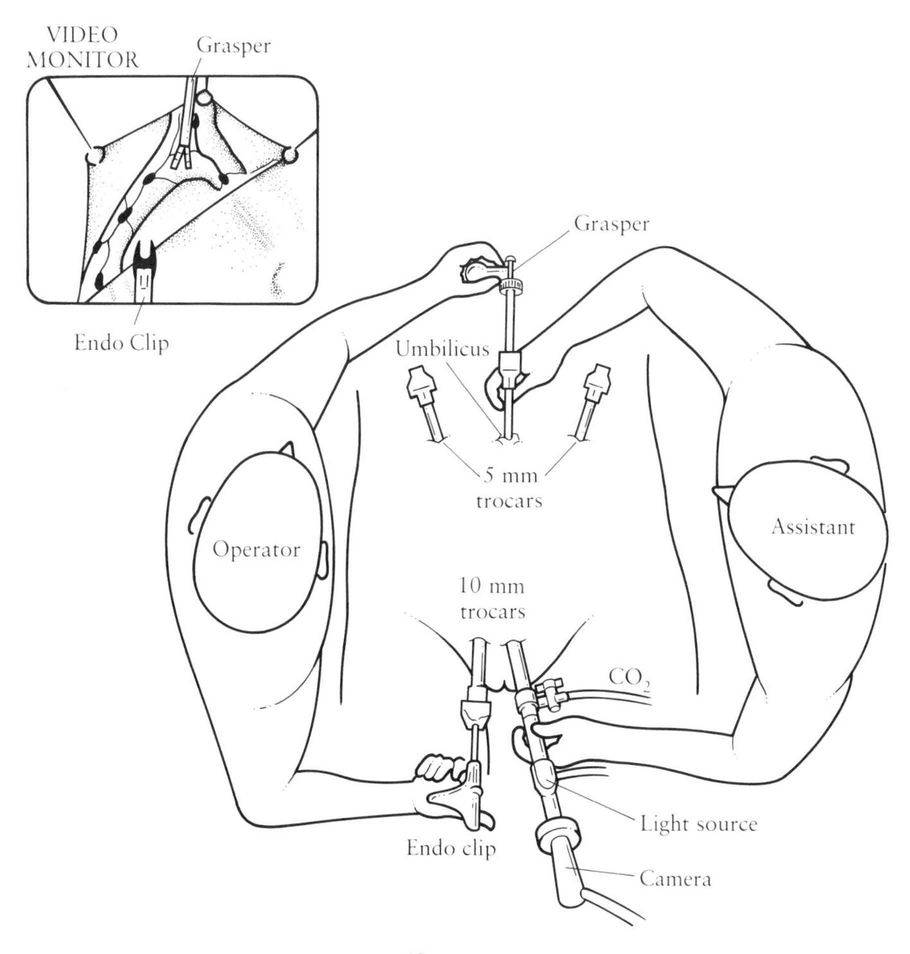

Figure 9.3: Technique of Herd *et al.*[15] for approaching the retroperitoneum laparoscopically.

ligature is maintained under tension extracorporeally and additional ties are placed at short intervals and brought under tension. This is repeated on the left side, with the ties brought out through the left lateral trocar. The result is a tenting of the peritoneum which effectively retracts the small bowel (Figure 9.3). The trocars through which the ligatures pass may still be used to introduce instruments, although there may be some loss of pneumoperitoneum. The nodal tissue is then removed using traction and electrocautery with clips placed as needed.

Additional efforts to localize nodal involvement may be realized through the technique of radioimmunolocalization using monoclonal antibodies to colorectal tumor antigens. A 1992 report[10] describes the use of radiolabeled CC49 (a second-generation monoclonal antibody directed against tumor associated glycoprotein) and a hand-held gamma-detecting probe during open abdominal exploration in the detection of primary and recurrent colorectal cancer[10]. They succeeded in detecting 18 of 21 primary, and 29 of 30 recurrent tumors. In at least 14 specimens the tumor was occult, and in many cases, was discovered in gastrohepatic, iliac or celiac nodes. Of particular interest, six of 15 specimens, which were considered CC49 positive and histologically negative, were found on re-examination to have tumor foci. In addition, the authors stated that their findings altered management in nearly half of their patients. Application of this technique to laparoscopic staging awaits the development of an appropriately modified gamma probe.

Celiotomy

Following laparoscopic investigation, a variety of situations mandate progressing on to formal celiotomy. The first would be the finding of local invasion by a primary tumor requiring en bloc resection. Another is the identification of potentially resectable hepatic metastases. The third situation arises when laparoscopic staging is completely negative and the primary lesion is easily resectable. This area will remain controversial for several years since the argument against pursuing laparoscopic resection at this point is the newness of the procedure and the lack of even short-term data on recurrence. On the other hand, if there is laparoscopic evidence of significant hepatic or distal nodal spread, then open resection offers no theoretical benefit, and laparoscopic colectomy may be a reasonable option to achieve palliation.

Results

Although the literature contains no reports of laparoscopic staging of colorectal carcinoma, the technique has been applied with some success to the staging of lymphoma and esophageal, gastric, pancreatic, prostate and ovarian cancer. In 1989, Watt and coworkers[16] discussed the evaluation of 90 patients who had endoscopically diagnosed carcinoma of the esophagus or gastric cardia. They compared laparoscopy, ultrasound and computed tomography in the detection of hepatic, nodal and peritoneal metastases, and found laparoscopy to be superior to imaging studies in identifying hepatic and peritoneal metastases, and equivalent to computed tomography regarding nodal metastases.

In a study of 40 patients with documented gastric carcinoma and negative abdominal ultrasound and computed tomography, Kriplani and Kapur[17] laparoscopically identified five patients with metastases and 11 patients who were considered unresectable due to local extension. Twenty-three of the remaining patients were explored; only three had further findings obviating resection.

Warshaw and colleagues[18] evaluated two groups of patients with pancreatic cancer using a laparoscopic approach. In 1986 they reviewed 40 patients deemed resectable following endoscopic retrograde cholangiopancreatography, ultrasound, computed tomography and mesenteric and celiac angiography, and who subsequently underwent laparoscopy. In this manner, they obtained histologic proof of metastasis in 14 (six hepatic, seven peritoneal and one omental). Three of the 26 remaining patients who underwent celiotomy were also discovered to have metastases. A second study published in 1990[19] demonstrated the value of multiple diagnostic modalities in avoiding unnecessary celiotomy. Individually, angiography, computed tomography, and laparoscopy were approximately 50% successful in predicting resectability of a pancreatic malignancy. However, in combination, this rose to 87.5%.

Parra and colleagues[20] compared the results of open and laparoscopic staging pelvic lymphadenectomy in 24 men with prostate cancer and found them to be equivalent in assessing nodal tissue. Rosenhoff and coworkers[21] evaluated seven patients referred to them with ovarian cancer and noted to have disease localized to the pelvis (stage I and II) at diagnostic celiotomy. They performed staging laparoscopy prior to initiating local therapy, and found that six had developed extra-pelvic disease.

The utility of laparoscopy in the identification and biopsy of hepatic lesions continues to be debated. Studies have been published supporting all views[22–4], yet all are lacking in objective evidence. Probably the most realistic assessment is that expressed by Fornari *et al.*[25] who found that a combination of ultrasound-guided fine-needle aspiration followed by laparoscopy resulted in a diagnostic accuracy of 98.4% and a sensitivity of 97.5% in the diagnosis of hepatic lesions. This does not change the fact that there is a very low yield for ultrasound and CT in the primary evaluation of colorectal cancer, and that their routine use is not recommended.

Follow-up

Despite resection for cure, nearly half of all colorectal carcinomas will recur[26], most frequently within two years of operation. Patterns of recurrence differ markedly between colon and rectal carcinomas after 'curative' resection. Willett and colleagues[27] discussed recurrence patterns five years after curative resection of colon malignancies with a typical distribution of stages. Of 533 patients, 163 (31%) developed recurrence during that period with metastatic disease in 25% and local disease in 19%. Six percent had local disease only, while 71 patients (13%) had extra-abdominal metastases. Michelassi and colleagues[28] reported an 8% overall local recurrence rate with a median time to diagnosis of 18 months and with all but 16% presenting within five years. In those patients who underwent resection of a rectal lesion, the incidence of local recurrence was 12%. Metastatic lesions were not addressed in that study. Stipa *et al.*[29] recently examined recurrence retrospectively in 469 patients who had undergone resection of colorectal cancer with curative intent. At a median follow-up of 42 months, 31.1% showed evidence of relapse (10% local only, 3.4% local and metastatic, and 17.5% metastatic only). Rectal cancers recurred locally with an incidence of 18.3% as opposed to 8.9% for colon cancer. McDermott and coworkers[30] examined a series of 1008 patients following curative resection of rectal carcinomas, of whom 934 were available for analysis. They found relapse in 38% of their subjects (11% local only, 17% metastatic only, and 9% with both) (Table 9.1). It is now recognized that, if

	Overall recurrence	Local recurrence only	Distant recurrence only	Local and distant recurrence
Willett *et al.*[27], colon and rectal	163/533 (31%)	32/533 (6%)	61/533 (11%)	70/533 (13%)
Stipa *et al.*[29], colon and rectal	146/469 (31%)	48/469 (10%)	82/469 (17.5%)	14/469 (3.4%)
McDermott *et al.*[30], rectal only	364/934 (38%)	107/934 (11%)	173/934 (19%)	84/934 (9%)

Table 9.1: Recurrence of colorectal cancer following 'curative' resection.

identified early, aggressive resection of recurrent local disease, as well as limited metastatic disease, may result in long-term survival[31]. The key word is 'early', opening up the question of what constitutes ideal follow-up.

In the past, patients underwent reoperation only for signs or symptoms of recurrent disease and depending on the aggressiveness of the surgeon. By this time tumors were usually far advanced and surgery was palliative at best. In 1951, Wangensteen and colleagues[32] advocated routine 'second-look' abdominal exploration at six to eight months postoperatively in all patients with gastrointestinal malignancies resected for cure with repeat laparotomies performed until no residual tumor was found. This led to an unacceptably high number of negative explorations, with attendant morbidity and mortality. The results were particularly dismal in patients with gastric cancer treated in this manner: only one of 22 patients who had a positive second exploration remained cancer-free 31 months after the fourth operation[33]. The results in subjects with rectal tumors were no better, with only one of 15 positive second-look subjects free of disease 12 months after the final procedure. The numbers were somewhat better (4/14) for colon lesions. Overall, 52 of 93 initial re-explorations were negative, yet 11 of these developed recurrent disease. Thankfully, means have been developed to reduce the number of negative explorations. If these could be eliminated, a salvage rate of 29% for recurrent colon cancer would be more than acceptable.

Histopathologic stage has been used to identify a population at risk for recurrence. In most studies, Duke's stage A lesions recurred in less than 5% of cases[26]. The percentage increases rapidly with advancing stage. This information, along with a directed history, physical examination and various diagnostic tests, could theoretically be used to identify patients likely to have recurrent disease early enough to offer the possibility of salvage through second-look laparotomy.

In 1987, Sugarbaker and colleagues[34] published the results of a prospective study begun in 1978 which examined this concept in detail[34]. They studied 66 patients deemed to be at high risk on the basis of stage (Duke's C/TNM stage III), perforation, invasion of adjacent organs, locally recurrent disease, or age less than 30 years. All underwent resection with no apparent residual disease, and were followed for a median of four years with all modalities available at the time. Follow-up included:

- a review of symptoms and physical examination at every visit
- carcinoembryonic antigen (CEA) assays
- abdomino-pelvic CT scanning } monthly
- complete lung tomograms
- liver-spleen scintigraphy every four months
- intravenous pyelography
- barium enema } annually
- bone scintigraphy.

Thirty-one patients (47%) developed recurrences. A serial increase in CEA levels was the first indication in 22 (67%), while symptoms or examination provided the first indication in seven (21%). Abdominal CT uncovered two recurrences and corroborated disease in 17 of 20 cases; however, this record is marred by a 50% false-positive rate. The other studies were useful only for corroboration and localization of relapse.

Second-look procedures

Several groups have applied the concept of second-look surgery directed only by an increase in CEA in an attempt to intervene in recurrent cancer at an early (and potentially curable) stage. The best results are those from studies by the Society of Surgical Oncology and a group from Ohio State University in which CEA levels were closely followed and secondary resections were aggressively performed, for the most part, by specialists in surgical oncology. In 1985, Martin *et al.*[35] reported a study of 146 patients who underwent second-look laparotomy on the basis of rising CEA alone. Their criterion for exploration was a steadily rising CEA level greater than 7.5 ng/ml. Of these 139 had demonstrable disease, and recurrence later became evident in six of the remaining patients. Resections were considered possible in 81 (65%). Of the 45 patients followed for five years or more, 14 (31%) remained alive.

In 1978, Minton *et al.*[36] began a prospective, non-randomized study of 400 patients following curative resection of colon or rectal cancer: 130 recurrences were documented (32%), and 75 (19%) underwent second-look laparotomy. A rising CEA level greater than 2.5 ng/ml was the primary indication in 43, and 23 (59%) of these were considered resectable. Of those patients followed for more than five years, 37% of those undergoing curative resection for a rising CEA remained alive without disease, compared with 28% directed by clinical information.

On a more sobering note, Fucini *et al.*[37] followed 64 patients prospectively and detected 90% of 22 recurrences with CEA determinations. However, of 12 patients undergoing second-look celiotomy, only one was still alive with metastases at the time of publication. Four of the five patients undergoing celiotomy solely for rising CEA levels had no detectable disease and one had unresectable carcinomatosis.

Even in the best circumstances and with thorough preoperative staging, a large number of patients are found to be unresectable at second-look laparotomy and suffer needlessly. Laparoscopy may be utilized to reduce this number, and may in the future offer therapeutic benefit as well. It must be remembered that a negative examination in no way rules out recurrence, and therefore it may be followed by celiotomy.

Second-look laparoscopy has been reported in the gynecologic literature. In 1984, Xygakis et al.[38] reported on 46 asymptomatic women who underwent laparoscopy 10–18 months after surgical, radiation or chemical therapy for ovarian cancer. Findings in 20 obviated laparotomy; 16 of the remainder underwent laparotomy, at which time three were found to have recurrence. No major morbidity was reported.

Marti-Vicente et al.[39] performed 44 second-look and 28 third-look laparoscopies in 52 women with ovarian cancer in clinical remission. Nearly 50% of these examinations demonstrated recurrent tumor, yet a 31% false-negative rate was discovered at laparotomy. Neither of these studies addressed the benefits of surgical debulking in the treatment of this disease.

Currently the indications and opportunities for second-look laparoscopy remain limited. If recurrence is suggested on the grounds of a rising CEA level or clinical findings, evidence of unresectable disease should be sought using roentgenograms, computed tomography, ultrasound, magnetic resonance imaging and possibly scintigraphy using radiolabeled monoclonal antibodies. The presence of distal metastases, if unresectable, would make further evaluation unnecessary except for histologic confirmation. The extent of locally recurrent disease is difficult to appraise using noninvasive imaging studies due to scar formation, alteration of the normal anatomy and possible reactive lymphadenopathy. Therefore the suggestion of recurrence by history, examination or rising CEA levels, even where imaging has given negative or equivocal results, would justify invasive evaluation. Laparoscopy may represent the next stage in the evolution of the second-look evaluation with a goal of performing celiotomy only in patients with resectable disease. A major obstacle to this goal is the prevalence of adhesions in the previously operated abdomen. These are frequently present to such a degree as to limit severely or even prevent inspection by this method. However, the careful insertion of trocars using an open technique, followed by patient adhesiolysis, will permit laparoscopic examination in most patients. Visual examination may be augmented by laparoscopic ultrasound and radioimmunolocalization techniques in the near future. A finding of peritoneal carcinomatosis or unresectable hepatic metastases would obviate further surgical intervention, but other findings may be more difficult to interpret. In general, a finding of potentially resectable recurrence or lack of evidence of unresectable disease would warrant a subsequent celiotomy with aggressive resection of all malignant tissue in the low- or moderate-risk patient.

Future concepts

There may be a therapeutic role for laparoscopy in the near future as well. Several recent studies have demonstrated prolonged remission in as many as 22% of patients with multiple hepatic metastases from colorectal cancers[40] and in 37.5% of patients with unresectable hepatocellular carcinoma[41] following ultrasound-guided hepatic cryosurgery. Instruments are now being developed for the laparoscopic application of this technique.

Conclusion

The treatment of cancer is an emotional issue for all involved, including the surgeon. On the one hand we have a strong desire to do something to offer our patients the chance of a cure; on the other we are reluctant to add what may prove to be unnecessary pain and disability to what the patient is already suffering. In some instances, minimal access techniques may offer a means of achieving both of these goals.

The diagnosis of colorectal cancer still rests on endoscopic or radiologic demonstration of tumor, and laparoscopy will probably continue to play a very restricted role. The real strength of laparoscopy in the treatment of this disease lies in its potential ability to stage primary and recurrent malignancy accurately, coupled with a real and growing potential for therapeutic intervention.

References

1 Nagy AG, Poulin EC, Girotti MJ *et al.* (1992) History of laparoscopic surgery. *Can J Surg.* **35**:271–4.

2 Moertel CG, O'Fallon JR, Go VLW *et al.* (1986). The preoperative carcinoembryonic antigen test in the diagnosis, staging, and prognosis of colorectal cancer. *Cancer.* **58**:603–10.

3 Lieberman DA (1990) Colon cancer screening: the dilemma of positive screening tests. *Arch Intern Med.* **150**:740–4.

4 Winnan G, Berci G, Panish J *et al.* (1980) Superiority of the flexible to the rigid sigmoidoscope in routine proctosigmoidoscopy. *N Engl J Med.* **302**:1011–12.

5 Howard ML and Greene FL (1990) The effect of preoperative endoscopy on recurrence and survival following surgery for colorectal carcinoma. *Am Surg.* **56**:124–7.

6 Schlinkert RT (1991) Laparoscopic-assisted right hemicolectomy. *Dis Colon Rectum.* **34**:1030–1.

7 Corbitt JD Jr (1992) Preliminary experience with laparoscopic-guided colectomy. *Surg Laparosc Endosc.* **2**:79–81.

8 Phillips EH, Franklin M, Carroll BJ *et al.* (1992) Laparoscopic colectomy. *Ann Surg.* **216**:703–7.

9 Shimi S, Banting S and Cuschieri A (1992) Laparoscopy in the management of pancreatic cancer: endoscopic colecystojejunostomy for advanced disease. *Br J Surg.* **79**:317–19.

10 Arnold MW, Schneebaum S, Berens A *et al.* (1992) Intraoperative detection of colorectal cancer with radioimmunoguided surgery and CC49, a second-generation monoclonal antibody. *Ann Surg.* **216**:627–32.

11 Bonhof JA, Linhart P, Bettendorf U *et al.* (1984) Liver biopsy guided by laparoscopic sonography. *Endoscopy.* **16**:237–9.

12 Okita K, Kodama T, Oda M *et al.* (1984) Laparoscopic ultrasonography: diagnosis of liver and pancreatic cancer. *Scand J Gastroenterol.* **19** (Suppl. 94):91–100.

13 Salky BA, Bauer JJ, Gelernt IM *et al.* (1988) The use of laparoscopy in retroperitoneal pathology. *Gastrointest Endosc.* **34**:227–30.

14 Chiders JM and Surwit EA (1992) Laparoscopic para-aortic lymph node biopsy for diagnosis of a non-Hodgkin's lymphoma. *Surg Laparosc Endosc.* **2**:139–42.

15 Herd J, Fowler JM, Shenson D *et al.* (1992) Laparoscopic para-aortic lymph node sampling: development of a technique. *Gynecol Oncol.* **44**:271–6.

16 Watt I, Stewart I, Anderson D *et al.* (1989) Laparoscopy, ultrasound, and computed tomography in cancer of the oesophagus and gastric cardia: a prospective comparison for detecting intra-abdominal metastases. *Br J Surg.* **76**:1036–9.

17 Kriplani AK and Kapur BML (1991) Laparoscopy for pre-operative staging and assessment of operability in gastric carcinoma. *Gastrointest Endosc.* **37**:441–3.

18 Warshaw AL, Tepper JE and Shipley WU (1986) Laparoscopy in the staging and planning of therapy for pancreatic cancer. *Am J Surg.* **151**:76–80.

19 Warshaw AL, Zhuo-yun G, Wittenberg, J *et al.* (1990) Preoperative staging and assessment of resectability of pancreatic cancer. *Arch Surg.* **125**:230–3.

20 Parra RO, Andrus C and Boulier J (1992) Staging laparoscopic pelvic lymph node dissection: comparison of results with open pelvic lymphadenectomy. *J Urol.* **147**:875–8.

21 Rosenhoff SH, Young RC, Anderson T *et al* (1975) Peritoneoscopy: a valuable staging tool in ovarian carcinoma. *Ann Int Med.* **83**:37–41.

22 Brady PG, Peebles M and Goldschmid S (1991) Role of laparoscopy in the evaluation of patients with suspected hepatic or peritoneal malignancy. *Gastrointest Endosc.* **37**:27–30.

23 Jeffers L, Spieglman G, Reddy R *et al.* (1988) Laparoscopically directed fine needle aspiration for the diagnosis of hepatocellular carcinoma: a safe and accurate technique. *Gastrointest Endosc* **34**:235–7.

24 Gandolfi L, Muratori R, Solmi L *et al.* (1989) Laparoscopy compared with ultrasonography in the diagnosis of hepatocellular carcinoma. *Gastrointest Endosc.* **35**:508–11.

25 Fornari F, Rapaccini GL, Cavanna L *et al.* (1988) Diagnosis of hepatic lesions: ultrasonically guided fine needle biopsy or laparoscopy. *Gastrointest Endosc.* **34**:231–4.

26 Beahrs OH (1986) Staging and prognostic features of cancer of the colon and rectum. In: Beahrs OH, Higgins GA and Weinstein JJ (Eds) *Colorectal tumors.* J.B. Lippincott, Philadelphia. p115.

27 Willett CG, Tepper JE, Cohen AM *et al.* (1984) Failure patterns following curative resection of colonic carcinoma. *Ann Surg.* **200**:685–90.

28 Michelassi F, Vannucci L, Ayala JJ *et al.* (1990) Local recurrence after curative resection of colorectal adenocarcinoma. *Surgery.* **108**:787–93.

29 Stipa S, Nicolanti V, Botti C *et al.* (1991) Local recurrence after curative resection for colorectal cancer: frequency, risk factors, and treatment. *J Surg Oncol.* Suppl. 2: 155–60.

30 McDermott FT, Hughes ESR, Pihl E *et al.* (1985) Local recurrence after potentially curative resection for rectal cancer in a series of 1008 patients. *Br J Surg.* **72**:34–7.

31 Schiessel R, Wunderlich M and Herbst F (1986) Local recurrence of colorectal cancer: effect of early detection and aggressive surgery. *Br J Surg.* **73**:342–4.

32 Wangensteen OH, Lewis FJ and Tongen LA (1951) The 'second look' in cancer surgery. *Lancet.* **71**:303–7.

33 Wangensteen OH, Lewis FJ, Arhelger SW *et al.* (1954) An interim report upon the 'second-look' procedure for cancer of the stomach, colon, and rectum and for 'limited intraperitoneal carcinosis'. *Surg Gynecol Obstet.* **99**:257–67.

34 Sugarbaker PH, Gianola FJ, Dwyer A *et al.* (1987) A simplified plan for follow-up of patients with colon and rectal cancer supported by prospective studies of laboratory and radiologic test results. *Surgery.* **102**:79–87.

35 Martin EW Jr, Minton JP and Carey LC (1985) CEA-directed second-look surgery in the asymptomatic patient after primary resection of colorectal carcinoma. *Ann Surg.* **202**:310–17.

36 Minton JP, Hoehn JL, Gerber DM *et al.* (1985) Results of a 400-patient carcinoembryonic antigen second look colorectal cancer study. *Cancer.* **55**:1284–90.

37 Fucini C, Tommasi SM and Rosi S (1987) Follow-up of colorectal cancer resected for cure: an experience with CEA, TPA, Ca19-9 analysis and second-look surgery. *Dis Col Rect.* **90**:273–7.

38 Xygakis AM, Politis GS, Michalas SP *et al.* (1984) Second-look laparoscopy in ovarian cancer. *J Reprod Med.* **29**:583–5.

39 Marti-Vicente A, Sainz S, Soriano G *et al.* (1990) Utilidad de la laparoscopia como metodo de second-look en las neoplasias del ovario. *Rev Esp Enf Digest.* **77**:275–8.

40 Onik G, Rubinsky B, Zemel R *et al.* (1991) Ultrasound-guided hepatic cryosurgery in the treatment of metastatic colon carcinoma. Preliminary results. *Cancer.* **67**:901–6.

41 Zhou X-D, Tang Z-Y, Yu Y-G *et al.* (1988) Clinical evaluation of cryosurgery in the treatment of primary liver cancer: report of 60 cases. *Cancer.* **61**:1889–94.

10

Ultrasonography for Preoperative and Intraoperative Staging of Colorectal Malignancies

ARMIN BRUEGGEMANN

Introduction

The ultimate aim of surgical therapy for colorectal malignancies is the tumor-free long-term survival of the patient. It can be demonstrated that exact staging and a staging-correlated therapy lead to a significantly higher rate of tumor-free long-term survival and a reduction of local tumor recurrence[1,2]. In planning surgical therapy, especially in rectal cancer, exact tumor staging should be performed before surgical therapy by imaging procedures. Ideally, restaging must be possible preoperatively with a minimum of patient discomfort. Sonography has proved to be an accurate diagnostic imaging procedure, causing no harm or discomfort to the patient, and when performed and interpreted by a surgeon it is a well accepted tool in pre-, intra- and postoperative diagnosis[3]. The goal of a sonographic examination in patients with colorectal malignancies is:

- the localization of the tumor
- its staging
- the detection of lymph node and liver metastases.

Tumor complications, such as intestinal obstruction, ascites due to peritoneal seeding or dilatation of the renal pelvis should also be assessed.

Ultrasonic examination is possible percutaneously, endoluminally, intraoperatively and, more recently, during laparoscopic surgery. This chapter deals with the technical aspects, results and typical findings of ultrasound staging.

Percutaneous ultrasound

The initial diagnostic procedure for histologically proven colorectal malignancies is percutaneous ultrasound (PUS). The examination should be performed using a frequency between 3.5 and 5 MHz. Sector or convex arrays are suitable, while the use of linear arrays may cause some difficulties in the adjustment of the scanner. All abdominal organs, including the kidneys and the extra-peritoneal lymph node regions, must be examined. Examination should be performed on the fasting patient. Further preparation for routine sonography of the abdomen is not necessary. In constricting tumors the proximal colon can be extremely gaseous, rendering the examination more difficult.

Liver metastases

Due to the cascade hypothesis, hematogenous metastases from colorectal cancer will first be found in the liver and, in most cases, no further metastases can be detected[4,5]. Finlay and Mc Ardle[1] reported that liver metastases can be found in 24% of the patients at the onset of surgical therapy. Since the presence of liver metastases is known to determine the long-term survival of the patients[6], it is necessary to scan the liver for metastases prior to surgical therapy in order to adapt the therapeutic and operative strategy if liver metastases can be confirmed.

Sonographic examination of the liver should be performed during deep inspiration to shift the liver down towards the lower aperture of the thorax. To ensure that the entire organ is examined, scans must be done parallel to the costal arch. The parts of the liver close to the diaphragm can only be examined if the scanner is angled toward the abdominal wall. Sagittal scans through the liver will be done afterwards and the examination should include scans through the right intercostal spaces. Through this examination, further information can be obtained about the presence of cirrhosis, fatty degeneration, liver cysts and hemangiomas. Liver metastases larger than 1–1.5 cm can be detected by PUS[3,7] and, regarding the vascular anatomy of the liver, can be allocated to the liver segments.

Liver metastases present themselves as hyper- or hypoechoic ball-shaped masses, often displacing the liver vessels (Figure 10.1**a**). In colorectal malignancies, metastases are mostly hyperechoic to the echo-pattern of the liver with a small hypoechoic halo (bulls-eye-sign, Figure 10.1**b**). In large metastases, central necrosis may occur making the center look like a nearly anechoic cyst (Figure 10.1**b**). In some cases, multiple metastases or a diffuse tumorous seeding can only be detected due to the displacement of the liver vessels (Figure 10.1**c**).

According to the literature, scanning will show up between 34 and 100% of liver metastases (Table 10.1). The sensitivity of the sonographic detection of liver metastases depends on the quality of the ultrasound unit used, anatomical features of the patient and, most of all, on the experience of the examiner. Furthermore, it should be pointed out that ultrasound may yield no histologic diagnosis. Metastases can be suspected on the basis of specific

(a)

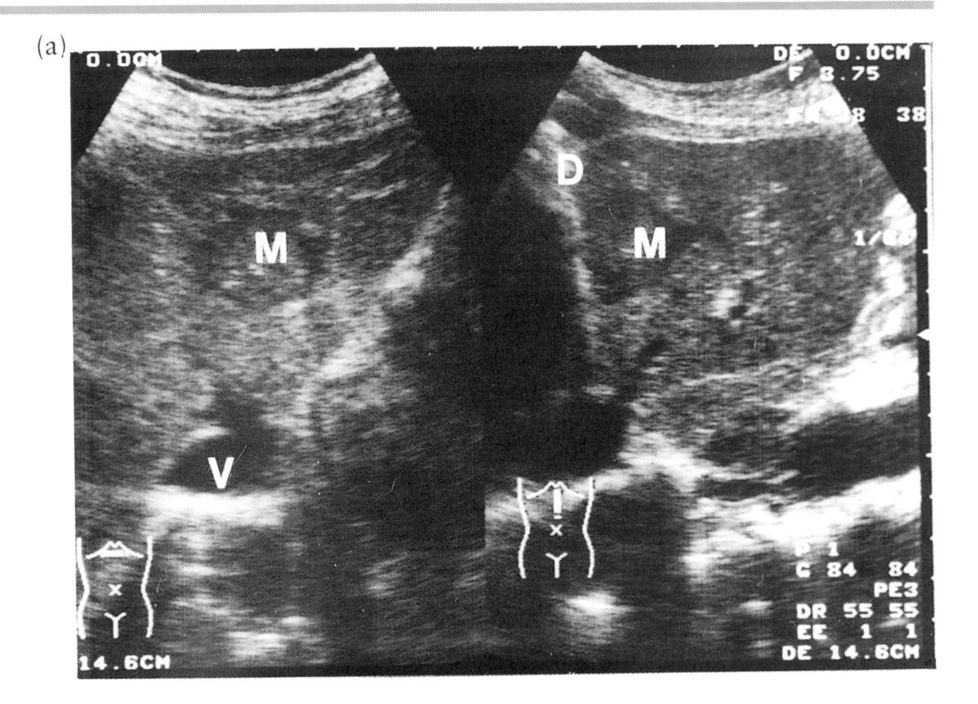

(b)

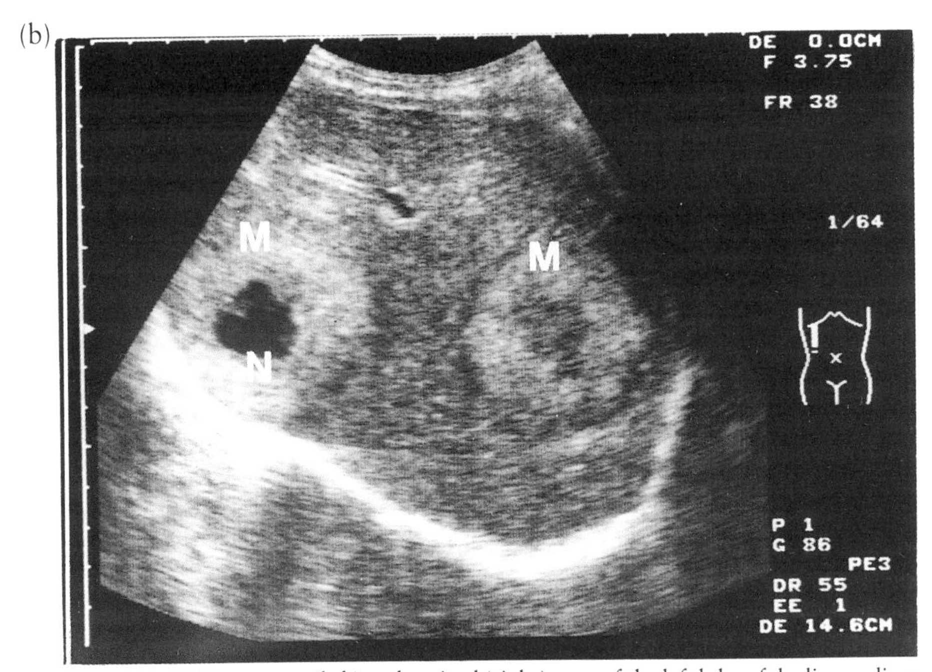

Figure 10.1: (**a**) Transverse (left) and sagittal (right) scan of the left lobe of the liver: a liver metastasis (M) with a typical hypoechoic halo can be detected in segment II (Couinaud) close to the diaphragm (D). V, inferior vena cava. (**b**) Sagittal scan in the midclavicular line: two large liver metastases (M) can be seen. Both show the typical hypoechoic halo. The central necrosis (N) appears similar to anechoic cyst. This type of liver metastasis was named 'bulls-eye-lesion' due to its appearance.

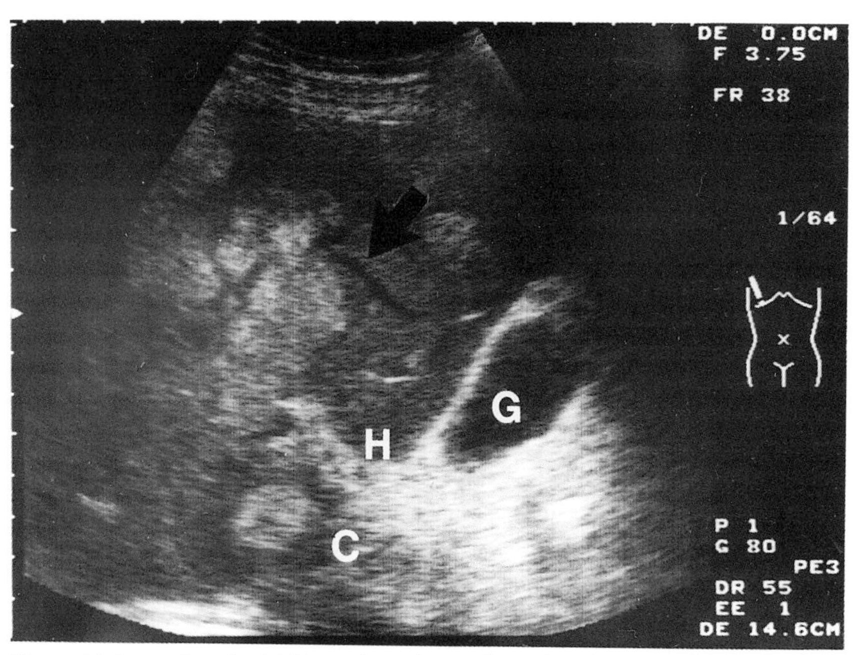

Figure 10.1: *continued* (c) Ventrolateral scan through an intercostal space: several hyperechoic liver metastases in the center of the right lobe of the liver close to the hilum (H) and the caudate lobe (C). The metastases are surrounded by a small halo. The vascular architecture of the liver is disturbed (arrow). G gall bladder (curved array scanner, 3.75 MHz).

	Sonography (%)	CT scan (%)
Alderson *et al.*[8]	82	91
Boldrini *et al.*[9]	76	76
Castaing *et al.*[10]	68	67
Charnley *et al.*[11]	34	69
Clarke *et al.*[12]	76	61
Gozzetti *et al.*[13]	81	74
Rifkin *et al.*[14]	62	42
Schreve *et al.*[15]	85	88
Snow *et al.*[16]	85	91
Vlachos *et al.*[17]	100	100
Zocholl *et al.*[18]	64	83

Table 10.1: Comparison of sonography and computed tomography in the evaluation of liver tumors. Accuracy is as reported by the authors. Differences may be due to different study designs, different technical devices and the experience of the examiners.

findings and depending on the experience of the examiner. The diagnosis should then be confirmed by ultrasound-guided biopsy.

Localization of tumors

The next factor to be assessed by PUS is the localization and the extent of the tumor. Although the intestinal tract is normally thin-walled and often air-filled, some authors have reported good results in the localization of colorectal malignancies using PUS[9–21,41].

The examination should be performed using a 3.5 or 5 MHz scanner. Linear or convex arrays are preferred. Starting at the cecum, the large bowel must be investigated following its anatomic position by transverse and longitudinal scans. The fixed parts (cecum, ascending and descending colon, right and left colic flexure) can normally be visualized without any problems. Some difficulties may occur in localizing the transverse and sigmoid colon.

Normal colonic wall thickness is about 3–5 mm. Using PUS, normally three different layers can be differentiated at a frequency of 3.5 MHz. A 5 MHz scanner can depict five different layers under ideal conditions (Table 10.2, Figure 10.2a). At 3.5 MHz, the 'entrance echo', mucosa and submucosa form the inner hyperechoic layer. The following hypoechoic layer represents the muscularis propria. The outer hyperechoic layer is known to correlate to the peritoneal cover. At a higher frequency, the colonic wall can be divided into five different layers, with the inner hyperechoic being the 'entrance echo'. A small inner hypoechoic layer, representing the mucosa, follows. The connecting broad middle hyperechoic layer is the correlate of the submucosa. The broad outer hypoechoic layer resembles the muscularis propria, and the small outer hyperechoic layer the peritoneal cover.

	Sonographic correlate	
Anatomical structure	5 MHz	3.5 MHz
'Entrance echo'	Inner hyperechoic	Inner hyperechoic
Mucosa	Inner hypoechoic	Inner hyperechoic
Submucosa	Middle hyperechoic	Inner hyperechoic
Muscularis propria	Outer hypoechoic	Hypoechoic
'exit echo' (Peritoneal cover)	Outer hyperechoic	Outer hyperechoic

Table 10.2: Sonographic appearance of the colonic wall. At 3.5 MHz, the 'entrance echo', mucosa and submucosa will form the inner hyperechoic layer. A five-layer differentiation can be seen at 5–8 MHz. At 10 MHz, the outer hypoechoic layer of the rectal wall can be divided into two by another small hyperechoic layer, representing the inner circular and the outer longitudinal muscular layers.

Measurement of tumor size

Malignancies of the colon present themselves as hypoechoic thickenings of the colonic wall in the longitudinal scans, allowing the measurement of the tumor size. Following transverse scans, the circular extent of the tumor can be estimated. This typical appearance on sonography is called the 'target sign' or 'pseudo-kidney sign'. In evaluating colonic cancer in PUS, attention must be given to the differentiation of the outer hyperechoic layer. If this layer can be delineated over the entire extent of the tumor, a staging 'uT2' can be estimated (Figure 10.2**a**). In a uT3-tumor, hypoechoic infiltration of the surrounding tissue occurs with a penetration of the outer hyperechoic layer (Figure 10.2**b**). Using PUS, 81–94% of colonic tumors can be detected and localized. Small tumors and colonic polyps will be missed. For anatomical reasons, the evaluation of rectal tumors is more difficult. If the urinary bladder is full, it is often possible to detect malignancies of the rectum (Figure 10.2**c**). Although rectal tumors are visible on PUS under certain circumstances, PUS is not the first choice in the evaluation of rectal tumors, as it is impossible to define the distance of the tumor to the anocutaneous line.

The detection of colonic lesions can be improved by having a fluid-filled large intestine. To achieve a completely fluid-filled colon, about 1500 ml of water must be instilled retrograde after subcutaneous injection of 20 mg of N-butyl-scopolamine. The retrograde filling of the colon is made possible by changing the patient's position. Sonographic examination should be performed retrograde from the sigmoid to the cecum, while filling the large intestine with water. Each examination takes about 20 minutes and in 90% of patients the large intestine can be evaluated from the sigmoid to the cecum[22]. Using a high-resolution 5 MHz scanner, 96% of the tumors and 91% of the polyps larger than 7 mm can be detected[23].

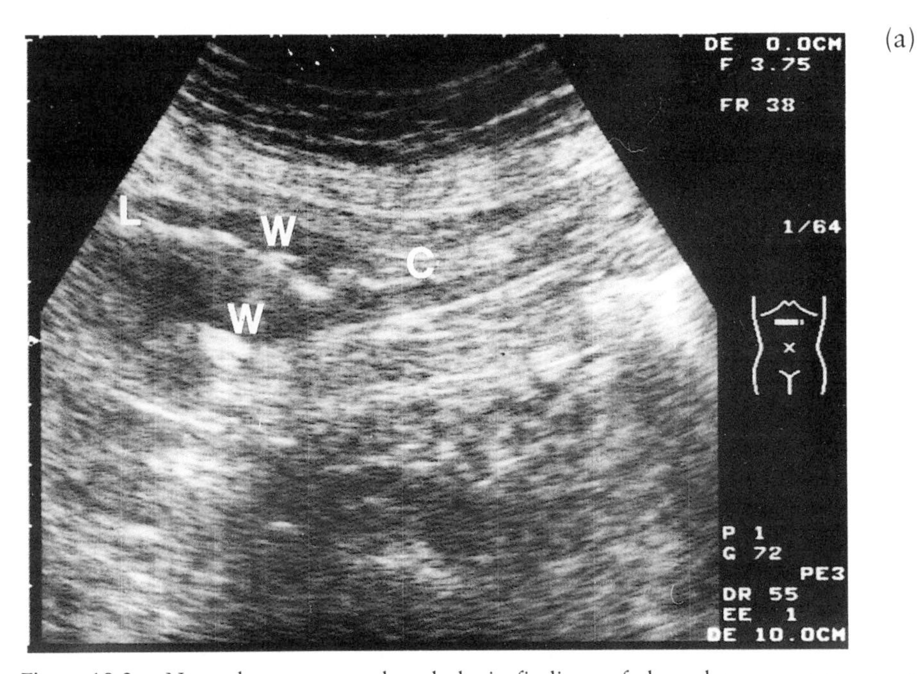

Figure 10.2: Normal anatomy and pathologic findings of the colon on percutaneous ultrasound. (**a**) Transverse scan in the middle of the upper abdomen. Due to a malignant tumor, the wall (W) of the transverse colon is thickened and hypoechoic, surrounding a small, air-filled lumen (L). The different layers of the normal colon (C) are too small to be differentiated. Note that the wall can be clearly delineated from the surrounding tissue (uT2).

(b)

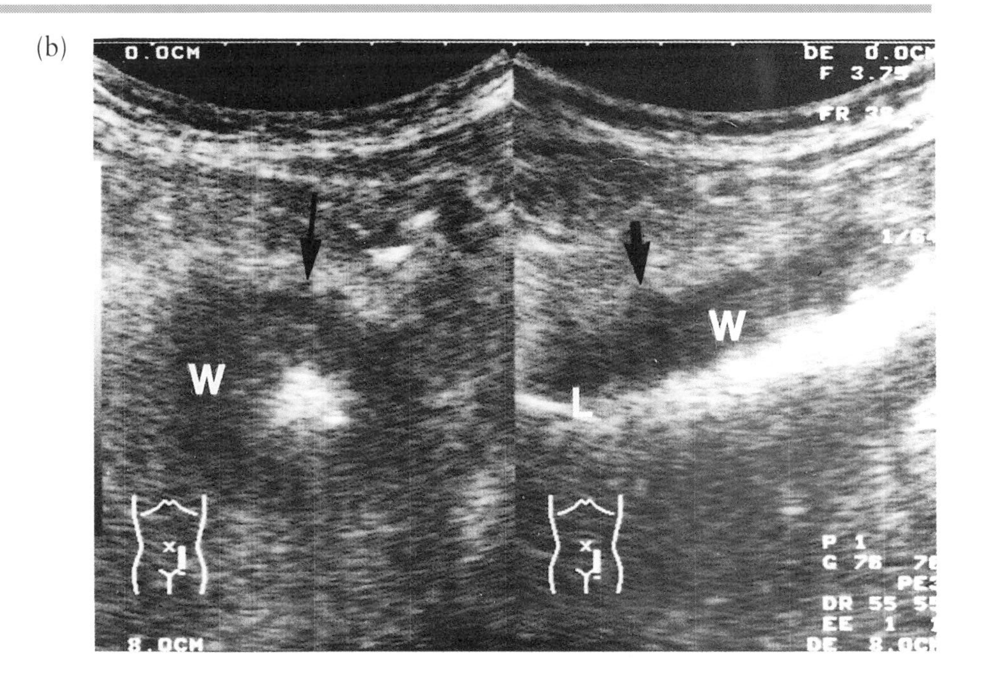

(c)

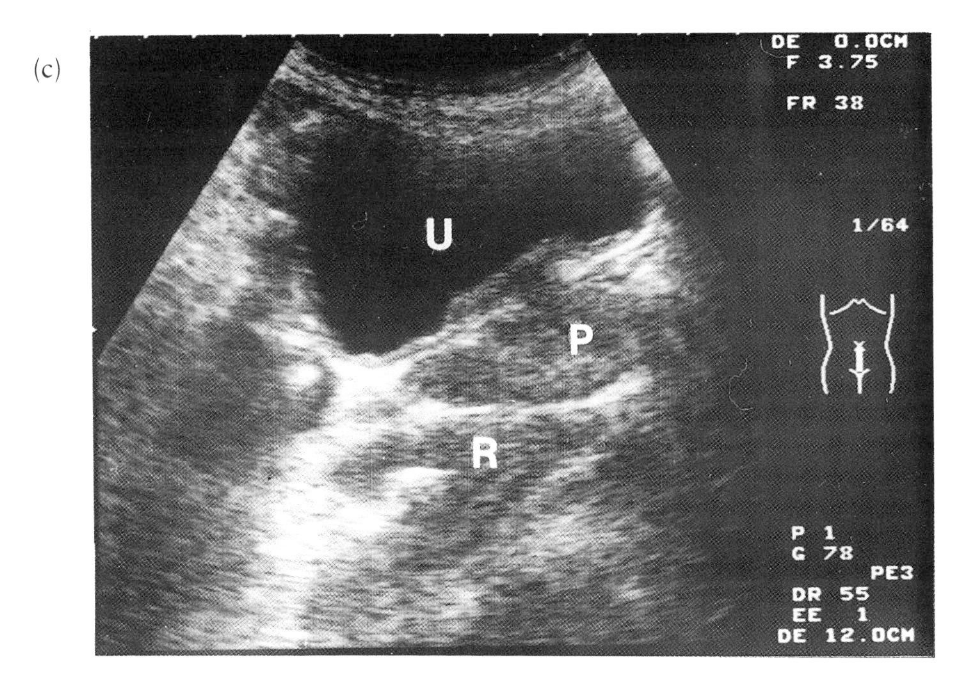

Figure 10.2: *continued* (**b**) Longitudinal (left) and transverse scan (right) of the left lower abdomen: this large tumor of the sigmoid leads to extensive hypoechoic thickening of the wall (W) leaving only a small air-filled lumen (L). The infiltration of the tumor into the surrounding fatty tissue is indicated by arrows (uT3). (**c**) Sagittal scan in the middle lower abdomen: the rectal wall (R) is hypoechoic thickened in a patient with extensive rectal cancer. The enlarged prostate gland (P) is compressing the wall of the urinary bladder (U) (curved array scanner, 3.75 MHz).

Although the results are good, it must be noted that ultrasound is unable to differentiate between tumorous, inflammatory and traumatic lesions. Furthermore, the examination is time-consuming (taking about 20 minutes) and the rectum can be examined only cursorily. In routine diagnostic procedures, a classification of the tumor as presented in Table 10.4 will not normally be obtained by PUS.

Reviewing the literature, only one report could be found which investigated regional lymph node metastases by PUS[24]. Using a 3.5 or 5 MHz scanner, lymph nodes in the mesentery larger than 10 mm could be detected. Every pathologically altered lymph node observed was hypoechoic and ball-shaped. Compared with the histologic findings, metastastic and inflammatory altered lymph nodes could not be differentiated with sufficient specificity. From these data it can be stated that PUS is an inefficient procedure in the detection of mesenteric lymph node metastases due to colorectal malignancies.

In colorectal malignancies, PUS should not only be used to detect the primary tumor, liver or lymph node metastases. Sonographic examination of the abdominal and retroperitoneal organs can also offer much information on secondary or independent pathologies. For this reason, sonographic examination must include a complete scanning of all abdominal and retroperitoneal organs. A specification of the diagnostic pathologies by PUS will not be included in this chapter.

Endoluminal ultrasound

The correct staging of colorectal malignancies depends on the detection of tumor invasion into the different anatomic layers of the colonic wall. On sonography, a high resolution is associated with a high frequency of the scanner on a physical basis. On the other hand, the higher frequency diminishes the penetration into the tissue. This physical limitation requires a close contact of a high-frequency scanner to the structures to be examined. For rectal malignancies, this problem was first solved by Dragstedt and Gammelgaard[25] using a rigid endorectal probe with a rotating scanner. Numerous investigations utilizing different probes followed and, especially for planning the local excision of rectal tumors, endorectal ultrasound (ES) has become a necessary tool in the preoperative staging of colorectal malignancies[26].

Probes

Different probes are available for ES. Most of them are rigid probes without an optical device, which have to be inserted blind or through a rectoscope. The ultrasound scanner is located at the tip of the probe. The current favorite is a rotating sector scanner with frequencies between 5 and 10 MHz. The rotating scanner is covered by a latex balloon. By filling this balloon with normal saline or water, an acoustic coupling between probe and rectal wall can be achieved and damage to the rectal wall from the rotating scanner can be avoided. Scanner rotation yields a stationary circular image of the rectal wall and the surrounding tissue. The extent and the depth of invasion can be examined. The longitudinal extent of the tumor can be measured by withdrawal or further insertion of the probe. Other probes use linear scanners: longitudinal extent and depth of invasion can be assessed after insertion of the probe. To estimate the localization and the circular extent of a tumor, the linear scanner must be rotated on its axis. These probes are more difficult to handle than on the rotating scanner. Today, a combination of both types is available.

For ES, the fasting patient is given an enema about 15 minutes prior to the examination. To perform rectoscopy and sonographic examination, the patient should be placed in the lithotomy or left lateral decubitus position. Rectoscopy is done first to measure the distance of the lesion from the anocutaneous line and to obtain a macroscopic evaluation. Having localized the tumor, the endorectal ultrasound probe is inserted through the rectoscope or blindly after removing the scope. The tip of the probe should be positioned proximal to the tumor to ensure the complete sonographic examination of rectal wall, tumor and surrounding tissue. In some cases it is impossible, even after bouginage, to pass a constricting tumor. If a probe with multiple frequencies (eg 5 and 7 MHz) is used, the examination should start at 5 MHz to get an overview and then sweep to the higher frequency for assessing the tumor invasion of the colonic wall.

Evaluation of tumors

At a frequency of about 7 MHz, normal rectal wall can be differentiated into five different layers (Table 10.2, Figure 10.3**a**). An inner hyperechoic layer, the entrance echo, represents the acoustic interface between the water-filled balloon and the mucosa. For this reason, the innermost layer is not part of the rectal wall. The following hypoechoic layer is the sonographic correlate of the mucosa. The middle hyperechoic layer represents the submucosa and the connecting outer hypoechoic layer the muscularis propria. Using higher frequencies (eg 10 MHz), this layer can be divided into two by a very small hyperechoic layer. These two layers represent the inner circular and the outer longitudinal muscular layer. The outer hyperechoic layer (exit echo) is the acoustic interface of rectal wall and surrounding fatty tissue of the peritoneal cover. A proper differentiation of these five layers will be seen only if the scanner is positioned at a right angle to the rectal wall. Since the rectum is not a stiff tube, it may be that these layers will not be completely visualized over the entire circumference. When using endorectal ultrasound to evaluate malignant tumors, the neighbouring organs as well the vagina, prostate gland and urinary bladder should also be investigated.

Rectal tumors appear mostly as hypoechoic masses. The sonographic staging assesses the hypoechoic infiltration of the rectal wall. A sonographic staging of rectal tumors has been defined according to the TNM classification (Table 10.3). To determine the sonographic staging, the prefix 'u' should be used according to a proposal by Hildebrandt and Feifel[27]. A tumorous infiltration of mucosa and submucosa (pT1) will appear on sonography as a hypoechoic thickening of the inner hypoechoic and the connecting middle hypoechoic layer. A small hyperechoic zone will delineate the tumor from the adjacent

(a)

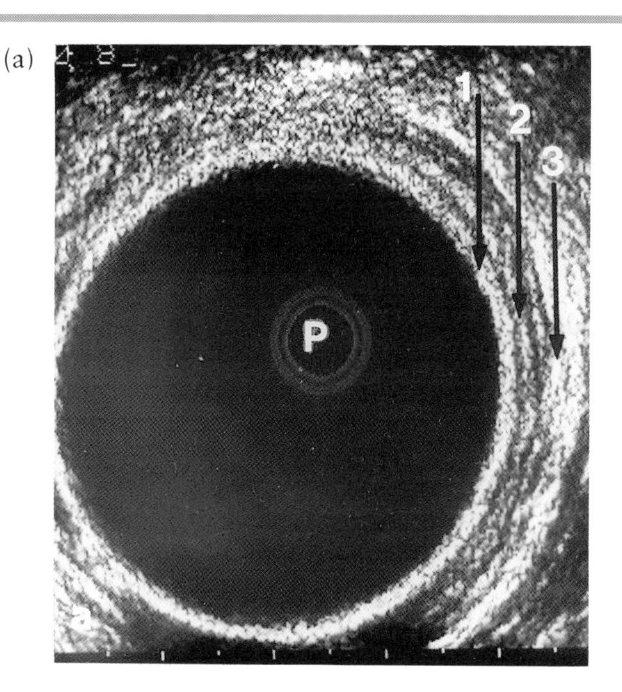

Figure 10.3: Sonographic anatomy and pathology of the rectum on endoluminal ultrasound (rotating sector scanner, frequency 7 MHz). (**a**) Normal anatomy of the rectal wall: the inner hyperechoic layer (1) represents the 'entrance-echo', the following hypoechoic layer the mucosa. The middle hyperechoic layer (2) is known to be the submucosa. The outer hyperechoic layer (3, 'exit-echo') delineates the muscularis propria from the surrounding tissue. In this case, the muscularis propria is divided by a small hyperechoic layer into two parts, representing the inner circular and the outer longitudinal muscle layer. P probe.

puT0	No tumor detected by ultrasound
puT1	Inner hypoechoic and connecting hyperechoic layer are hypoechoic thickened by the tumor. Outer hypoechoic layer can be clearly delineated.
puT2	Colonic wall is totally infiltrated by the tumor. Outer hyperechoic layer can be clearly delineated.
puT3	Tumor infiltrates the pericolic fatty tissue. Outer hyperechoic layer cannot be delineated.
puT4	Tumor infiltrates surrounding organs.

Table 10.3: Sonographic staging of rectal malignancies by endorectal ultrasound with regard to the TNM classification

hypoechoic muscularis propria (uT1, Figure 10.3**b**). A pT2-tumor shows an infiltration of the rectal wall without invading the perirectal fat. Sonography demonstrates a hypoechoic tumorous mass invading the outer hypoechoic layer. This layer must be visually undamaged to estimate a tumor as uT2 (Figure 10.3**c**). According to the TNM classification, a hypoechoic infiltration through the outer hyperechoic layer can be observed in a uT3 tumor

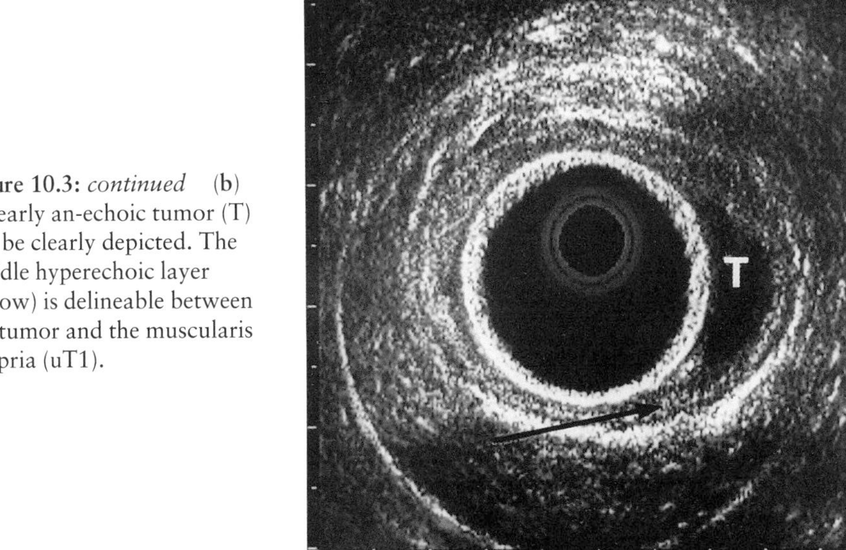

Figure 10.3: *continued* (b) A nearly an-echoic tumor (T) can be clearly depicted. The middle hyperechoic layer (arrow) is delineable between the tumor and the muscularis propria (uT1).

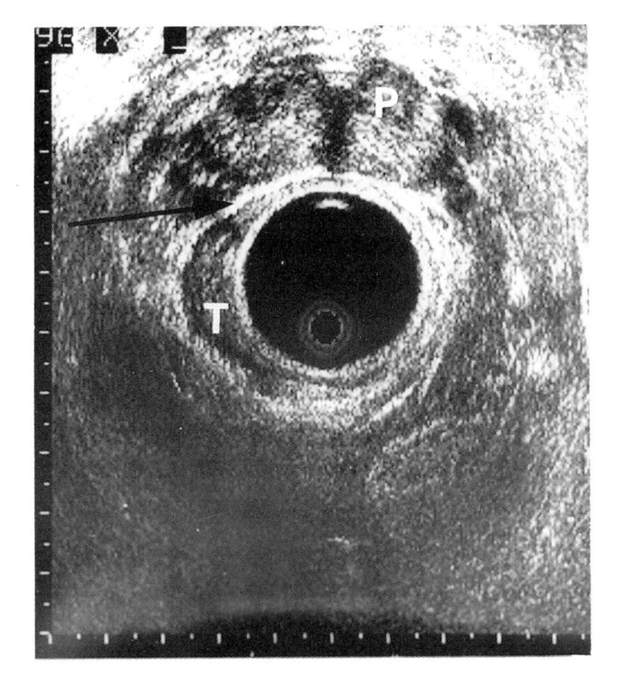

(c) The hypoechoic tumor (T) is infiltrating all layers of the rectal wall. It is clearly set off from the surrounding tissue and the prostate gland (P) by the outer hyperechoic layer (arrow) (uT2).

(Figure 10.3**d**). In a uT4-tumor, hypoechoic infiltration of the neighbouring organs can be noted. Compared with pathologic findings, the assessment of tumor invasion in rectal cancer is specific (Table 10.4). From the data presented, it can be seen that an overstaging of the tumor will occur more often than an understaging. This may be due to edema caused by the tumor. Edema will lead to a hypoechoic alteration of the tissue, and in rectal cancer it will enlarge the tumorous mass on sonography.

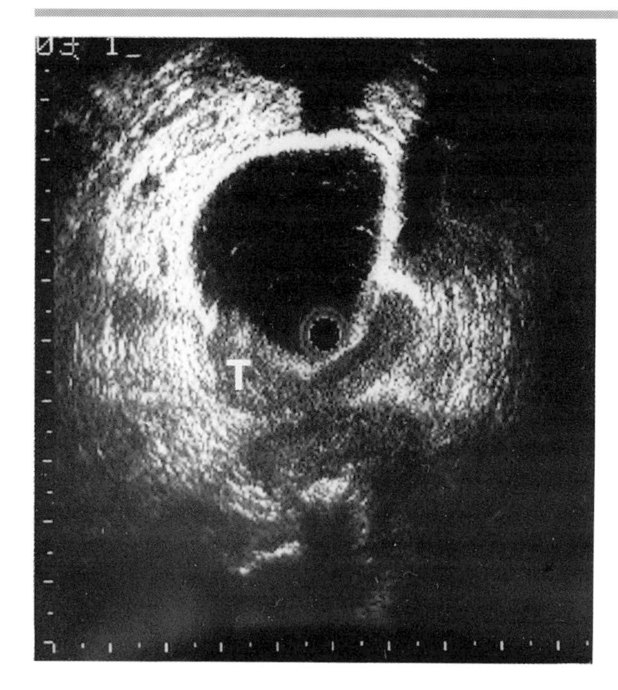

Figure 10.3: *continued* **(d)** A large hypoechoic tumor invading the perirectal fat. Normal structures of the rectal wall cannot be distinguished. Due to the reduced scale, even the layers of the non-infiltrated rectal wall are not visible (uT3).

Sonographic staging	Pathologic classification			
	pT1	pT2	pT3	pT4
uT1	111	7	2	–
uT2	14	95	2	–
uT3	–	25	172	2
uT4	–	–	–	18

Table 10.4: Accuracy of sonographic staging of colorectal malignancies with regard to the TNM-system (cumulative data drawn from the literature cited, n = 448). Results of studies using comparable ultrasound devices and the TNM-classification have been compounded.

	Pathologic staging	
Sonographic staging	pN+	pN–
uN+	153	41
uN–	21	95

Table 10.5: Accuracy of sonographic lymph-node staging (cumulative data drawn from the literature cited, n = 310)

Especially when planning sphincter-preserving surgery in rectal cancer, information about local lymph-node metastases must be obtained. Endorectal ultrasound offers the opportunity to detect local lymph-node metastases with a great degree of accuracy (Table 10.5). As described above, lymph-node metastases will be hypoechoic and ball-shaped. In most cases they can be clearly

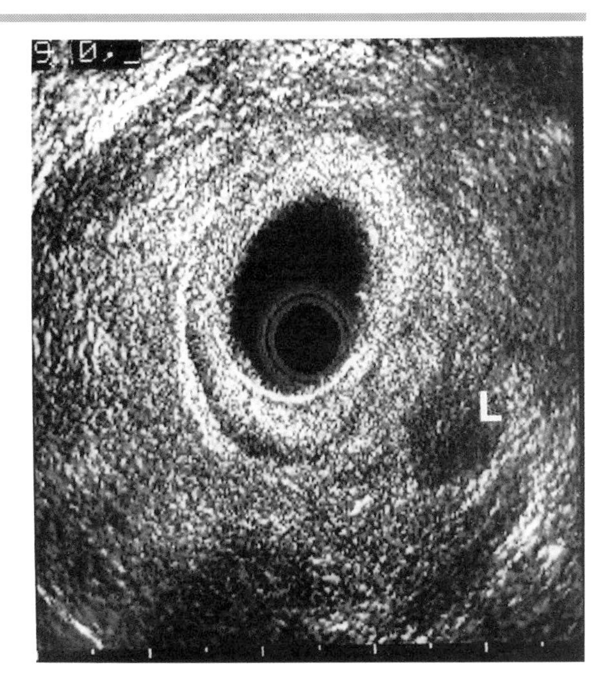

Figure 10.3: *continued* (e) Hypoechoic lymph-node metastasis (L) in the left pararectal fat. The lymph-node is distinctly separate from the surrounding fatty tissue.

distinguished from the surrounding fatty tissue (Figure 10.3e). Differentiation from a transverse scan of a vessel can be reached by moving the scanner head: a vessel will show its tubular structure. Normal non-altered lymph-nodes are hyperechoic and cannot be differentiated from the surrounding fat. Changes in lymph nodes due to infections may cause a hypoechoic pattern. In most cases, such lymph-nodes are more ovoid and their margins are not too readily discernible from the surrounding fatty tissue.

Although most tumors of the colon occur in the rectum and the sigmoid, only about two-thirds of all colorectal malignancies can be detected using a rectoscope or by palpating with a finger. The assessment of tumor invasion in the proximal large intestine has been difficult. PUS offers the opportunity of detecting and localizing colonic tumors, but an assessment of the depth of invasion can not be achieved with any great accuracy.

Ultrasound coloscope

Recently the first results using an ultrasound coloscope have been reported[28,29]. This coloscope has a forward-viewing optic and a rotating sector scanner offering an ultrasound image of 320°. Coloscopy and sonographic examination of the colon can be performed simultaneously. After enema-cleaning of the large intestine, the examination is performed in the left lateral position. Acoustic coupling of the transducer to the colonic wall can be achieved by filling a latex balloon as in endorectal sonography. If the diameter of the large intestine exceeds that of the balloon, acoustic coupling can be achieved by local instillation of water and by changing the patient's position. Preliminary reports refer to good practicability in assessing the large intestine: in 55% of the patients complete examination up to the cecum could be performed. The disadvantage is that this examination is very time-consuming taking an average of 58 minutes, one-third of which is needed for positioning the scanner into the cecum. Further investigation will have to prove the feasibility of this new method for daily practice.

Intraoperative ultrasound

As described above, the existence of liver metastases will determine the long-term survival of patients suffering from colorectal malignancies[6]. Metastases greater than 1–1.5 cm can be detected on PUS, but small metastases will be missed in a high percentage of cases. By pathologic definition, a small metastasis is about 0.6 cm in diameter. Following colorectal malignancies, the ratio between large and small liver metastases is about 1 : 1.6[30]. From this data it is evident that high-resolution ultrasound is necessary to detect small liver metastases. As described above, high-resolution sonography requires higher frequencies. As the higher frequencies have a diminished tissue penetration, the probe must be placed on the liver surface to achieve good imaging.

To perform intraoperative ultrasound (IOUS), high-resolution scanners with a frequency of 5–7.5 MHz are needed. They should also be narrowly focused to detect lesions close to the liver surface. Furthermore, distorted imaging of the liver anatomy must be avoided. Due to these demands, only linear arrays are suitable for IOUS. These arrays are normally small and flat. To be guided by the palpating fingers of the surgeon, the scanners should be T- or I-shaped.

To avoid infections by IOUS, the scanner must be sterile if used in the open abdomen. One alternative is gas-sterilization of the scanner. The advantage of gas-sterilization is that no further preparation of the scanner is needed when it is used for IOUS. Its disadvantages are that frequent sterilization may cause some damage to the probe, and that the interval between gas-sterilization and reuse is long so that a probe can be used only once a day. In centers where more than one daily operation for colonic cancer or liver metastases is performed, two or more scanners must be available. The second alternative for IOUS utilizes a sterile cover over a non-sterile probe. This sterile cover must be waterproof. To ensure the acoustic coupling, some water-soluble jelly must be deposited into the tip of the cover prior to insertion of the probe. The advantage of this procedure is that one probe can be used as often as necessary in one day. The disadvantages are that it may take as long as five minutes to prepare the probe and the cover, and that infections may occur if the sterile covering is compromized.

IOUS is performed after opening the abdomen. Even from lower abdominal incisions, a complete liver scan is possible analogous to a palpating examination. Mobilization of the liver is not needed. Due to moisture in the peritoneal cavity, the scanner can be attached to the liver surface without using a coupling medium. The liver is scanned in longitudinal and transverse sections, beginning at the convex surface. For an organ of this size, the liver must also be scanned from the abdominal surface if a 7.5 MHz scanner is used. If using a 5 MHz scanner, examination via the abdominal surface should be performed. A complete examination of the liver takes about 10 minutes.

Since the surface of the liver offers no orientation points, the intrahepatic vessels are used to assign the liver segments. As in PUS, branches of the portal venous system and the hepatic veins can be exactly differentiated. The portal venous system can be identified by its broad hyperechoic surrounding tissue (Figures 10.1**a** and 10.4). Close to the larger branches a second tubular system can be detected, representing the intrahepatic biliary ducts. Hepatic veins are usually not surrounded by a hyperechoic wall. Using these vessels as a guide, the liver segments can be precisely determined and lesions can be located. As in PUS, the general echogenity of the liver should be estimated and focal lesions judged by their echo-pattern. Small liver metastases from colorectal cancers are normally ball-shaped and hyperechoic. A small hypoechoic halo as a sign of malignancy can also mostly be visualized (Figure 10.4). Large metastases can appear in IOUS as described above. In order to verify the sonographic suspicion of liver metastases ultrasound guided biopsy can be performed.

Even early IOUS investigations using a 5 MHz sector scanner demonstrated good results in detection of occult liver metastases compared to necropsy findings[31]. It could be shown that metastases smaller than 0.4 cm were not visible. Sixty-five percent of metastases 0.5–0.9 cm in size could be detected. Since then, the use of linear scanners has enabled better imaging. Numerous investigators have referred to supplementary information about liver metastases by IOUS and adapted their surgical procedure in several patients accordingly (Table 10.6).

Although IOUS is a well accepted tool for detecting liver metastases due to colorectal malignancies, it is not yet practicable in minimal access surgery, since the available probes can not currently be introduced into the abdomen via a laparoscopic trocar.

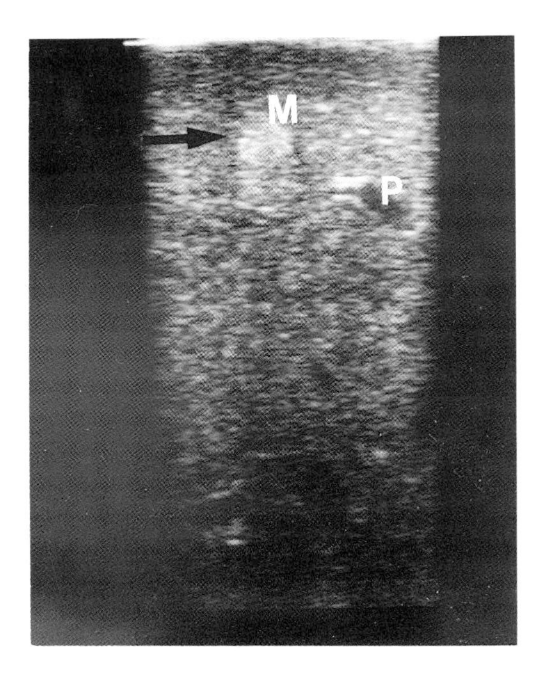

Figure 10.4: This intraoperative sonogram shows a non-palpable tiny (4 mm) hyperechoic metastasis (M). A small hypoechoic halo (arrow), which often surrounds malignant lesions, can be noted. An adjacent small branch of the portal venous system (P) can also be seen. (Linear array, frequency 7.5 MHz)

	n	Additional information	change in tactics
Boldrini *et al.*[9]	86	5	NR
Castaing *et al.*[10]	98	NR	19
Charnley *et al.*[11]	99	9	NR
Clarke *et al.*[12]	54	22	17
Gozzetti *et al.*[13]	37*	20	20
Klotter *et al.*[3]	58*	19	10
Machi *et al.*[32]	84	10	NR
Rifkin *et al.*[14]	49	16	9
Traynor *et al.*[32]	123	44	19

Table 10.6: Additional information regarding liver metastases by intraoperative ultrasound and resulting change in surgical tactics (NR, not referred to by the authors.*includes only patients with preoperatively confirmed metastases).

Laparoscopic ultrasound

As described above, IOUS can detect occult liver metastases and lead to a change in the planned surgical procedure. Furthermore, laparoscopic surgery for colorectal malignancies requires an exact tumor localization. This may cause difficulties if the tumor is too small to be visible (eg a small pT2-tumor). In these cases, the localization can be determined by intraoperative colonoscopy or by IOUS. For these reasons, laparoscopic ultrasound (LUS) is likely to become an important diagnostic instrument in minimal access surgery for colorectal malignancies in the future.

There have been several reports on LUS since the early 1980s, most of them describing the technical equipment. Kodama *et al.*[34] used a flexible linear scanner in combination with a forward-viewing optic. Ota *et al.*[35] reported using a scope in combination with a 7.5 MHz radial scanner. A further improvement could be achieved by using a linear scanner connected to a rigid shaft[36]. In the mid-1980s, Frank *et al.*[37] examined intraabdominal and retroperitoneal organs with good results. Even ultrasound-guided biopsies were performed laparoscopically[38]. It remains unclear why this diagnostic instrument has been abandoned.

There was a revival of LUS in 1989: Fornari *et al.*[39] reported good results in liver imaging using a flexible ultrasound endoscope with a rotating 7.5 MHz sector scanner. Roethlin *et al.*[40] referred to the advantage of LUS in detecting common bile-duct stones during laparoscopic cholecystectomy. A rotating 5.5 MHz sector scanner at the tip of a rigid probe without an optical device was used.

Brueggemann *et al.*[41] used a 7.5 MHz linear scanner. As described on IOUS, this array does not lead to distorted imaging of the anatomic features. Preliminary results indicate that LUS will be useful in minimal access surgery for colorectal cancers: localization of not readily visible tumors and the detection of lymph-node metastases can be achieved. LUS also allows the differentiation

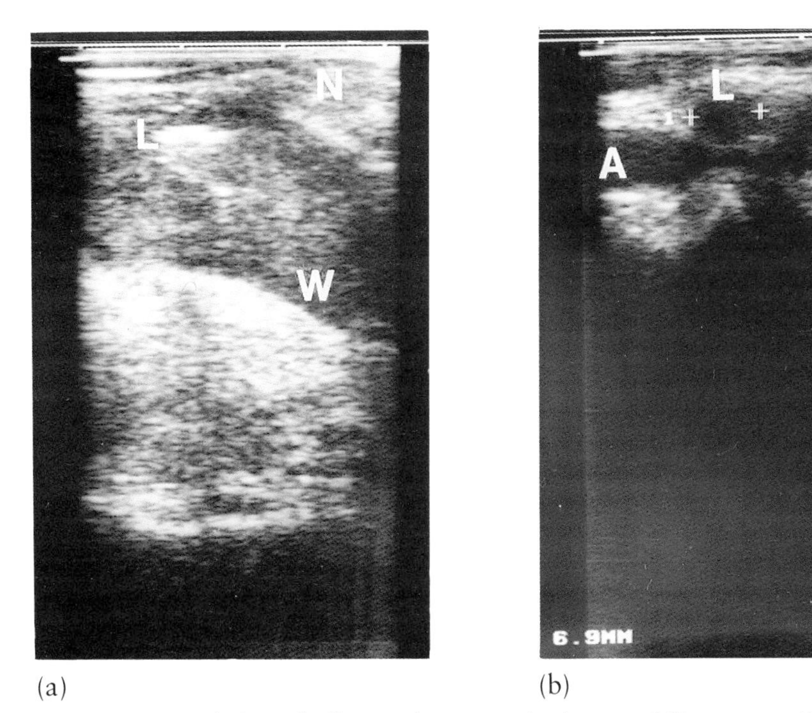

(a) (b)

Figure 10.5: Pathologic findings on laparoscopic ultrasound (linear array, 7.5 MHz) (**a**) Sonographic localization of a malignant tumor of the sigmoid: the hypoechoic thickened wall (W) can be clearly differentiated from the surrounding tissue (uT2). A small air-filled lumen (L) can be found. The tumor is hidden by normal small intestine (N). (**b**) A hypoechoic lymph-node metastasis (L) with a diameter of 6.9 mm could be detected close to the iliacal artery (A) in a patient with rectal cancer.

of five layers of normal intestine. Tumors will appear as hypoechoic alterations of the different layer (Figure 10.5**a**). Lymph-node metastases are hypoechoic, ball-shaped structures which can be exactly demarcated from the surrounding tissue (Figure 10.5**b**). Further investigation is necessary to prove the feasibility of this method for daily practice.

References

1 Finlay IG and McArdle CS (1986) Occult hepatic metastases in colorectal carcinoma. *Br J Surg.*, **73**:732–53.

2 Gall FP and Hermanek P (1992) Wandel und derzeitiger Stand der chirurgischen Behandlung des colorectalen Carcinoms. *Der Chirurg.* **63**:227–34.

3 Klotter HJ, Foerster R, Zielke A *et al.* (1990) Wertigkeit der intraoperativen Sonographie in der Chirurgie von Lebermetastasen. *Hessisscbes Aerzteblatt.* **5**:226–30.

4 Weiss L, Grundmann E, Torhorst J *et al.* (1986) Haematogenous metastatic patterns in colonic carcinoma: an analysis of 1541 necropsies. *J Pathol.* **150:** 195–203.

5 Eder M and Weiss M (1991) Haematogene Lebermetastasen – human-pathologische Grundlagen. *Der Chirurg.* **62**:705–9.

6 Mueller JM Schmidt A, Strauss JM *et al.* (1991) Resektion von Lebermetastasen kolorektaler Karzinome. Anspruch und Wirklichkeit. *Deutsche Medizin Woch.* **116**:681–8.

7 Kremer B and Henne-Bruns D (1989) Surgical techniques. In: *Hepatobiliary and pancreatic malignancies. Diagnosis, medical and surgical management.* Thieme Medical, New York. pp. 195–6.

8 Alderson PO, Adams DF, McNeil BJ *et al.* (1983) Computed tomography, ultrasound, and scintigraphy of the liver in patients with colon or breast carcinoma: a prospective comparison. *Radiology.* **149**:225–30.

9 Boldrini G, de Gaetano AM, Giovannini I *et al.* (1987) The systematic use of operative ultrasound for detection of liver metastases during colorectal surgery. *World J Surg.* **11**:622–7.

10 Castaing D, Edmond J, Kunstlinger F *et al.* (1986) Utility of operative ultrasound in the surgical management of liver tumors. *Ann Surg.* **204**:600–5.

11 Charnley RM, Morris DL, Dennison AR *et al.* (1991) Detection of colorectal liver metastases using intraoperative ultrasono-graphy. *Br J Surg.* **78**:45–8.

12 Clarke MP, Kane RA, Steele G *et al.* (1989) Prospective comparison of preoperative imaging and intraoperative ultrasonography in the detection of liver tumors. *Surgery*, **106**:849–55.

13 Gozzetti G, Mazziotti A, Bolondi L *et al.* (1985) Intraoperative ultrasonography in surgery for liver tumors. *Surgery.* **99**:523–9.

14 Rifkin MD Rosato FE, Branch HM *et al.* (1987) Intraoperative ultrasound of the liver. An important adjunctive tool for decision making in the operating room. *Ann Surg.* **205**:466–72.

15 Schreve RH, Terpstra OT, Ausema L *et al.* (1984) Detection of liver metastases: a prospective study comparing liver enzymes, scintigraphy, ultrasonography and computed tomography. *Br J Surg.* **71**:974–9.

16 Snow JH, Goldstein HM, Wallace S *et al.* (1979) Comparison of scintigraphy, sonography, and computed tomography in the evaluation of hepatic neoplasms. *Am J Radiol.* **132**:915–18.

17 Vlachos L, Trakadas S, Gouliamos A *et al.* (1990) Comparative study between ultrasound, computed tomography, intra-arterial digital subtraction angiography, and magnetic resonance imaging in the differentiation of tumors of the liver. *Gastrointest Radiol.* **15**:102–6.

18 Zocholl G, Kuhn FP, Augustin N *et al.* (1988) Diagnostische Aussagekraft von Sonographie und Computertomographie bei Lebermetastasen. *Fort Geb Roent Nuklearmed.* **148**:8–14.

19 Price J and Metreweli C (1988) Ultrasonic diagnosis of clinically non-palpable primary colonic neoplasms. *Br J Radiol.* **61**:190–5.

20 Federmann G (1991) Sonographische Beurteilung des Ausmasses von Kolonwandlaesionen am Beispiel von Kolontumoren. *Ultraschall Med.* **12**:169–71.

21 Worlicek H (1991) Sonographische Diagnostik des Kolonkarzinoms. *Ultraschall Med.* **12**:164–8.

22 Limberg B (1986) Diagnostik entzuendlicher und tumoroeser Dickdarmveraenderungen durch Kolonsonographie. *Deutsche Medizin Woch.* **111**:1273–6.

23 Limberg B (1990) Diagnostik von Dickdarmtumoren durch Kolonsonographie. *Ultraschall Med.* **11**:127–31.

24 Federmann G and Penschuck C (1990) Sonographische Darstellung mesenterialer Lymphknoten beim Kolonkarzinom. *Ultraschall Klin Praxis.* 5:104–7.

25 Dragstedt J and Gammelgaard J (1983) Endoluminal ultrasonic scanning in the evaluation of rectal cancer: a preliminary report of 13 cases. *Gastrointest Radiol.* 8:367–9.

26 Herfarth C and Hohenberger P (1992) Radikalitaet mit eingeschraenkter Resektion in der Carcinomchirurgie des Gastrointestinaltrakts. *Der Chirurg.* **63**:235–41.

27 Hildebrandt U and Feifel G (1985) Preoperative staging of rectal cancer by intrarectal ultrasound. *Dis Colon Rectum* **28**:42–6.

28 Lorenz R, Roesch T, Suchy R *et al.* (1990) Kolon-Endosonographie. Erste Erfahrungen in der klinischen Anwendung. *Medizin Klinik*, **85**:57–60.

29 Roesch T, Lorenz R, Classen M *et al.* (1990) Endoscopic ultrasonography in the evaluation of colon and rectal disease. *Gastrointest Endosc.* **36**:33–9.

30 Schulz W and Borchard F (1992) Groesse der Lebermetastasen bei geringer Metastasenzahl. Eine quantitative Studie an postmortalen Lebern. *Fort Geb Roentg Nuklearmed.* **156**:320–4.

31 Thomas DL, Morris DL, Hardcastle JD *et al.* (1987) Contact ultrasonography in the detection of liver metastases from colorectal cancer: an in vitro study. *Br J Surg.* **74**:955–6.

32 Machi J, Isomoto H, Yamashita Y *et al.* (1987) Intraoperative ultrasonography in screening for liver metastases from colorectal cancer: comparative accuracy with traditional procedures. *Surgery.* **101**:678–84.

33 Traynor O, Castaing D, Bismuth H *et al.* (1988) Peroperative ultrasonography in the surgery of hepatic tumours. *Br J Surg.* **75**:197–202.

34 Kodama T, Okita K, Oda M *et al.* (1982) Development and clinical investigation of ultrasonic laparoscopy. *Scand J Gastroenterol.* **17** (Suppl. 78):1.

35 Ota Y, Sato Y, Takatsuki K *et al.* (1982) New ultrasonic laparoscope: improvement in diagnosis of intra-abdominal diseases. *Scand J Gastroenterol.* **17**: (Suppl. 78):194.

36 Okita K, Kodama T, Oda M *et al.* (1984) Laparoscopic ultrasonography. Diagnosis of liver and pancreatic cancer. *Scan J Gastroenterol.* **19** (Suppl. 94):91–100.

37 Frank K, Bliesze H, Boenhof JA *et al.* (1985) Laparoscopic sonography: a new approach to intraabdominal disease. *J Clin Ultrasound.* **13**:60–5.

38 Boenhof JA, Frank K, Loch EG *et al.* (1985) Laparoscopic sonography. *Ann Radiol.* **28**:16–18.

39 Fornari F, Civardi G, Cavanna L *et al.* (1989) Laparoscopic ultrasonography in the study of liver diseases. Preliminary results. *Surg Endosc.* **3**:33–7.

40 Roethlin M, Schlumpf R, Largiader F *et al.* (1991) Die Technik der intraoperativen Sonographie bei der laparoskopischen Cholecystektomie. *Der Chirurg.* **62**:899–901.

41 Brueggemann A, Wuestner M, Klinge B *et al.* (1993**a**) Was Leistet die Sonographie des Kolons in der taeglichen Routine? *Ultraschall in Klinik und Praxis.* **8**:197.

42 Brueggemann A, Neufang T, Lepsien G (1993**b**) Laparoskopische Sonographie. *Ultraschall in Klinik und Praxis.* **8**:44–7.

Beynon J, Foy MA, Roe AM *et al.* (1986) Endoluminal ultrasound in the assessment of local invasion in rectal cancer. *Br J Surg.* **73**:474–7.

Beynon J, McC. Mortensen NJ, Foy DMA *et al.* (1989) Preoperative assessment of mesorectal lymph node involvement in rectal cancer. *British J Surg.* **76**:276–9.

Federmann G (1992) Einfluss der Tumor-Klassifikation (TNM-Klassifikation) auf die Praktikabilitaet sonographischer Tumordarstellung am Beispiel des Kolonakarzinoms. Tumordiagnostik und Therapie, **13**:34–6.

Feifel G, Hildebrandt U, Dhom G *et al.* (1987) Assessment of depth of invasion in rectal cancer by endosonography. Endoscopy. **19**:64–7.

Glaser F, Schlag P, Herfarth C *et al.* (1990) Endorectal ultrasonography for the assessment of invasion of rectal tumours and lymph node involvement. *British Journal of Surgery*, **77**:883–7.

Heintz A, Buess G, Junginger T *et al.*, (1990) Endorektale Sonographie zur praeoperativen Beurteilung der Infiltrationstiefe von Rektumtumoren. *Deutsche Medizinische Wochenschrift*, **115**:1083–7.

Hildebrandt U and Feifel G (1986) Endosonographische Bestimmung der Infiltrationstiefe und Beurteilung von Lymphknoten beim Rektumkarzinom. *Ultraschall in Klinik und Praxis*, **1**:89–94.

Rifkin MD *et al.* (1986) Endorectal sonographic prospective staging of rectal cancer. *Scandinavian Journal of Gastroenterologie*, **21** (Suppl. 123):99–103.

Saitoh N, Okui K, Sarashina H *et al.* (1986) Evaluation of echographic diagnosis of rectal cancer using intrarectal ultrasonic examination. *Diseases of Colon and Rectum*, **29**:234–42.

Strunk H, Frank K, Kuntz C *et al.* (1988) Endorektale Sonographie beim Rektumcarcinom. *Fortschritte auf dem Gebiete der Roentgenstrahlen und der Nuklearmedizin*, **149**:420–2.

UICC. TNM-Klassifikation maligner Tumoren. (ed.: Hermanek P. *et al.*). 4th edition. Springer-Verlag, Berlin, 1987.

11

Laparoscopic Resection of Left Sigmoid Colon Lesions, Low Anterior Resections and Abdomino-perineal Resections

MORRIS E FRANKLIN

Introduction

Colon surgery is a very common type of open surgery. It is estimated that more than 160,000 colonic procedures are performed in the USA every year[1], and that numbers in the developed world are broadly commensurate. Procedures vary from polyp removal and elective resections for carcinoma, diverticular disease and familial polyposis, to emergency procedures for bleeding, perforation, obstruction and trauma. Each category of procedure carries its own inherent risks and complications[2], many of which are directly or indirectly related to the abdominal incision and its sequelae. Modifications of the incision[3] have been numerous, but none has been as dramatic as the laparoscopic approach to these very common procedures. Both general and colorectal surgeons have been slow to give recognition to the advent of laparoscopy into the world of abdominal surgery, and some centers remain slow to accept it[4]; but despite this, the wide acceptance of laparoscopic cholecystectomy[5–9] has opened the door to previously unthinkable procedures[10–15].

Historical review[16–28]

Transabdominal and transanal colonic procedures have gained acceptance all over the world particularly since the refinement of anesthesia. There have been few challenges to the need for these procedures, but the methods have varied, from minimal resections for benign disease to massive resections with extensive lymph-node dissection for carcinoma. Before the advent of antibiotics, multi-stage techniques were designed to prevent the mortality and other problems associated with infection. Techniques for the early isolation of carcinoma, keeping adequate control of the vascular supply of the removed segment while maintaining adequate blood supply to the remaining segment, have been extensively described and are generally accepted by surgeons worldwide. The physiology of the colon and the pathophysiology of colonic disease continue to be studied, and new theories are continually put to the test, but the basic premise of resection and reanastomosis has remained constant ever since its effectiveness was first demonstrated. Most surgeons accept that colonic resections and reanastomosis are necessary in certain circumstances. Only the technique and results appear to be in question.

Justification of minimal access laparoscopic techniques

While new equipment and techniques (eg advances in anesthesia, antibiotics, and devices for autotransfusion, blood salvage, reinfusion and stapling) have all improved survival and reduced morbidity in surgery of the colon[12,29], the inherent rates of wound infection[30,31], dehiscence[32–35], deep vein thrombosis[30,36–38], and pronounced pulmonary complications[39] from abdominal incisional pain continue to cloud the success of colon surgery. Severe cardiac and pulmonary disease frequently leads to stop-gap measures being taken instead of proper colonic surgery. Minimal access techniques, and laparoscopy in particular, are likely to bring about lower morbidity and mortality: but only if the equipment and techniques are fully understood.

Left-sided colon resections

For the vast majority of left-sided procedures, the authors favor a totally intracorporeal resection and anastomosis. While laparoscopically assisted techniques are certainly quicker and easier, we feel that certain basic principles remain intact when a totally intracorporeal technique is used. Among these are the no-touch technique for proximal and distal control of the bowel ends, early control of the vasculature, and non-contamination of the abdominal wall and abdominal cavity with cancerous cells in patients with carcinoma[43].

Positioning

Patient positioning is of paramount importance for successful visualization regardless of the technique utilized. An operating table with left and right lateral tilt as well as Trendelenburg and reverse Trendelenburg capabilities is virtually mandatory, and Lloyd Davis-type stirrups or other positional devices are desirable for anal access. The patient must be securely fixed to the table with arms by the side to allow maximum tilt and access by the operating team. Arms spread in the classic position may be an obstruction, and this position is no longer used in our operating theater.

Instrumentation

Special equipment includes the standard laparoscopic insufflator (high flow), high-resolution cameras and monitors, adequate suction and irrigation devices, colonoscope (with monitor if possible) and KTP laser. The latter instrument is not mandatory, but it certainly aids the procedure. Adequate needle holders and bowel-handling instruments such as laparoscopic Babcock, Glassman and Allys Clamps are also very helpful. Before embarking upon laparoscopic colon resection of any type, the surgeon must have a proper background in intracorporeal suturing, and intra- and extracorporeal knot-tying. Skills and experience with stapling devices will also enhance the surgeon's ability to perform these highly technical and complex procedures.

Trocar placement

Trocar placement depends not just on the procedure but also on the preferred technique. Umbilical placement of the laparoscope has been adequate for the vast majority of laparoscopic left-sided, sigmoid, low anterior and abdomino-perineal resections; however, movement of the laparoscope to alternative sites may be needed during the procedure, and 10 mm ports are therefore recommended at all sites. Figure 11.1 shows the typical trocar placement for sigmoid, low anterior and abdomino-perineal resections. Movement of the trocars, and/or placement of additional trocars for left and left transverse colon mobilization and resection, may be desirable in some instances. The monitors should be at the foot of the bed for low anterior, sigmoid and abdomino-perineal

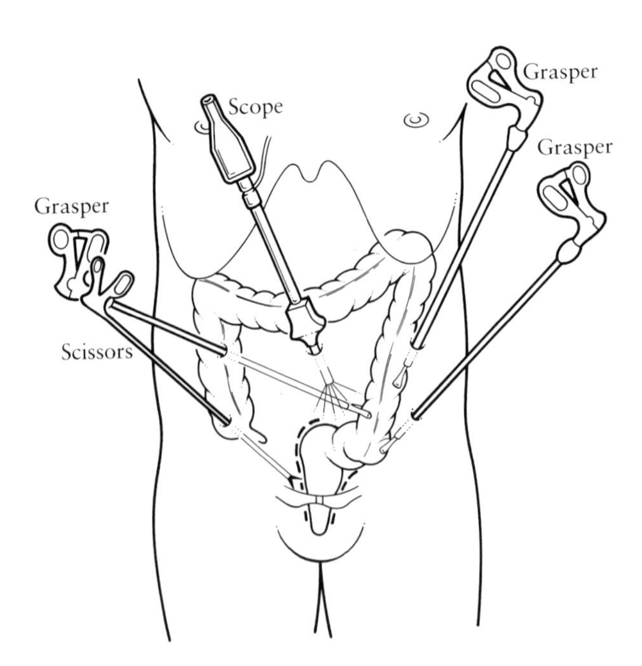

Figure 11.1: Instrument placement for low anterior and abdominal peritoneal resection.

resections, or at the midpoint umbilical level for left or transverse colon resections.

Technique

The technique for sigmoid, low anterior, abdomino-perineal and left colon resections are basically the same. The first step is identification of anatomy in the area which should include left and right ureters, left and right external iliac artery and veins, inferior epigastric arteries and veins, the bladder and the inferior mesenteric artery. In the case of low anterior and abdomino-perineal resections, it is vital to locate the internal iliac artery and vein, the middle hemorrhoidal veins bilaterally, and the course of the ureters along the pelvic wall.

The lesion in question must be clearly identified, and since the sense of touch is now for the most part gone, reliance upon radiographs and particularly the colonoscopic identification of the lesion and safe margins of resection are very important in these procedures. Guessing the location of a lesion is fraught with dangers. One or more members of the team must be skilled in colonoscopy, not only to locate the lesion but also to retrieve it, to monitor the adequacy of the bowel prep and check the anastomosis for bleeding and leakage after resection.

The next step is adequate mobilization of the involved segment and the distal and proximal margins to facilitate a tension-free anastomosis. Our preference is for the surgeon to be on the patient's right side along with the camera holder. Medial traction on the sigmoid is placed while freeing the lateral peritoneal connections of the sigmoid, upper rectal segment and left colon to and around the splenic flexure if needed. Early and precise identification of the ureter is mandatory and may be occasionally helped by the use of ureteral stents. After left lateral mobilization of the sigmoid has been accomplished, a mesenteric window is developed while avoiding injury to the ureters and vascular structures immediately adjacent to the left side of the pelvic wall. A readily developed space is almost always present just inferior to the bifurcation of the aorta allowing safe development of the window and rapid identification of the inferior mesenteric artery (IMA) and vein as well as the superior hemorrhoidal branches. Identification of the IMA at its origin from the aorta, and careful dissection along the pelvic wall posteriorly and laterally, will result in an adequate specimen for benign and malignant disease processes.

The next step is careful circumferential cleaning of the proximal and distal lines of resection of the colon. At this point of laparoscopic Glassman or other bowel-occluding clamp is placed across the proximal bowel and colonoscopy is routinely performed (except where there is obstruction) to ensure that the lumen of the bowel is clean. Irrigation with an antiseptic solution such as dilute (10%) betadine may also be carried out.

After circumferential cleaning of the proximal lines of resection (we recommend 1.5–2 cm minimal margins, but prefer 5 cm for carcinoma), and when proximal occlusion has been guaranteed, the proximal bowel is divided. The KTP 532 laser is an ideal cutting/coagulation device which causes little lateral damage; however, division with scissors or even cautery can be performed as long as bleeding is controlled and the lateral damage of the cautery is calculated when computing the viability of the anastomised segment ends. The proximal portions of the resected segment are then closed with a stapling device or an endoloop and the distal line of resection is divided. The distal end of the resected segment is controlled in a similar manner. The entire segment is then placed in a specimen bag and the bag is closed. Usually it can be removed through the rectal stump if the distal line of resection is below the sacral promontory, or placed out of the way and removed through an expanded infraumbilical incision at the completion of the anastomosis.

The proximal and distal ends of the colon are irrigated with an iodinated solution and a circular stapling device is introduced through the rectum. If the lower end of the resection is 8 cm or higher, a PDS endoloop is applied; the stapler is brought through the end of the colon and the endoloop tightened around a sufficient circumferential collar of tissue. If the distal line of resection is 8 cm or less from the anus we usually place a hand-sewn purse-string suture prior to placement of the stapling device. An Endo GIA stapling/cutting device can also be used for closure of distal segment. We have found that a removable anvil greatly facilitates this portion of the procedure, allowing instant inspection of the circumference of the closed end of the bowel. The anvil is then placed in the proximal end of the anastomosis and fixed in place with a PDS endoloop as previously outlined. Frequently a second endoloop is applied for additional security. Excess tissue is trimmed from each end with scissors or laser, the anvil is reattached to the head of the stapler, and the ends are reapproximated. Great care must be taken to prevent other portions of tissue, bowel, or other foreign material from being caught in the instrument, as this will result in an incomplete anastomosis. Proper tension is applied to the device, the colon is checked for adequate length and the instrument is fired. The anastomosis is then checked with underwater insufflation and direct inspection with the colonoscope. Small leaks can be repaired with simple 3-0 Vicryl sutures until there is no further leakage. Drains are routinely placed after thorough irrigation of the pelvis and all dissected areas is completed. Any ligated vessels are reinspected, bleeding is controlled and the specimen is removed through the expanded umbilical incision; then all trocar sites are reinspected for bleeding prior to removal of the last port trocar that houses the laparoscope.

Distal division of the bowel

An alternative technique is distal division of the bowel, enlarging a lateral or supraumbilical incision for removal and division of the diseased segment of bowel, placing the anvil extracorporeally, replacing the bowel and anvil intracorporeally, closing the abdominal defect, and completing the anastomosis as described above. Frequently the distal resection can be completed with a stapling/cutting device such as the Endocutter and the distal purse-string or Endoloop maneuver avoided. There are many variations of this type of anastomosis, but we feel that the totally intracorporeal dissection and anastomosis with early isolation of the diseased segment is a more aesthetically appealing and pure procedure. A wide variety of instruments are needed for this complex procedure, but most are now becoming readily available.

Clinical results

Since the inception of this procedure we have felt that it should be offered to each patient in a non-randomized, non-prejudicial way. In some patients, however, the procedure should either not be offered or it should be abandoned early in favor of the more classic open procedure. These patients are primarily those with more extensive disease where bladder or perhaps other organs are involved (additional loops of bowel, stomach, abdominal wall etc), and those who have massive adhesions from multiple previous surgical procedures. However, many of the patients in our series had already undergone procedures such as appendectomy, abdominal hysterectomy and aorto-bifemoral bypass, and if the adhesions were not too great the procedure could nevertheless be performed[43].

The personal details of our initial group of patients (age, weight and sex) are shown in Table 11.1. Table 11.2 shows the disease processes most commonly encountered, and Table 11.3 gives details of the hospital stay. Table 11.4 shows the complications encountered in this initial group. These results compare favorably with results of open procedures as well as the results of other laparoscopic series. The only main difference is that we have yet to see any intestinal obstructions in this current series. The one death was of a 96-year-old female who died of pneumonia 21 days postoperatively. This was felt to be unrelated to the primary surgical procedure.

	Mean	Range
Age (yrs)	68	22–96
Weight (lbs)	178	110–278
Sex		
Female	33	
Male	38	

Table 11.1: Age, weight and sex distribution.

Location	Malignant (N)	Inflammatory (N)
Right colon	8	0
Transverse colon	3	0
Left colon	9	0
Sigmoid colon	21	14
Low anterior resection	21	0
Abdominal perineal	9	0

Table 11.2: Disease processes and locations.

	Average (days)	Range (days)
Right colon resection	3.5	3–6
Transverse colon resection	3.8	3–6
Left colon resection	2.8	2–6
Sigmoid colon resection	3.8	1.7–30
Low anterior resection	3.6	2–13
Abdominal perineal resection	2.8	1.5–21

Table 11.3: Laparoscopic colon resection: postoperative hospital stay.

Wound infections	1*
Pneumonia	1
Deaths	1**
Anastomotic leak	1
Blood transfusion	1
Reoperation	2†
Cerebral vascular accident	1

Table 11.4: Complications. *Specimen removed transanally. **Same patient with pneumonia—95-year-old who died 3½ weeks postoperatively. †One patient with bleeding gastric ulcer; one patient with presumed anastomotic leak.

Discussion

It is doubtful that laparoscopic colon resection will ever completely replace open colon surgery, especially in some emergency cases, where bleeding, obstruction or massive contamination is present. Other contraindications have been discussed, but we feel that inflammatory bowel disease with friable tissue, and large abdominal aortic aneurysms and aorto-iliac aneurysms, are better handled open. As new equipment becomes available, these procedures will become less painful for the patients and less difficult for the surgeon.

The most impressive facet of laparoscopic colon resection is the rapid recovery time, particularly compared with that of the classic open procedures. Our patients have required a minimal amount of analgesia, usually less than 5 mg morphine sulphate or its equivalent in the first 24 hours. We have encountered very few pulmonary problems and almost no wound problems (*see* Table 11.4). The amount of ileus is dependent upon the amount of small bowel dissection required to free the colon but for the most part, except in extreme cases, this has been minimal and quite similar to that found by Jacobs and colleagues[40], Fowler and White[41] and Phillips (personal communication), and quite contrary to that experienced by Wexner and coworkers[42]. Our patients have all had bowel sounds within 24 hours, bowel movements within 30 hours, and were also taking food within 30 hours of surgery. One recent patient with a sigmoid resection and anastomosis for diverticulitis had bowel sounds in six hours, was fed 18 hours postoperatively, had a bowel movement at 27 hours postoperatively, was discharged 40 hours after his surgery and did well at home.

We have been impressed with the almost uniform well-being of patients within 24–30 hours: walking readily, coughing without pain and anxious to go home. This is in contrast to all but the rare patient in our elderly population who require much prompting to do more than minimal activity because of discomfort and pain.

The average time of dismissal seems to have been considerably shortened, with the vast majority of patients being ready for discharge in 48 hours and almost all being discharged within four days. Those who stayed longer did so mainly because of concurrent medical problems such as CVA (cerebral vascular accident), gastric bleeding or poor cardiac status, rather than complications of the surgical procedure. One patient, however, did have a suspected anastomatic leak and underwent a loop ileostomy during the initial hospitalization.

Conclusion

Although laparoscopic colon resection is in its very early stages, and is currently being performed by very few surgeons, it seems to offer great potential benefits to the patient: rapid recovery, minimal pain and faster return to full function. It offers many of the advantages that laparoscopic cholecystectomy has offered, but there is also a whole new range of unfamiliar and potentially life-threatening complications. Just as with open colonic procedures the margin of error is probably considerably less, but recognized problems can be rapidly corrected by opening up the patient and doing what all surgeons are trained to do. There is little doubt that skilled workers can perform exactly the same surgical maneuvers with colonic laparoscopy as with open surgery, with equally good or better results. It is doubtful, however, that every surgeon will be able to perform these highly technical and often time-consuming procedures. The applicability of laparoscopic colonic surgery will remain directly dependent upon the individual surgeon's laparoscopic skill and level of comfort with this more difficult but certainly rewarding approach to colon surgery. As caring surgeons, we must put the patient's well-being above our desire to perform new and exciting procedures for financial or other selfish motives.

References

1 Rutkow IM (1982) Rates of surgery in the United States: the decade of 1970s. *Surg Clin N Am.* **62**:559–78.

2 Hedberg S and Welch (1985) Complications in surgery of the colon and rectum. In: *Complications in surgery and their management*. W. B. Saunders, Philadelphia. pp. 620–64.

3 Kenady DE (1984) Management of abdominal wounds. *Surg Clin N Am*. **64**: 803–7.

4 Braasch JW (1992) Laparoscopic cholecystectomy and other procedures. *Arch Surg*. **127**:887.

5 Dubois F, Icord P, Berthelot L (1990) Celioscopic cholecystectomy. *Ann Surg*. **211**: 60–2.

6 Reddick EJ and Olson PD (1989) Laparoscopic laser cholecystectomy: Comparison with mini-lap cholecystectomy. *Surg Endosc*. **3**:121.

7 Soper JN, Stockman PT, Dunnegon DL *et al.* (1992) Laparoscopic cholecystectomy: the new 'gold standard'? *Arch Surg*. **127**:917–22.

8 Southern Surgeons Club (1991) A prospective analysis for 1,518 laparoscopic cholecystectomies performed by Southern US surgeons. *N Engl J Med*. **324**: 1073–8.

9 Schirmer BD, Edge SB, Dix J *et al.* (1991) Laparoscopic cholecystecomy: treatment of choice for symptomatic cholelithiasis. *Ann Surg*. **213**:665–77.

10 Semm K (1977) Atlas of gynecologic laparoscopy and hysteroscopy. W. B. Saunders, Philadelphia. pp. 141–2.

11 Schreiber JH (1990) Laparoscopic appendectomy in pregnancy. *Surg Endosc*. **4**:100.

12 Easter DW, Cushieri A, Nathanson LK *et al.* (1992) The utility of diagnostic laparoscopy for abdominal disorders. Audit of 120 patients. *Arch Surg*. **127**: 379–83.

13 Carroll BJ, Phillips EH, Daykhovsky L *et al.* (1992) Laparoscopic choledochoscopy: an effective approach to the common duct. *J Lap Endosc Surg*. **2**:15–21.

14 Schultz LG, Pietratly J and Hickok D (1990) Laser laparoscopic herniorraphy: a clinical trial of preliminary results. *J Lap Surg*. **1**:141, 1990.

15 Winfield HN, Donovan JF, See WA *et al.* (1991) Urological laparoscopic surgery. *J Urol*. **146**:941–8.

16 Corman ML (1989) *Colon and rectal surgery*. J. B. Lippincott, Philadelphia. pp. 387–578.

17 Ellis H (1985) Anterior resection and other procedure. In: Schwartz SI and Ellis H (Eds) *Maingot's abdominal operations*. Norwalk.

18 Blond KI and Copeland EM (1986) Malignant diseases of the colon and rectum in surgical treatment of digestive disease. In: Moody FG *et al.* Year Book Medical Publishers, Chicago. pp. 664–86.

19 Re RN (1992) New Paradigms of oncogenesis and their implications for surgery in the twenty-first century. *Dis Colon Rectum*. **35**:627–34.

20 Maron MR, James EC, Rothenberger DA *et al.* (1992) Prognostic value of positive lymph nodes in rectal cancer. *Dis Colon Rectum*. **35**:579–81.

21 Copeland EM, Miller LD and Jones RS (1968) Prognostic factors in carcinoma of the colon and rectum. *Am J Surg*. **116**:875–81.

22 Senogor A, Milsom JW, Walshaw R *et al.* (1992) Does a proximal colostomy affect colorectal anastomosic healing. *Dis Colon Rectum*. **35**:182–7.

23 Debos JT and Thomson FB (1972) A critical review of colectomy with anastomosis. *Surg Gynecol Obstet*. **135**:747–52.

24 Ware P, Sorensen K and Berg V (1981) Proximal fecal diversion: review of ten years experience. *Dis Colon Rectum*. **24**:114–19.

25 Kyzer S and Gordon PH (1992) Experience with the use of the circular stapler in rectal surgery. *Dis Colon Rectum*. **35**:696–706.

26 Gillen P and Peel AL (1986) Comparison of mortality, morbidity and incidence of local recurrence in patients with rectal cancer treated by either stapled anterior resection or abdomino-perineal resection. *Br J Surg*. **73**:339–41.

27 Coco C, Magistrelli P, Granone P *et al.* (1992) Conservative surgery for early cancer of the rectum. *Dis Colon Rectum*. **35**:131–5.

28 Sankar MY and Joffe SN (1988) Laser surgery in colonic and anorectal lesions. *Surg Clin N Am*. **68**:1447–69.

29 Daly JM and Decosse JJ (1983) Complications in surgery of the colon and rectum. *Surg Clin N Am*. **63**:1215–31.

30 Moossa AR, Lavelle-Jones MB and Scott M (1986) Surgical complications. In: *Sabiston Textbook of Surgery*. W. B. Saunders, Philadelphia. pp. 331–69.

31 Schwartz SI (1984) *Complications in Schwartz principles of surgery*. McGraw-Hill, New York. pp. 454–84.

32 Bartlett LC (1985) Pressure necrosis is the primary cause of wound dehiscence. *Can J Surg*. **28**:27–30.

33 Baggish MS and Lee WK (1975) Abdominal disruption. *Obstet Gynecol.* **46**: 530–4.

34 Efron G (1975) Abdominal wound disruption. *Lancet.* **1**:1287–90.

35 Mendoza GB, Postletwaite RW and Johnson WB (1970) The incidence of wound disruption following operation. *Arch Surg.* **101**:396–9.

36 Kakkar VV, Howe CT, Flanc C *et al.* (1969) Natural history of post-operative deep vein thrombosis. *Lancet.* **ii**:230–2.

37 Huber O, Bounameaux H, Borst F *et al.* (1992) Post-operative pulmonary embolism after hospital discharge, an underestimated risk. *Arch Surg.* **127**:310–13.

38 Scurr JH, Coleridge-Smith PD and Husty JH (1988) Deep venous thrombosis: a continuing problem. *B Med J.* **297**:28.

39 Van De Water JM (1980) Preoperative and postoperative techniques in the prevention of pulmonary complications. *Surg Clin N Am.* **60**:1339–72.

40 Jacobs M, Verdeja GD and Goldstein DS (1992) Minimally invasive colon resection. *Surg Lap Endosc.* **1**:144–50.

41 Fowler DL and White SA (1991) Laparoscopy-Assisted Sigmoid Resection. *Surg Lap Endosc.* **1**:183–8.

42 Wexner SD, Johonsen OB, Nagueras JJ *et al.* (1992). Laparoscopic total abdominal colectomy. A prospective trial. *Dis Colon Rectum.* **35**:651–5.

43 Franklin ME, Ramos R, Rosenthal D *et al.* (1993) Laparoscopic colonic procedures. *World J Surg.* **17**: 51–6

12

Right Hemicolectomy and Total Abdominal Colectomy and Proctocolectomy

MOISES JACOBS AND GUSTAVO PLASENCIA

Historical introduction

Traditional open colectomy has usually required nasogastric tube drainage for treatment of an expected ileus which usually lasts four to seven days (although not all surgeons routinely use this). After flatus has been passed, the nasogastric tube is removed and patients are fed liquids with slow advancement to solids. This was partly to protect the colonic anastomosis: it was thought that too early an oral intake could lead to increased anastomotic leaks.

With the advent of laparoscopic colon resection, these older traditions have been questioned. For example, only 10–15% of laparoscopic colectomy patients develop ileus, and most patients have had bowel movements by the third or fourth postoperative day, while tolerating regular diet, without an increase in anastomotic leaks.

Traditional oncologic principles are such that most surgeons, when doing open colectomies, dissect the feeder blood vessels at the base of the mesentery. With laparoscopic cases, again in keeping with traditional oncologic principles, devascularization of the mesentery should be done at the base. In fact it is easier to devascularize at the base of the mesentery during laparoscopy whether dealing with malignancy or not. The rationale behind dissecting blood vessels near the base of the mesentery lies in knowing the anatomy of the colon mesentery. The colon is supplied by seven major blood vessels:

- the ileocolic
- the right colic
- the right branch of the middle colic
- the middle colic
- the left branch of the middle colic
- the inferior mesenteric artery (IMA)

- the marginal artery of Drummond, which parallels the mesenteric colonic border.

If one imagines the blood supply of the colon as resembling limbs on a tree, one can begin to appreciate why it is easier to control the blood supply of each individual colonic segment near its base. For instance, the right colon is supplied by the superior mesenteric artery (SMA) which gives birth to the ileocolic, right colic and the right branch of the middle colic. If one thinks of the SMA as being the trunk of the tree and of the previously mentioned blood vessels as being direct limbs from the trunk, each of which in turn has its own smaller branches, one can see that the easiest, quickest and most efficient method of cutting the tree down (devascularizing the mesentery) is to cut down the major trunk (the SMA). However, ligating and transecting the SMA would be disastrous. Therefore the next biggest tributaries become the next level of branches (right colic, ileocolic, and right branch middle colic).

The tissue at the base of the mesentery between these named blood vessels is avascular; thus control of the mesentery of the right colon is easiest when done near the base of the right colic, ileocolic and right branch of middle colic. Only three vessels have to be ligated and divided when at the base of the mesentery. If one were to get closer to the bowel and away from the base of the mesentery, one would have to ligate and divide smaller and smaller branches—a much more cumbersome task.

For sigmoid lesions, the analogy of cutting down the main tree-trunk is even more appropriate. The IMA supplies the sigmoid colon and gives off several major tributaries. However, one can ligate only the IMA without any untoward effects, and devascularize the whole sigmoid colon. This makes sigmoid devascularization a much easier task when done at its base.

Not only is it easier and more efficient to devascularize bowel at the base of the mesentery: it also helps overcome the criticism that one cannot do an oncologic mesenteric resection laparoscopically. Indeed, at the base of the mesentery, this becomes an oncologic mesenteric resection.

Instrumentation

Although special instrumentation for laparoscopic colonic resection has only recently been developed, it has already reached a high level of sophistication. There are 10 mm instruments that mimic open conventional instruments and can also rotate 360°. These instruments include Babcock, Glassman, Allis, right-angle and Kelly clamps and scissors. The end-effectors of these instruments are large enough to allow for easy grasping and dissection of the bowel and its mesentery. In addition, since these are all 10 mm instruments, it is not necessary to use reducer caps or to change to 5 mm instruments.

Linear stapling devices are now available in 30 mm and 60 mm lengths, both for the bowel and the mesentery, and with or without cutting blades. Endoscopic circular staples, which are about 10 mm longer and prevent loss of pneumoperitoneum, are available for intracorporeal anastomosis. Larger cannulae for introduction of these staples range from 12 to 33 mm in diameter.

Technique

There are five steps to laparoscopic colon resection:

1 identification
2 mobilization
3 devascularization
4 resection
5 anastomosis.

Identification

When dealing with a neoplasm, one must be sure of its exact location. In open surgery, one can palpate the area in question and usually identify the lesion. If necessary one can open the bowel and inspect the area visually. In laparoscopic surgery, unless the disease process involves the serosa identification can be very difficult. Lesions can currently be localized either radiographically with a barium enema (BE) or colonoscopically. With colonoscopy one can identify the lesion preoperatively by placing a clip at the site or tattooing it with dye; alternatively one can obtain an abdominal X-ray with the colonoscope at the site. If there is any doubt as to the location of the lesions intraoperatively, one can perform an intraoperative colonoscopy.

Mobilization

There are three keys to the mobilization of the large bowel:

- the two-handed technique
- traction/countertraction
- the use of gravity as a second assistant

All three are routinely used in open surgery. The two-handed technique allows the surgeon to gain depth perception which is lost on the two-dimensional laparoscopic video monitor. Traction/countertraction allows easier mobilization and dissection of the tissue planes and blood vessels. Mobilization allows the bowel to reach the anterior abdominal wall easily.

Electrical operating tables enable patients to be tilted and positioned so that gravity can act as a retractor. Since cannulae and retractors are limited in laparoscopic surgery, one must be able to position the patient in such a fashion as to allow gravity to retract the small bowel away or to allow prominence of visualization of the colon segment involved. For right colectomies, therefore, when dealing with the cecum, the patient is placed in Trendelenberg to bring the cecum out of the pelvis into view, in left lateral decubitus to let the small bowel fall away.

Devascularization

For benign diseases, devascularization can be done extracorporeally by making a small incision (usually less than 6 cm) in the anterior abdominal wall. When dealing with a malignancy, devascularization should be done intracorporeally at the base of the mesentery as described above.

Resection and anastomosis

For right-sided lesions, bowel resection and anastomosis are usually done extracorporeally. A small counterincision is made in the anterior abdominal wall and the bowel is exteriorized. The margins of resection are chosen and the anastomosis is performed in the usual fashion. To complete the resection and anastomosis intracorporeally requires more time and dexterity as well as more complex instrumentation. There is still the problem of specimen retrieval, which would require at least a 3–4 cm incision in any case. In our experience, if the counterincision is limited to 6 cm or less, there is very little difference in patient's course vs a totally laparoscopic colectomy.

Right hemicolectomy

Operating room Set-up

Two monitors are used, both on the right side of the patient (Figure 12.1): one at the foot and one at the head. The surgeon and cameraman/assistant stand on the left side of the patient, opposite the side of the pathology. The cameraman can act as first assistant, or a second assistant may stand on the right side of the patient.

Patient positioning

The patient is placed in the left lateral decubitus position (right side up). When working on the cecum and ileum the patient is placed in Trendelenberg; when working on the transverse colon, the patient is placed in reverse Trendelenberg.

Trocar placement

Four 10/11 mm trocars are used, one in each of the following positions (Figure 12.2):

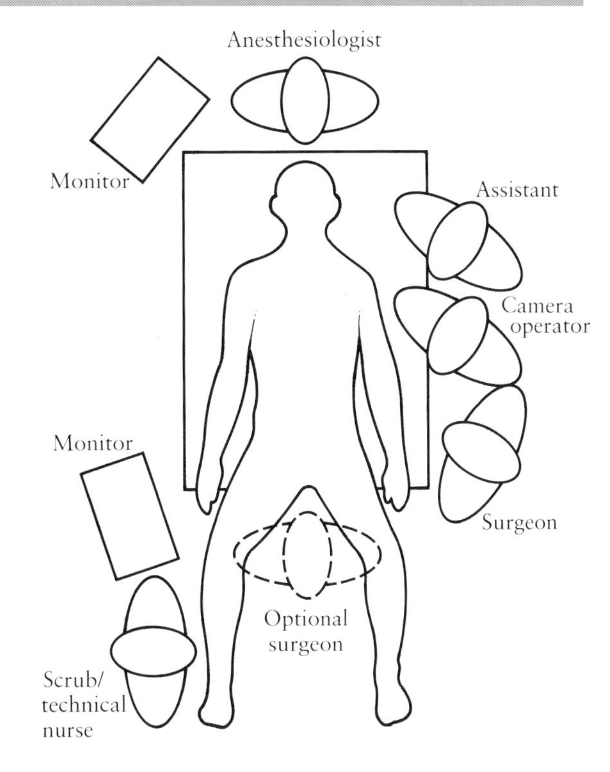

Figure 12.1: Operating room set-up for right hemicolectomy.

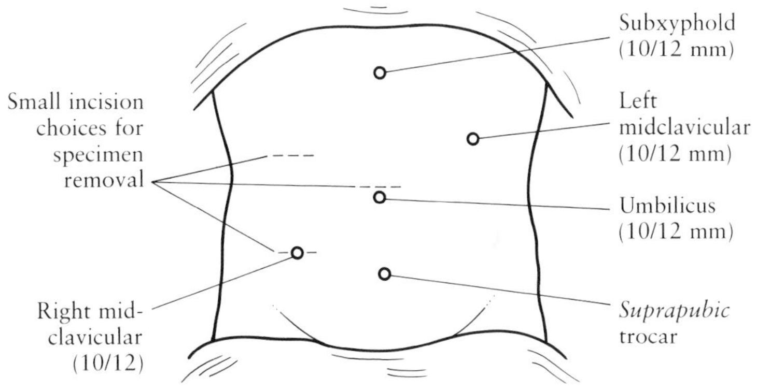

Figure 12.2: Trocar sites for right hemicolectomy.

- umbilicus
- suprapubic midline
- subxyphold to the left of the midline
- left midclavicular line halfway between the costal margin and umbilicus.

Technique

Both surgeon and cameraman use two-handed techniques. Using traction/countertraction, the ascending colon, cecum and white line of Toldt are

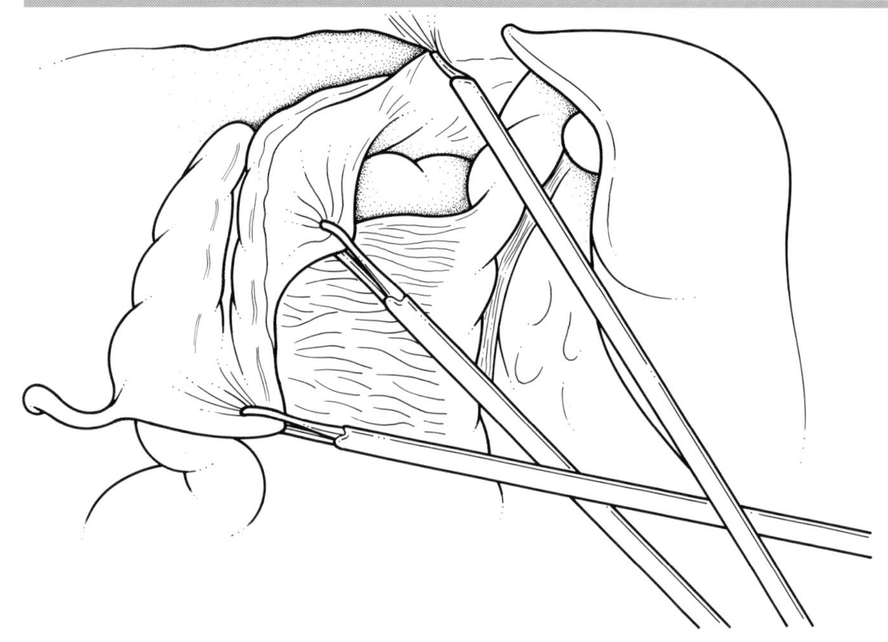

Figure 12.3: Mobilization of the white line of Toldt to the hepatic flexures. Medial traction using Babcock clamps.

mobilized medially to the hepatic flexure (Figure 12.3). Attention is then turned to the transverse colon, with the patient positioned in reverse Trendelenberg. The surgeon and cameraman may change position, with the camera (+ 30° angle scope) placed through the suprapubic cannula. The gastrocolic ligament is placed on traction and may be transected using electrosurgical scissors, while larger vessels may be clipped before being transected (Figure 12.4). This mobilization of the gastrocolic ligament continues down until the duodenum is exposed. Blunt and sharp dissection are then used to push the duodenum away from the adjacent colonic mesentery. Having completely mobilized the right colon to the midtransverse colon, devascularization is started. The patient is again placed in the Trendelenberg position and the mesentery is placed on traction so that the named blood vessels bow out like violin strings. The peritoneum is scored overlying these blood vessels and the ileocolic artery and vein are dissected out individually. They are ligated using two or three clips on the mesenteric side and one clip on the specimen side (Figure 12.5). When these vessels are too large for the clips, a technique is used whereby, after placing two clips, the vessel is only partially transected and then two more clips are used to completely ligate the whole vessel before transecting it completely. Other methods of ligating vessels include pretied Roeder loops or endovascular staples (Figure 12.6). Once the ileocolic artery and vein have been transected, a window is created in the mesocolon. This window is enlarged using electrosurgical scissors (until the next named vessel is identified—the right colic artery). At the base of the mesentery the tissue between the named blood vessels is avascular and can usually be transected without clips. The process continues until the right branch of the middle colic has been transected. At this point the whole right colon has been mobilized and devascularized. A 6 cm counterinci-

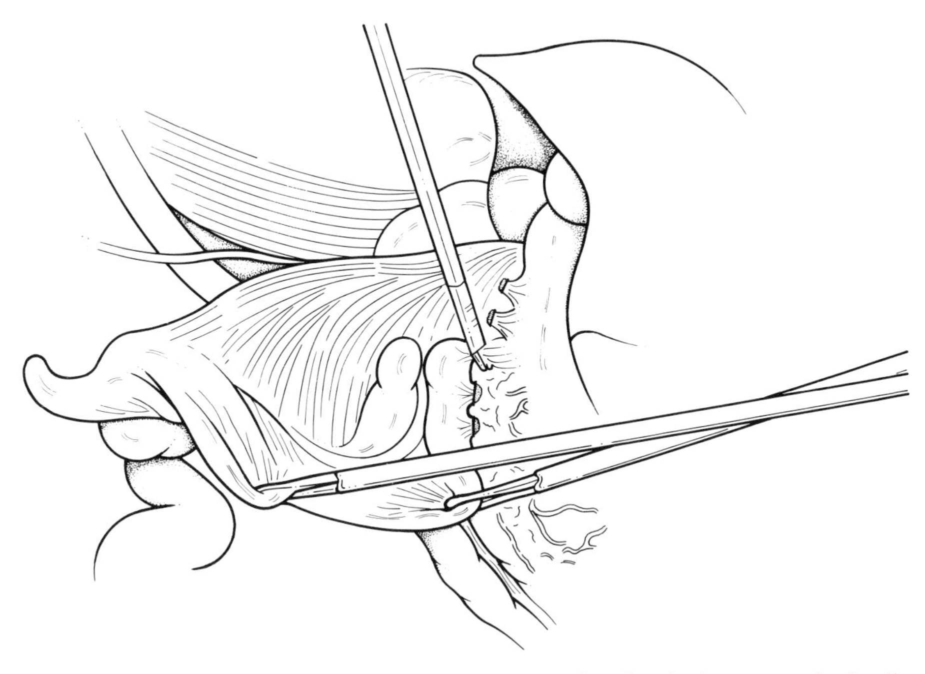

Figure 12.4: Division of gastrocolic omentum using clips for the larger vessels. Smaller vessels can be cauterized.

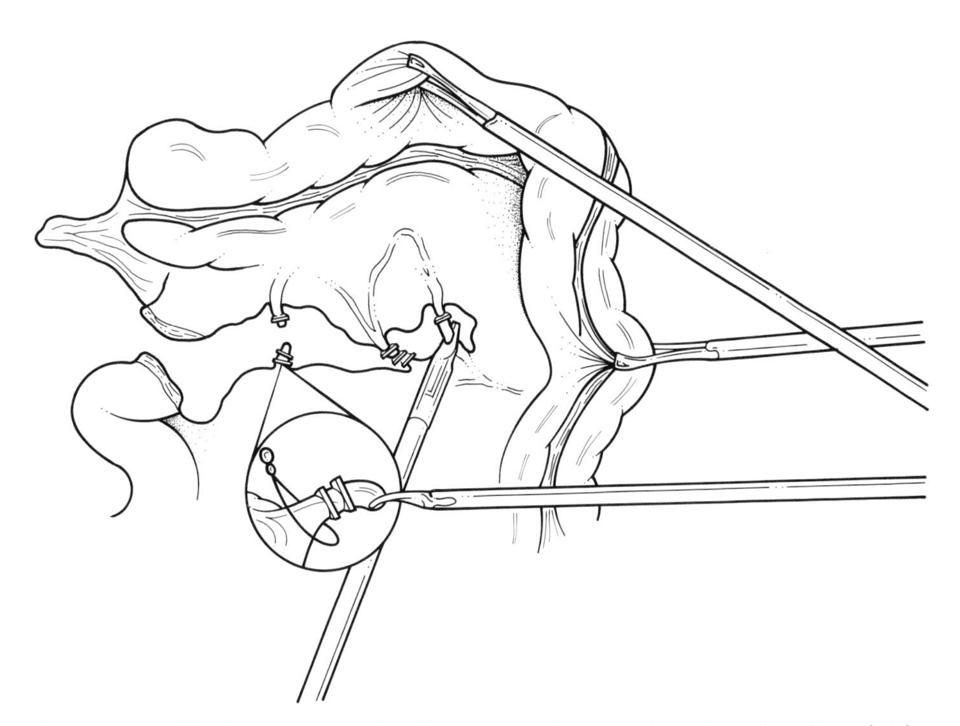

Figure 12.5: Windows are created in the mesentery between ileocolic, right colic and right branch of the middle colic. The vessels can be clipped or endolooped for control. The tissue between these vessels at the base of the mesentery is avascular.

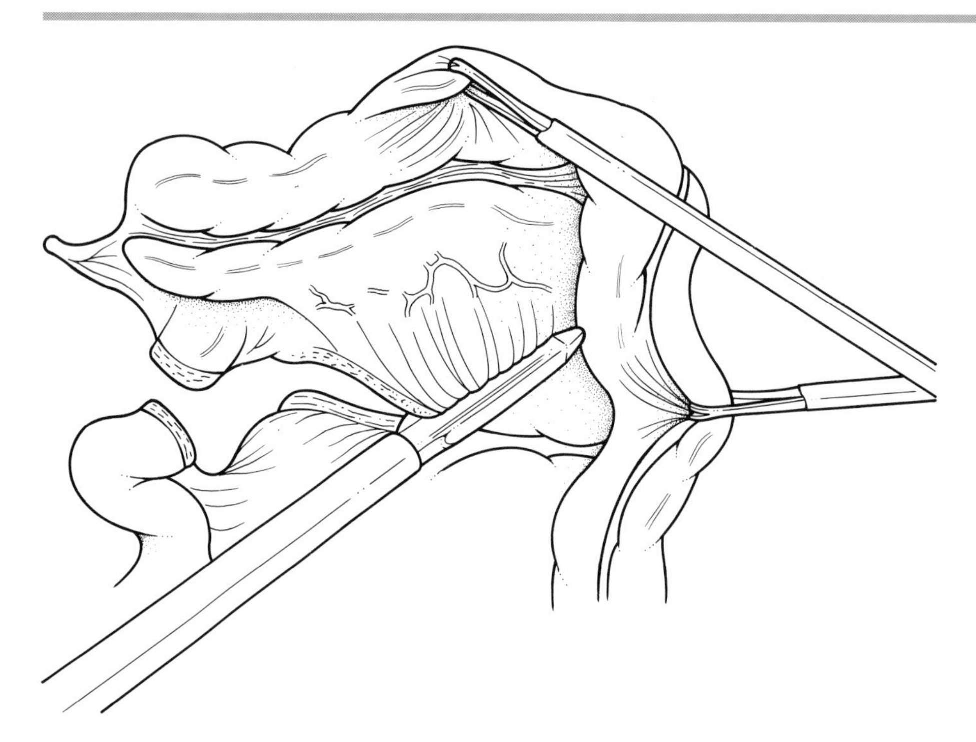

Figure 12.6: Alternative method for controlling the mesentery, using vascular endostaples.

sion is made in the anterior abdominal wall, usually to the right of the umbilicus or at the level of the umbilicus (incorporating the umbilical cannula).

The bowel is exteriorized, the resection and anastomosis are done in the surgeon's usual fashion, and the bowel is returned to the abdominal cavity (Figure 12.7).

Alternative techniques include intracorporeal anastomosis which can be done using either laparoscopic linear cutter staplers and/or endoscopic circular staplers. However, there is still the problem of specimen removal. Although theoretically it can be overcome by transanal extraction via colonoscopy, currently it requires the creation of an abdominal wall incision.

Total abdominal colectomy and proctocolectomy

Ileoanal pouch is increasingly becoming popular in the treatment of ulcerative colitis and familial polyposis. The majority of these patients are young and at the most productive stage of life. The laparoscopic approach offers a new alternative to speed recovery and return to normal life. Other conditions such as slow transit constipation may also be indications for this procedure.

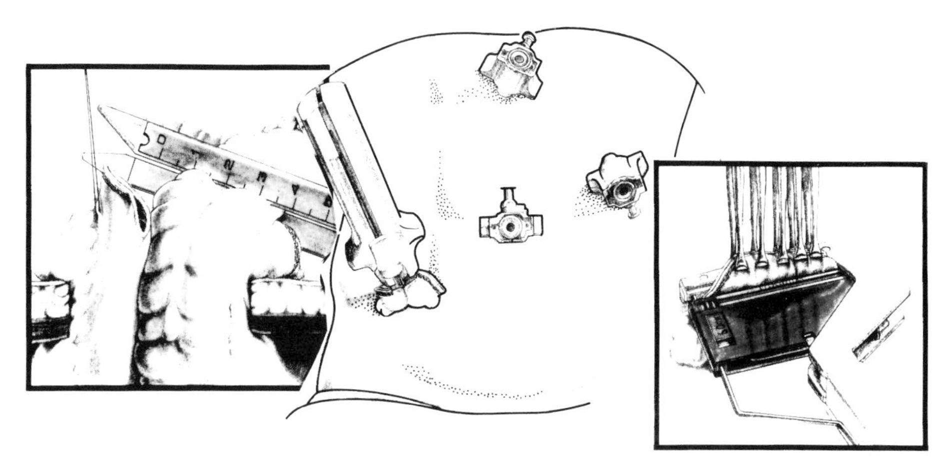

Figure 12.7: A small incision is made (either in the right upper or lower quadrant or in the umbilicus). The bowel is exteriorized and resected, and an ileocolic anastomosis is created using staples.

Technique

The patient is placed in the decubitus supine position with strapped arms at the side. General anesthesia is required. If an ileorectal anastomosis is contemplated, lithotomy is usually not needed as it would be in the case of ileal pouch or total proctocolectomy.

Closed pneumoperitoneum is initiated through the umbilicus and three trocars are then placed under direct vision: one in the epigastric and two in the right and left suprapubic area (this being the most cosmetic alternative). In moderately obese patients, the last two trocars could be placed lateral to the rectus muscle at the level of the umbilicus, in the right and left side. Dissection is begun at the right side at the ileocecal level. The camera is switched to the level of the suprapubic port and the ileocecum is held medially through the umbilical and epigastric ports.

The surgeon and assistant will be on the left, looking at the video monitor located at the right side towards the patient's head. The right peritoneal reflection is incised utilizing the right suprapubic cannula, and dissection continues proximal to the level of the hepatocolic ligament, which is transected by scissors and electrosurgery.

The greater omentum is then reflected superiorly and the avascular plane between this and the transverse colon is incised. Traction is placed on the omentum superiorly through the epigastric port by the assistant who is also holding the camera in the left lateral quadrant. The surgeon holds the transverse colon through the right lower-quadrant port and uses the scissors through the umbilical port. The omentum is progressively detached, working towards the splenic flexure. When this is reached it is usually necessary to reverse positions, switching the camera to the right lower-quadrant cannula. The assistant and surgeon change to the right side and view the video monitor at the left upper side. The assistant provides countertraction through the epigastric port and the surgeon continues to operate through the umbilical cannula, providing traction and performing the dissection through the left lower-quadrant port. Once the splenic flexure is mobilized and reflected medially and inferiorly, it is frequently necessary to transect the splenocolic ligament between clips.

The left upper-quadrant video monitor is then brought down towards the left flank and left lower quadrant, as dissection progresses towards the descending and rectosigmoid junction. Once this level of mobilization is obtained, the transverse colon and both flexures are held with Babcock clamps and a test of adequate mobilization is performed before the abdomen is opened. This is done by bringing the flexures and transverse colon down towards the pelvis to see if they easily reach the suprapubic area. If this is the case, the abdomen is entered through a Pfannenstiel's incision usually joining the two suprapubic ports, which include the right and left lower quadrants. If a more superior port location was utilized, a suprapubic transverse incision is made without incorporating any port sites. If the test of bringing the flexure down reveals inadequate mobilization, further dissection is done until this is accomplished.

Occasionally it is necessary to perform some mesenteric devascularization intraabdominally. To achieve this, the abdomen is entered and extracorporeal devascularization of the colon is performed to the level of the rectosigmoid, if ileorectal anastomosis is contemplated. If ileoanal pouch or total colectomy are being considered, it is then carried down to the levators.

In the case of proctocolectomy, combined perineal excision is done and a right lower-quadrant ileostomy is fashioned. (The right lower quadrant could also be the site of a trocar.) For ileoanal pouch procedures, a rotating or linear stapler is applied in the pelvis, 2 cm proximal to the dentate line. The anal canal is transected above the staple line. The colon is removed, the pouch (usually a J pouch) is constructed externally possibly with a double staple anastomosis technique. Mucosectomy is seldom done. The procedure is completed by creation of a covering loop ileostomy.

Results

Since June 1990 we have attempted more than 200 laparoscopic colonic procedures, including right, transverse, left and sigmoid colectomies, low anterior and abdominoperineal resections, total colectomy with ileoanal pouch, posterior rectopexy and Hartmann's procedure. Cancer accounted for 107 resections, including 35 right colectomies, two transverse colectomies, 10 left colectomies, 23 sigmoid colectomies, 23 low anterior resections and six abdominoperineal resections. In 17 cases we converted to an open procedure: because of bulky tumor in eight cases (one patient had a transected ureter) because of bleeding in three (including an iliac artery injury in one case), because of prior colectomy in three (two had previous radiation), and because the tumor was not in the specimen in three cases. There were 14 postoperative complications, including four small bowel obstructions, three urinary retentions, two cases of pneumonia, one case of bleeding, one stricture, one leak, one wound infection and one retrograde ejaculation. There were no tocar site recurrences. The operative mortality was 1%. The average length of stay for these patients, including those with complications, was 5.7 days.

In all these patients we adhered to strict principles of cancer management, including devascularizing at the base of the mesentery (see above). We compared the specimen lengths of colons removed with both open and laparoscopic approaches. The average specimen length for laparoscopic right colectomies was 30 cm, compared with 25 cm for specimens removed with the open technique. For patients undergoing sigmoid colectomy, the average length was 28 cm for open surgery and 26 cm for laparoscopic resection. Lymph node counts were also similar. In patients undergoing right colectomy, an average of eight nodes were retrieved with laparoscopic resection compared with an average of nine found when the open technique was used. For sigmoid colectomies the average numbers of nodes retrieved were seven and 7.5 respectively.

During this same period, 93 patients underwent laparoscopic colonic procedures for benign diseases. In this subset of patients the complication rate was 8%, the conversion rate was 16%, and operative mortality was 1%. The overall complication rate for the entire series of 200 patients was 11%, with a conversion rate of 16% and mortality of 1%. On average in the postoperative period, patients were started on clear liquids one day postoperatively, started taking oral analgesics on day 2 and a regular diet by 3.5 days, and had bowel movements by day 4. The average hospital stay was five days. The average hospital cost for laparoscopic colon procedures was $20 900, compared with $23 400 for open cases.

Conclusion

We believe that laparoscopic colonic surgery is currently one of the most advanced laparoscopic procedures and one of the most technically demanding. Only experienced laproscopists should perform this surgery. The high conversion or complication rates that have been reported in the literature may stem from surgeon inexperience.

Suggested reading

Bailey RW (1991) Complications of laparoscopic general surgery. In: Zucker KA (ed.) *Surgical Laparoscopy*. Quality Medical Publishing, St Louis. pp. 311–42.

Clayman RV *et al.* (1992) Laparoscopic nephrectomy: a review of 16 cases. *Surg Laparosc Endosc*. **2**:29–34.

Coller JA (1991) Laparoscopic assisted right hemi-colectomy. *Dis Colon Rectum*. **34**:1030–1.

Corbitt JD (1992) Preliminary experience with laparoscopic-guided colectomy. *Surg Laparosc Endosc.* **2**:79–81

Fowler DL and White SA (1991) Laparoscopic assisted sigmoid resection. *Surg Laparosc Endosc.* **1**:183–5.

Fowler DL and White SA (1992) The use of a Doppler probe for identifying the cystic artery during a laparoscopic cholecystectomy: a pilot study. *Surg Laparosc Endosc.* **2**:117–20.

Fitzgibbons RJ Jr *et al.* (1991) Open laparoscopy. In: Zucker KA (ed.) *Surgical Laparoscopy.* Quality Medical Publishing, St Louis. pp. 87–97.

Jacobs M *et al.* (1991) Minimally invasive colon resection (laparoscopic colectomy). *Surg Laparosc Endosc.* **1**:144–50.

Pezet D *et al.* (1992) Parietal seeding of carcinoma of the gallbladder after laparoscopic cholecystectomy. *Br J Surg.* **79**:230.

Saclarides TJ *et al.* (1991) Laparoscopic removal of a large colonic lipoma. *Dis Colon Rectum.* **34**:1027–9.

Zucker KA (ed.) (1991) *Surgical Laparoscopy.* Quality Medical Publishing, St Louis. pp. 143–82.

13

Principles of Stapling in Operations on the Small and Large Bowel by Laparoscopic Techniques

FELICIEN M STEICHEN, JOSEPH C IRACI, JEAN-MICHEL LOUBEAU, MARK B ANDERSON AND ROGER WELTER

Introduction

As interest in the laparoscopic approach to the abdominal cavity has spread from gynecologists to general surgeons, the indications for the various procedures have widened, and now include an assortment of pathologic conditions in the female and male pelvis and upper abdomen[1].

It takes time to design and produce new instruments for new procedures, and all our initial efforts were directed toward diagnostic, remedial and ablative procedures, in which a possible specimen could be retrieved through the available trocars. As proficiency grew, however, and surgeons attempted new procedures—vaporization of endometrial implants, tubal ligation and section, various ovarian and subserosal uterine procedures and then cholecystectomy, appendectomy, vagotomy, Nissen fundoplication and inguinal hernia repairs—expectations soared because of the generally favorable results: diminished postoperative pain, a decrease in the number of infections, reduced hospital stays and the earlier resumption of normal activities. With the surgeons' desire and temperament to improve operative efficiency and safety to benefit the patients, and the drive behind a new technology by both the public and the 'lobbying' surgical instrument industry, it became soon obvious that intraabdominal operations requiring not only correction or excision but also restoration would soon be considered. This class of operation presents two major additional steps, specimen retrieval and visceral reconstruction, which can seriously compromise the various technical features of a smooth successful laparoscopy.

Laparoscopic resection and reconstruction

The first operation at this level of complexity was the laparoscopically guided or assisted vaginal hysterectomy. However, the technical challenge is somewhat reduced here by the fact that the evacuation of the specimen and the reconstruction of the vaginal cuff can both be performed through a natural orifice: the vagina.

As resections of small and large bowel were planned and accomplished, the new level of complexity became more pressing: evacuation of the specimen and reconstruction of bowel continuity. Since in most instances the specimen had to be removed through a 'utility' or 'contingency' incision at the end of the ablative stage, in order to preserve the pneumoperitoneum during the earlier phase of laparoscopy, many surgeons placed this incision in an anatomical location that would favor access to both bowel ends. The anastomosis is then performed, either manually or mechanically by an extracorporeal approach. However, this technique requires additional liberation of both bowel ends in order to exteriorize them at or beyond the abdominal wall, a feat not always possible in the obese patient with a stiff mesocolon. The need for a larger incision, often in an anatomically unorthodox manner, would then negate the advantages of the extended laparoscopic prelude. In some specific cases one could also argue that the utility incision is not much smaller than the right transverse flank incision required to remove the cecum and ascending colon, for instance, and perform ileo–transverse colostomy. All of these factors have to be considered with this approach, and an early decision taken on the mode of reconstruction, if laparoscopy is chosen for the initial access to the abdomen[2,3,4].

The utility incision is not necessary in case of a rectosigmoid resection, where the specimen can be retrieved and reconstruction accomplished through another natural orifice, the anus (although many surgeons have an aversion to drawing a malignant specimen through a narrow passage like the anorectal canal). In addition, if the double-stapling technique is used with the circular stapler, there would still be the need for an incision to place the anvil and a purse-string suture into the proximal bowel end and optimally close the rectal stump and join the anvil rod into the transanally advanced hollow central shaft of the circular cartridge[5].

Manual sutures

In an effort to preserve the purity of the laparoscopic approach, other surgeons have developed manual suture techniques that allow the closure of an occasional accidental bowel rent, the completion of the gastric collar in a Nissen fundoplication, the closure of the sero-myotomy of a posterior truncal vagotomy and interruption of individual anterior fibers as they penetrate the gastric wall inside the lesser curvature. This expertise has now been expanded to include the manual construction of various bowel anastomoses, an extremely painstaking procedure even in the hands of experts, and certainly not part of the repertory of the average solid craftsman.

Conceptually, apart from some of the objections previously mentioned, the need for a contingency incision or the personal (somewhat romantic) preference for manual sutures represents a return to more traditional methods.

Our efforts should be directed to developing operative techniques that are in tune with the advances of the laparoscopic and thorascopic approach and exploration of abdomen and chest. Since this expansion will not occur in parallel or tandem, some compromises—such as the incision to evacuate the specimen—will probably always be necessary.

Stapling in minimal access surgery

Surgical stapling, even in open operations, has always represented a gentler and less traumatic invasion of tissues than the placement of the equivalent amount of manual sutures. The length of time that bowel ends are left open is reduced and the potential for peritoneal soiling is diminished. Furthermore, discrepancies in intestinal caliber are easily handled either by the linear, functional end-to-end anastomosis (if the bowel ends are relatively mobile) or by the circular triple-stapled anastomosis in the rectosigmoid or rectocolic anastomoses. All of these favorable characteristics go hand-in-hand with a safety record in bowel closure and anastomosis that is the equivalent of and often better than the results obtained with manual sutures, together with a background of continued simplification of the various operative steps.

Therefore the use of stapling instruments would seem to have a natural application in laparoscopic operations. In fact with the transformation of existing instruments and the continued development of new ones, capable of being introduced through small ports of entry and then efficiently deployed within the abdomen, this challenge has been brilliantly met. At the same time, existing stapling techniques have been modified and adapted, and new ones developed, to become laparoscopically compatible.

It is almost certain that the near future will see the development of other 'laparoscopy-friendly' instruments for bowel closure and anastomosis: eg a button for compression anastomosis, with two halves that collapse during transabdominal introduction and expand into rigid cones inside opposite bowel lumina like an umbrella. The two halves inside the lumina of the facing bowel ends can then be coupled and firmly anchored to each other, producing an end-to-end anastomosis by compression of the invaginated bowel edges held together by the framework of the consolidated button. A composition of biodegradable material or simple fragmentation of the button, after its task has been accomplished, will assure its elimination via normal intestinal passages.

High-grade biological glues will soon become available to reinforce circular compression and stapled anastomoses. They will be developed to a level of total tissue compatibility, to prevent microbial and viral contamination and provide an optimal degree of adhesiveness, so as to become the sole agent of a reliable, naturally healing anastomosis. While laser soldering of wounds and other similar techniques of cell mobilization and bridging are only in their early experimental stages, such techniques in conjunction with biological glues will ultimately come to fruition.

In operations on the small and large bowel we distinguish at present the following stapling techniques that permit total or near-total integrity of the laparoscopic approach:

- lateral, tangential excision and linear bowel closure, eg appendectomy, Meckel's diverticulectomy[6]
- bowel resection and linear functional end-to-end anastomosis, eg right colectomy (also small bowel loop, transverse and descending colon)[7]
- resection and circular end-to-end triple-stapled anastomosis through natural orifice (anus), eg rectosigmoidectomy[8].
- resection and circular side-to-end double-stapled anastomosis through a contingency anterior perineotomy, eg low anterior rectal resection.

Positions of surgical team members

Although in the USA the positioning of the operating team and monitoring instruments around the operating table was rigidly defined early on in laparoscopic cholecystectomy, it soon became obvious that different countries adhered to different guidelines. This may be a sign that the desire for safety during the early days of laparoscopy required a reproducible OR discipline that left little or no place for improvisation.

While the overall role of each participant is clearly defined, general concepts have evolved to facilitate adaptation to changing circumstances during complex operations such as the various bowel resections.

Placement of monitoring equipment and abdominal ports

In general we place laparoscope and camera through the umbilicus, so as to ensure complete visual access to the entire abdominal cavity, since usually at least half of the cavity (and sometimes all of it) will be involved in the various manipulations and the dissection. The working ports for handling, liberating, isolating and reconstructing bowel should be spaced sufficiently to allow for latitude of movement and yet permit convergence of instruments to a given area without creating duels or interference between them.

These conditions seem to be satisfied by placing ports in the right lower quadrant and suprapubic area for appendectomy, and in all four quadrants for colectomy, with an optional fifth suprapubic position for sigmoid and rectal resections. However, these are general recommendations only. Basing their decisions on visual intracavitary assessment and possibly intraoperative colonoscopy and delineation of a lesion by transmural illumination (an additional method it is wise to have available), the members of the team may concentrate several ports near a given area, and switch viewing and working ports (in which case reducing diaphragms should be available and an angled scope should be used). If a good flexible scope becomes available in the near future, further options may arise.

Additional ports may be necessary, but the total length of port site incisions should not exceed the length of a reasonably effective traditional incision. The preference of the surgeon, based on previous experience and operative habits, also plays a definite role.

The instruments for bowel retraction and exposure have longer work limbs than those used for cholecystectomy. Additionally, the mobilization of the specimen requires more space for the various maneuvers necessary to isolate and interrupt the vascular supply. Therefore the instruments for holding and handling the bowel are best placed through ports in the abdominal wall opposite the designated colon segment (eg left side for right colectomy, right side for descending and sigmoid colon, lower quadrants for transverse colectomy).

This places the surgeon and the ports that accept the instruments for the dissection and vascular isolation of the specimen, as well as reconstruction of bowel continuity, on the side of the colon segment to be removed. In case of a transverse colectomy the side chosen depends on whether the surgeon is right- or left-handed. But again it is important to realize that these recommendations are not written in stone and that there is a place for sound imagination, as in all other surgical endeavors.

Positioning of monitors

It is important that the viewing arrangement enables the surgical team to observe and work in a coordinated way. The viewing monitors should be placed in the prolongation of the projected flow of dissection and area of reconstruction. They should be at the right height, somewhat diagonal to the viewers. In a right colectomy, the monitor should be at the patient's left shoulder for the surgeon and his right shoulder for the assistant. In a left colectomy or rectosigmoidectomy the monitors should be in the opposite and reversed positions, with the surgeon's monitor placed at the patient's right thigh and the assistant's at the patient's left thigh.

In the figures, we have not indicated the positions of monitors and all the other laparoscopic equipment because there are wide personal and regional variations. Furthermore, the continued development of operating and visual equipment, the advent of three-dimensional pictures and other innovations might make such drawings obsolete before their publication.

We have shown port sizes as needed by currently available instruments. The release of the Endo-GIA 60, for instance, will make the use of 15 mm trocars a necessity. For holding the bowel, Babcocks are only stand-ins for other Endo-instruments: bowel clamps, holders, retractors, clip appliers etc.

It is hoped that the basic operative steps demonstrated here—all proven experimentally and some confirmed by our clinical experience in appendectomy and diverticulectomy—will have a half-life that justifies the efforts of the medical artist.

As for all laparoscopic procedures, the patient is prepared for both laparoscopy and laparotomy and told about possible intraoperative conversion. S/he should give informed consent to both. Perioperatively s/he is given three doses of a broad-spectrum antibiotic.

Laparoscopic operative techniques

Lateral, tangential excision and linear bowel closure

Appendectomy (Figure 13.1a, e–g).

Acute appendicitis mostly affects children and young adults, but it can threaten almost any age group. The treatment is appendectomy as soon as diagnosis can be established with a reasonable degree of certainty. However, establishing such 'reasonable certainty' is the real challenge, since the clinical picture of appendicitis can mimic and be mimicked by almost any known acute intraabdominal condition, and indeed by some acute extraabdominal infectious diseases in childhood.

Laparoscopy is therefore helpful in the diagnosis of abdominal pain, especially in women where it has now been used for over 20 years. The diagnostic laparoscopy is then converted to treat the condition that causes the pain, especially removal of the appendix if this turns out to be the culprit. The first laparoscopic appendectomy was done by Dr Semm in Germany in 1982.

Gastric decompression by naso–gastric tube and complete bladder drainage by Foley catheter should precede the creation of an adequate pneumoperitoneum. Pregnancy is a contraindication to pneumoperitoneum, mostly for medico–legal reasons.

Following the establishment of a satisfactory pneumoperitoneum a 10 mm port is placed at the umbilicus, through which the laparoscope with camera is advanced (Figure 13.1**a**). The entire abdomen is visually explored. If appendectomy is indicated, a 5 mm port is placed above the pubis and a 12 mm port into the right lower quadrant, inside the iliac spine, above the cecum. Both placements are done under direct vision.

If necessary, a fourth trocar may be placed into the left lower quadrant, to facilitate the manipulation of the cecum and exposure behind it in case of an inflamed retrocecal appendix.

The appendix is held taut with a grasper placed through the suprapubic port, and a small window is made at the base of the appendix (between it and the mesoappendix) with a dissector advanced through the lateral 12 mm port (Figure 13.1**e**).

The dissector is replaced by the Endo-GIA loaded with a vascular cartridge. The open cartridge is placed across the entire width of the mesoappendix and closed to compress the meso and vessels between anvil and cartridge proper. The instrument is activated to transect the entire mesoappendix between two triple lines of hemostatic staples. Any blood-oozing sites can be stopped by a clip or electrocautery.

The base of the appendix is now exposed, and the Endo-GIA instrument loaded with regular gastrointestinal staples is applied across the cecal base of the appendix in the same way as it was placed around the mesoappendix (Figure 13.1**f**).

Following activation of the Endo-GIA instrument, the base of the appendix and its cecal insertion are closed separately with two triple staple lines (Figure 13.1**g**).

The appendix is then evacuated through the 12 mm trocar or, if necessary, with the help of a specimen bag placed through the umbilical port that can be enlarged to net a thick inflamed appendix. This is followed by switching the camera to the right lower quadrant, and closure of the large port sites under vision. Postoperative care is much the same as with standard appendectomy, with early permission to take oral fluids and food, and discharge to home often within 24 hours.

Meckel's diverticulectomy (Figure 13.1a–d)

The diagnosis of a Meckel's diverticulum, with a clinical picture of inflammation rather than bleeding, will only be made incidentally, as in one of our patients: a 26-year-old female who presented with a 12 hour complaint of periumbilical pain, fever of 102° F, anorexia, periumbilical tenderness, no guarding and white blood cell count of 10 000. During a 24 hour clinical observation, fever, abdominal tenderness and elevated white count persisted. Diagnostic laparoscopy revealed a Meckel's diverticulum, normal appendix, ovaries, tubes and uterus, and no other visible lesions to explain the symptoms and signs.

Diverticulectomy was performed and histologic examination showed autolysis of intestinal tissue compatible with Meckel's diverticulitis. Appendectomy was also done. This seemed justified by the presence of three tell-tale puncture sites, which could later confuse the picture if there was recurrent lower abdominal pain.

Since most Meckel's diverticula will be discovered during the course of laparoscopy for suspected appendicitis, preparation of the patient and placement of abdominal ports will usually be the same as shown in Figure 13.1**a**.

The diverticulum is rotated to expose its posterior ileal wall from the mesentery to the tip of the diverticulum (Figure 13.1**b**). A window is created between the vessels and the base of the diverticulum, to accommodate the vascular Endo-GIA. The vessels and the mesentery surrounding them are hemostatically stapled on each side of their simultaneous transection. Often the vascular arcade to the diverticulum is narrow and can be severed between one distal and two proximal clips at this level.

The diverticulum is turned so as to present its base in an antero–posterior direction (Figure 13.1**c**). The visceral Endo-GIA is then placed through the 12 mm right lower quadrant port and applied to the base of the diverticulum at a right angle to the long axis of the ileum. Usually two or three such maneuvers are necessary with a wide-mouthed diverticulum. The Endo-GIA 60 may reduce the number of such applications. Care is taken to avoid including the vascular staples or clips in the closed Endo-GIA. Following complete closure of the base and site of implantation of the diverticulum, the specimen is removed through the 12 or 15 mm trocar (Figure 13.1**d**). The bowel

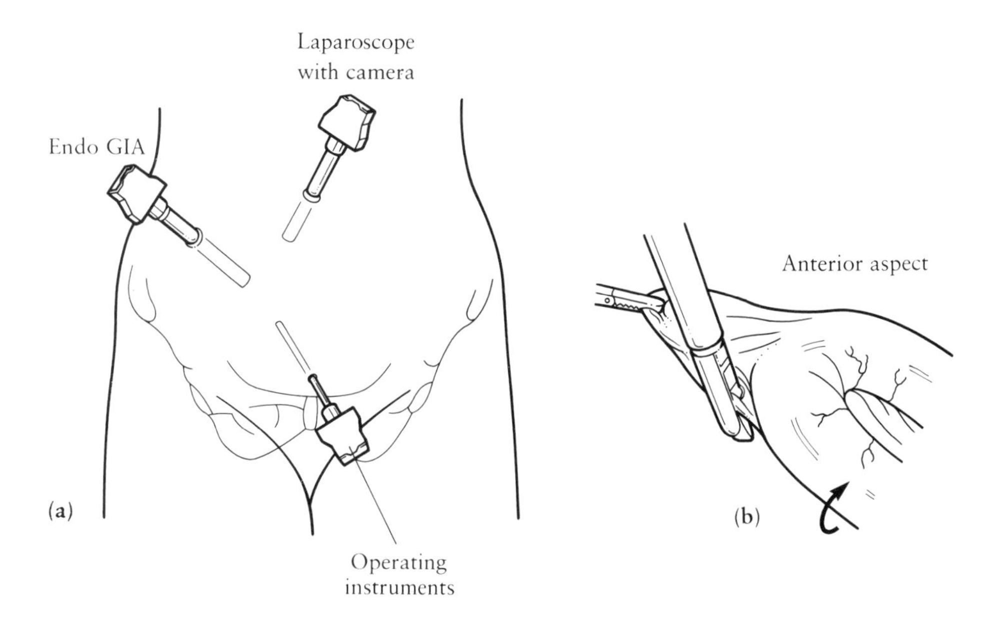

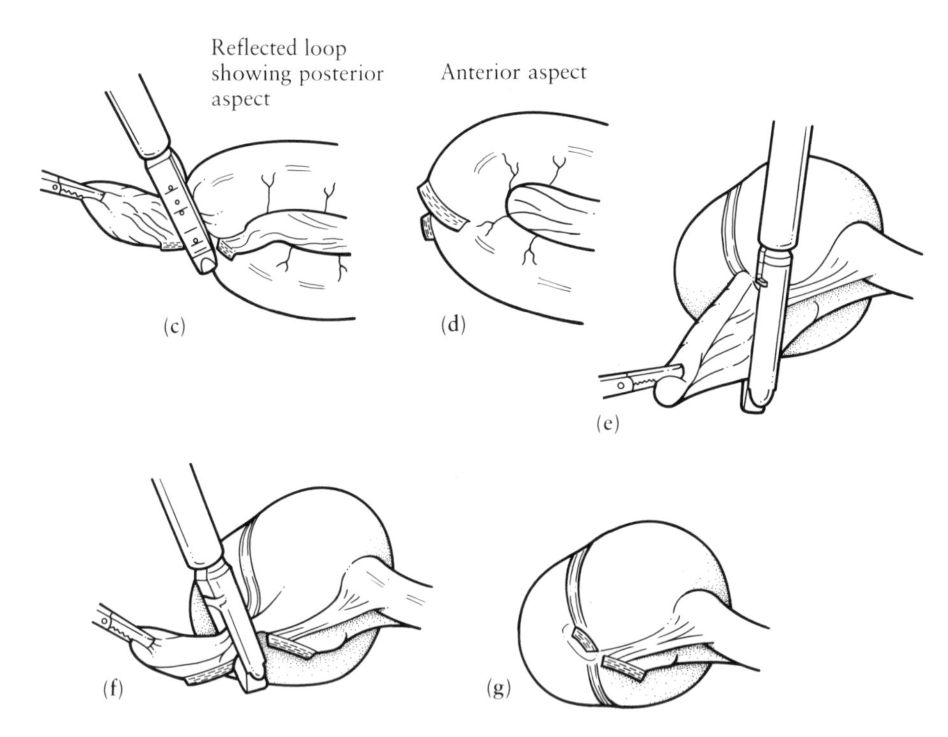

Figure 13.1: (**a**) Placement sites of laparoscope and working ports for appendectomy and Meckel's Diverticulectomy. (**b**) Stapled closure and division of mesentery and vessels to diverticulum. (**c**) Stapled closure and transection of the base of the diverticulum at right angle to the long axis of the bowel. (**d**) After removal of the specimen, the bowel closure and patency are inspected. (**e**) Stapled closure and division of the mesoappendix and appendical vessels. (**f**) Stapled closure and transection of the cecal base of the appendix. (**g**) Closure of cecum and base of appendix with triple staple lines.

closure, at strict right angles to the long axis of the ileum, does not obstruct or narrow the bowel lumen.

The postoperative management and hospital course are similar to those after an appendectomy. The patient described here left the hospital soon after diverticulectomy and appendectomy, symptom-free and eating a regular diet.

Bowel resection and linear, functional end-to-end anastomosis

The old-fashioned linear, anatomical side-to-side and functional end-to-end bowel anastomosis lends itself particularly well to an intraabdominal anastomosis, with preservation of the pneumoperitoneum. This is the case after resection of bowel segments where reconstruction with the circular end-to-end anastomosing instrument cannot take place through a natural orifice such as the anus or conceivably an open vaginal cuff after combined hysterectomy–sigmoidectomy or a man-made anterior 'contingency' perineotomy. By definition the functional end-to-end anastomosis is therefore potentially useful in all bowel resections between the first jejunal loop and the proximal sigmoid colon.

After satisfactory creation of the pneumoperitoneum, five ports are placed: one in the umbilicus for the laparoscope and camera, two on the left side for the holding, handling and exposing instruments and two on the right side for the dissecting, isolating and reconstructing instruments (Figure 13.2**a**). Additional ports may be needed as special intraoperative conditions develop: a port above the pubis and a 12 mm (Endo-GIA 30) or 15 mm (Endo-GIA 60) port in the right upper abdomen, closer to the projected functional end-to-end anastomosis than the original 12 mm port may have been placed.

Babcock clamps or blunt graspers are used to hold and pull the cecum and ascending colon to the left (Figure 13.2**b**). The liberation of the specimen is started by incising the lateral peritoneal reflection, through both right-sided ports, from below-up and above-down. During this dissection the right ureter should be clearly identified and preserved. The hepatocolic ligament at the right colon flexure can be transected between two triple vascular staple lines (not shown here).

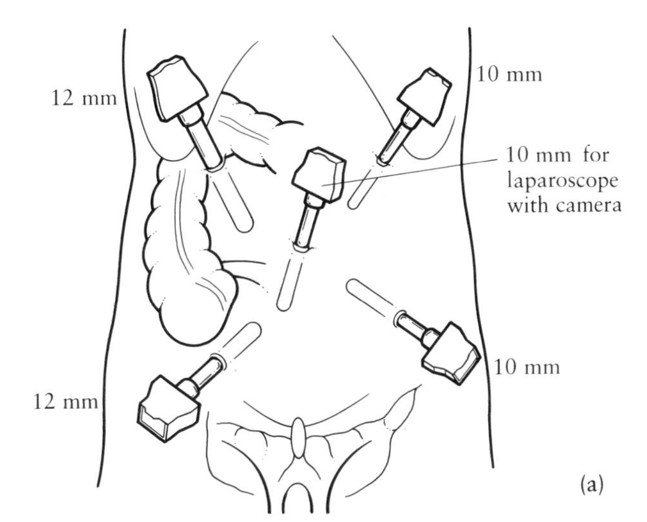

Figure 13.2: (**a**) Placement sites of laparoscope and working ports.

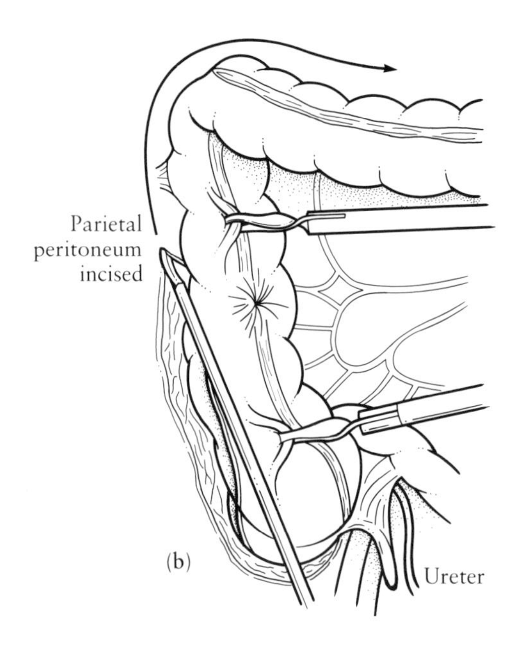

Figure 13.2: *continued* (**b**) Lateral liberation of cecum and ascending colon.

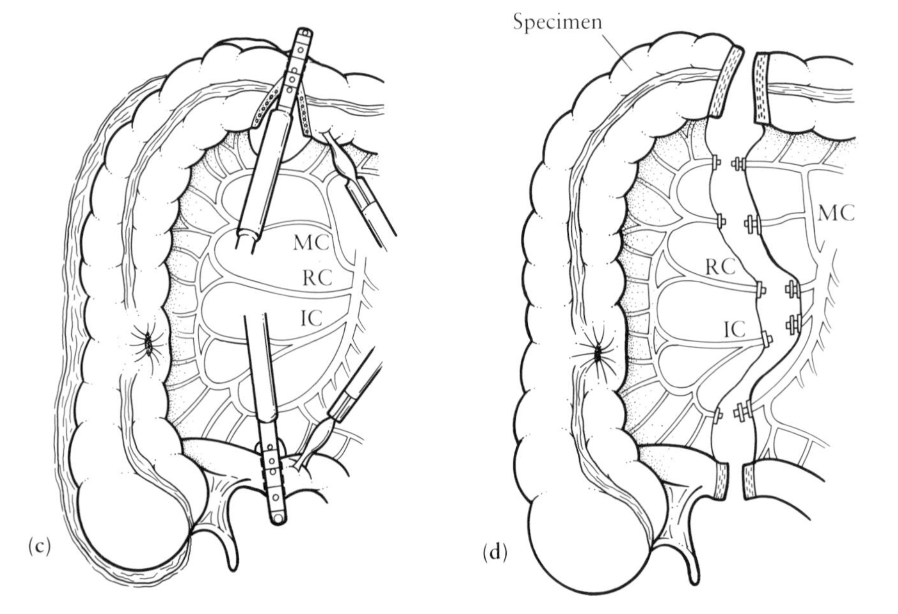

Figure 13.2: *continued* (**c**) Stapled closure and transection of distal ileum and proximal transverse colon. (**d**) Transection of right mesocolon and division of vessels between hemostatic clips.

Following complete liberation and elevation of the right colon and corresponding mesocolon, windows are created near the bowel walls, at the levels selected for resection (Figure 13.2**c**). The colon is temporarily replaced in its bed, and transection of the terminal ileum is done either (1) with the Endo-GIA

30 introduced through the right upper port, followed by transection of the proximal transverse colon with several GIA 30, or (2) by advancing one GIA 60 application through the right lower port. For each one of these maneuvers the bowel is held and identified with instruments placed from the left, so as to preclude inclusion of any other structures.

The isolation of the specimen is then continued by transecting the mesocolon and the vessels serving the right colon, between one distal and two proximal clips placed with the clip applier through either right-sided port (Figure 13.2**d**).

Alternatively, vascular control and mesocolic transection can be obtained by several applications of the vascular GIA instrument (Figure 13.2**e**). Following complete liberation of the specimen, it is 'bagged' and temporarily 'parked' in the empty right lower quadrant.

Next the two bowel ends are placed parallel to each other in the right upper quadrant and held in position with Babcocks introduced from the left side (Figure 13.2**f**). The stapled antimesenteric corners of the bowel ends are excised with instruments advanced from the right side: scissors from above and holder from below for the colon and the reverse of this for the ileum.

By carefully holding both bowel ends in position with Babcocks from the left side, the anvil arm of the GIA 30 is introduced into the large bowel through its excised corner (Figure 13.2**g**). At this point it is often necessary to close the instrument without firing it, in order to hold onto the colon, while the ileal end is prepared for placement around the anvil arm of the GIA. While holding the GIA steady and with the colon in the previously obtained position (with the upper left Babcocks), the ileal end is grasped at the staple line with a right lower holder and at a point some 6–7 cm upstream with left lower Babcocks. With both a pulling and pushing motion, the small bowel is brought around the anvil, separated from the cartridge to the open position just minutes before. The antimesenteric position of the GIA in both bowel ends is checked, then the instrument is closed and fired.

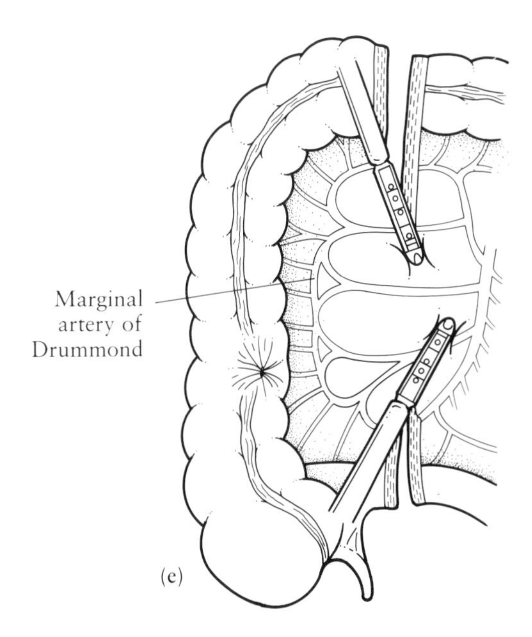

Figure 13.2: *continued* (e) Stapled closure and division of mesocolon and vessels.

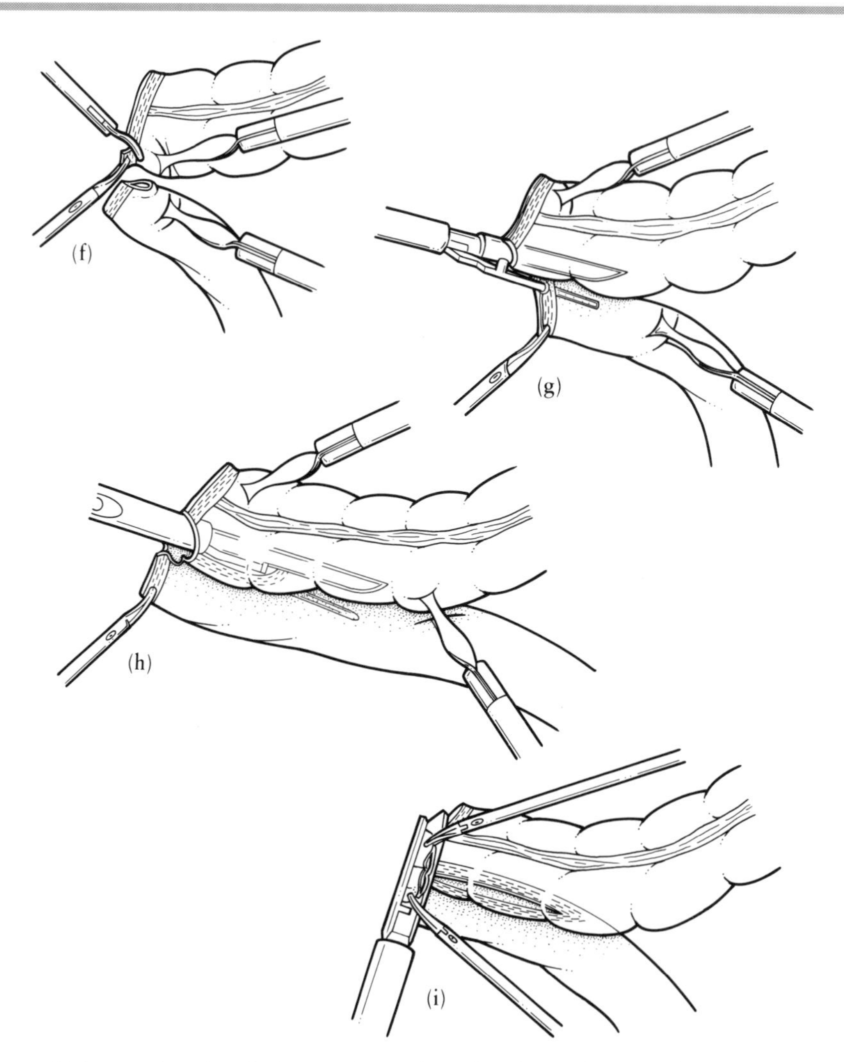

Figure 13.2: *continued* (**f**) Positioning of bowel ends for functional end-to-end anastomosis.(**g**) First application of the Endo GIA 30 for the side-to-side colo-ileostomy. (**h**) Second application of the Endo GIA 30 instrument. (**i**) Closure of the Endo GIA 30 opening with the Endo TA instrument.

If the GIA 30 has been used, a second application is necessary in order to obtain a satisfactory anastomotic cross-section (Figure 13.2**h**). For this purpose the crotch of the reloaded instrument is advanced against the crotch of the first linear anastomosis. Care is taken to continue in the same antimesenteric axis as before, by holding the bowel walls together at the tip of the anastomotic prolongation with left lower Babcock clamps.

If the GIA 60 has been used, then this second GIA 30 application is not necessary.

Following the side-to-side anastomosis, the now common bowel opening is closed with the Endo TA instrument and the excess tissue is excised using the stapler as a guide (Figure 13.2**i**). The specimen, protected by the bag, is then removed through a McBurney incision.

Resection and circular end-to-end triple-stapled anastomosis through a natural orifice

With the surgeon positioned initially on the patient's left side, the assistant on the right side and the monitors at the level of both thighs, diagonally across from surgeon and assistant, five ports are placed as shown in Figure 13.2**a**. In addition a sixth, suprapubic port may be necessary to work on the rectum in an antero–posterior direction. However, the lateral ports are used differently. While the two left lateral ports help mostly with the dissection and liberation of the specimen, the right lateral ports are used to introduce holding and handling instruments, but also to place the Endo-GIA 60 and Endo-PTA 60. The ports are not clearly dedicated to the same purpose throughout the entire operation, as the surgeon may have to work from the patient's right side for the mesocolic and retro-rectal dissection.

With the holding instruments brought in from the right side, the descending and sigmoid parts of the colon are elevated and the white line of Toldt is incised through the left-sided ports, from above-down and vice versa (Figure 13.3**b**). The vascular supply is interrupted between proximal and distal clips or with the vascular GIA (as shown in Figure 13.2**e**) at the origin of the sigmoid vessels and at the level of proximal bowel transection, for the marginal artery of Drummond. The left ureter is identified and preserved.

Following elevation and isolation of the specimen, the bowel is closed proximally (1) and distally (2) with the Endo-PTA 60, at a safe distance from the sigmoid tumor (Figure 13.3**c**). For this maneuver the holding instruments are placed through the left ports and the PTA 60 instruments through the right ports.

As shown in Figure 13.3**d**, a longitudinal colotomy is performed proximal to the cephalad colon closure (1) and a transverse rectotomy distal to the caudad rectal closure (2).

The CEEA anvil with a flat head and the attached rod are then advanced through the anus and rectotomy into the peritoneal cavity (Figure 13.3**e**), from where they are transported to the proximal colotomy (2) and inserted into the lumen of the descending colon ('intraperitoneal portage').

Following this maneuver, the rectum is closed and transected with the Endo-GIA 60, caudad to the distal rectotomy (Figure 13.3**f**–1). The head of the anvil is prevented from proximal drifting, by a half closed Babcock that is grasping around three quarters of the large bowel circumference. The descending colon is closed and transected cephalad to the proximal colotomy (2) with the Endo-GIA 60 instrument.

The completely liberated specimen is then bagged and parked into the left lower quadrant.

An alternative approach consists in the removal of a benign, average-sized lesion through the anorectal canal (Figure 13.3**g**). In this case all the steps at the cephalad level remain the same, but the distal anterior rectotomy is completed into a circumferential transection of the rectum.

Just as for the previous steps, holding and transecting instruments are advanced in a variety of ways according to the task at hand.

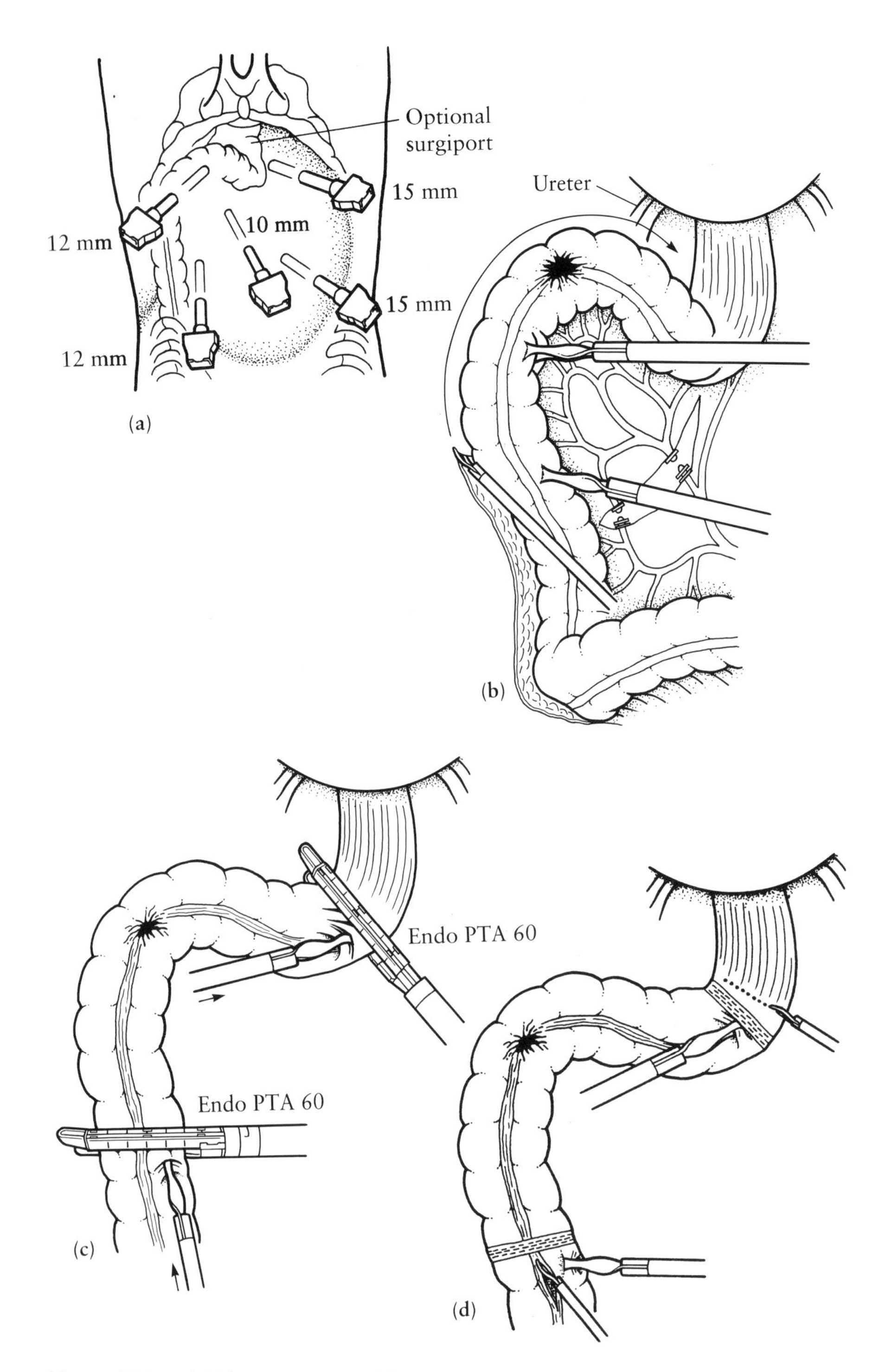

Figure 13.3: (**a**) Placement sites of laparoscope and working ports. (**b**) Lateral liberation of descending and sigmoid colon. Control of vascular supply with clips. (**c**) Temporary stapled closures on preselected proximal and distal sites of the specimen. (**d**) Proximal colotomy and distal rectotomy.

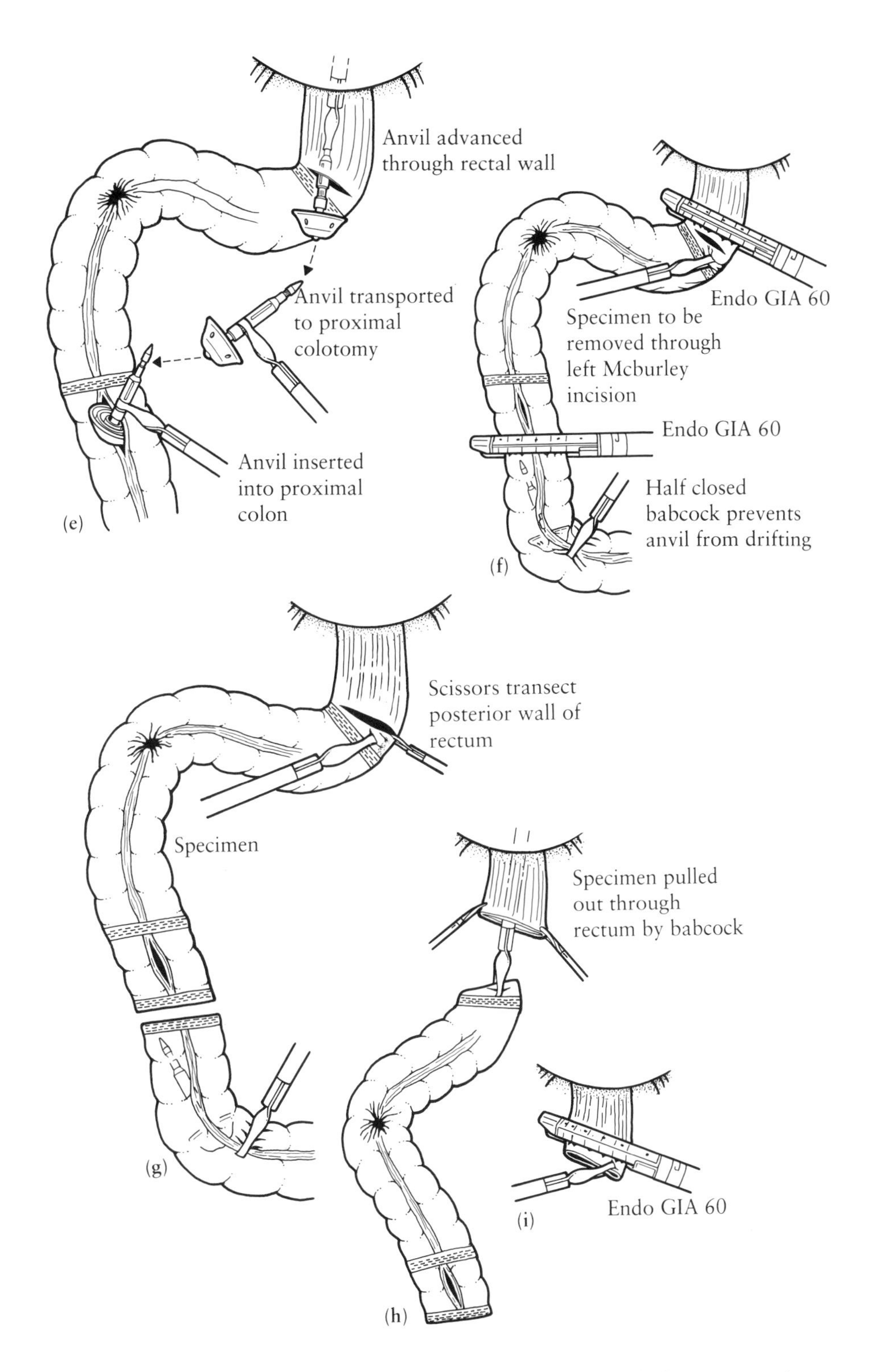

Figure 13.3: *continued* (**e**) Intraperitoneal portage of PCEEA anvil. (**f**) Permanent closure and transection of rectum and descending colon. (**g,h**) Transrectal evacuation of specimen (alternate approach). (**i**) Closure of the rectal cuff after transrectal evacuation of specimen (alternate approach).

The specimen is pulled onto the perineum with Babcock clamps advanced through the anorectal canal (Figure 13.3**h**). The rectum is held and pulled cephalad, to prevent invagination and prolapse of the cuff.

The rectal cuff is now closed with the GIA 60 and the excess separated tissue is removed through the left lower port (Figure 13.3**i**).

Steps to reconstruct bowel continuity are now initiated (Figure 13.3**j**). The anvil head is maintained in position with a half-closed Babcock and the center of the proximal colon staple line is incised over the sharp tip of the anvil shaft.

An empty, open PTA 60 is then applied around the colon, proximal to the CEEA anvil, and used as a backstop (Figure 13.3**k**).

Two Babcock clamps, advanced from the lower ports, are used to compress the colon against the PTA 60 and slip the anvil shaft through the opening in the staple line.

The anvil shaft is grasped beyond the staple line, pulled entirely through, so as to position the anvil firmly against the staple line, inside the proximal colon (Figure 13.3**l**).

The cartridge of the CEEA is placed through the anus and the hollow central rod—without its sharp trocar—is advanced against the rectal staple line. The center of this line is incised over the rod.

The anvil shaft and central rod are joined and anchored to each other (Figure 13.3**m**). The CEEA instrument is closed, joining colon and rectum in an X-shaped configuration.

Following completion of this triple-stapled anastomosis, the specimen is evacuated through a left McBurney incision, if it has not already been removed transanally (Figure 13.3**n**). The competence of the anastomosis is checked. If a leak is discovered, repair will be done by conversion to an open operation.

Resection and circular side-to-end double-stapled anastomosis through a contingency or utility anterior perineotomy, eg low anterior rectal resection.

Figure 13.4**a** shows the general arrangement of the abdominal ports and positioning of operative team and equipment. The white line of Toldt is incised along the sigmoid colon (Figure 13.4**b**).

The peritoneal reflection, to the left of the rectum and between bladder or uterus and rectum, is incised from the left. The inferior mesenteric artery is divided either between one distal and two proximal clips, or preferably between vascular GIA staple lines as shown in Figure 13.2**e**. The left ureter is identified and preserved. The figures do not show the dissection along the right side of the pelvis, which is done from the right side of the patient, with holding instruments brought in from the left—a mirror image of the left-sided dissection. The right ureter is identified and preserved. The mesorectum is identified by blunt dissection into the pelvis. It is transected and doubly stapled with an Endo-GIA placed along the hollow of the sacrum.

Following satisfactory liberation of the rectosigmoid from above through a laparoscopic approach, the technique of Welter—originally described for open transabdominal dissection and anterior perineal low colorectal anastomosis—is used with its perineal component (Figure 13.4**c**). The anterior perineal

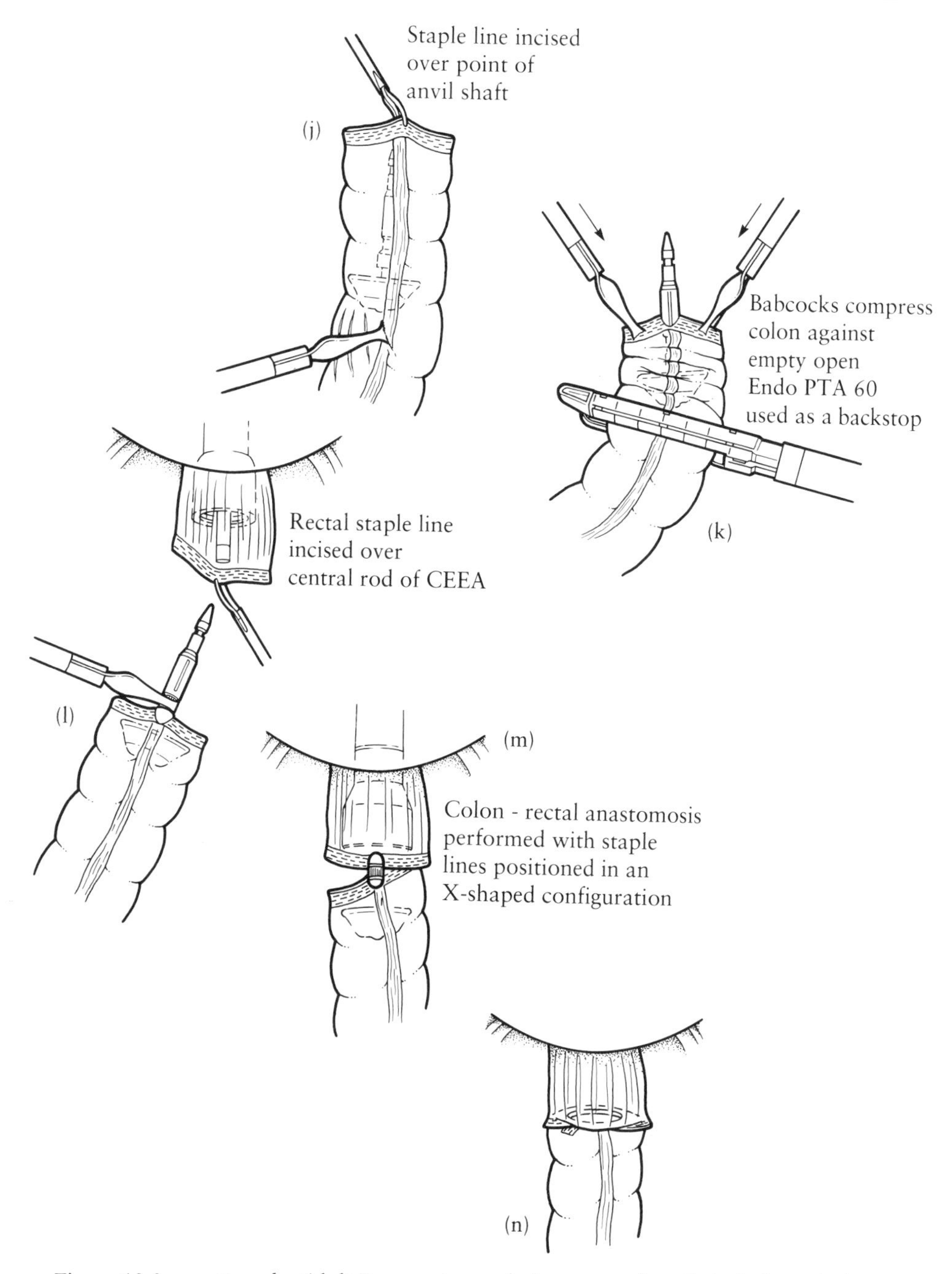

Figure 13.3: *continued* (**j,k,l**) Preparation and placement of anvil shaft through the proximal staple line. (**l**) Transanal placement of the cartridge and advancement of its central rod through the rectal staple line. (**m**) Mating of anvil and cartridge. (**n**) Triple stapled colo-rectal anastomosis.

incision serves as an approach to complete the dissection from below, to remove the specimen and to accomplish side-to-end anastomosis. It is the equivalent of an abdominal incision for extracorporeal anastomosis and more, yet produces less morbidity.

The patient, previously prepared for lithotomy position, is now placed in the Trendelenburg position and the legs and thighs are flexed into the pelvis and hyperabducted. A transverse incision is performed between genitourinary tract and anus, and brought through the subcutaneous tissue and central raphe to the rectum.

The rectum is dissected circumferentially and proximally into the abdomen, if any attachments persisted from the laparoscopic stage of the operation (Figure 13.4**d**).

The specimen is then pulled through the anterior perineotomy. If the tumor extends lower than was previously appreciated, abdominoperineal resection without oncological compromise is possible at this stage. If resection and anastomosis are possible, the specimen is resected between a cephalad purse-string placement and a caudad closure of the anorectal canal, just above the sphincter muscles, with the TA 55 roticulator.

The flat CEEA anvil with shaft is inserted into the opening of the proximal colon and brought out through the antimesocolic wall, some 10–15 cm cephalad to the bowel opening (Figure 13.4**e**).

The CEEA cartridge is placed into the anal canal and the center of the anorectal staple closure is pierced by the hollow rod. The anvil shaft and cartridge rod are joined and the instrument is closed.

The purse-string at the open end of the proximal colon is tied (Figure 13.4**f**). The excess of colon, beyond the side-to-end anastomosis, is excised peripheral to a TA 55 closure.

With the anastomosis accomplished, the CEEA is removed and the anastomosis and closure are checked for competence. The incision is then closed in layers (Figure 13.4**g**).

Reflections and results

The stapling techniques shown here—tangential closure, functional end-to-end anastomosis, triple and double stapling techniques for circular end-to-end anastomoses—are all well established methods experimentally and clinically in the classical, open operative procedures. Except for appendectomy and Meckel's diverticulectomy using tangential closures, we have demonstrated so far the intracorporeal feasibility of the various anastomotic techniques only experimentally. We plan to introduce their clinical use cautiously and progressively, in thin or normally built patients with benign lesions at first. While we would accept the removal of a narrow benign specimen through the anorectal canal, we are reluctant to do so with bulky and/or malignant lesions. Besides, placing the specimen in a bag before removing it through a utility incision is a safety measure that has never been used during open operations, although the incision was always protected by drapes and more recently by plastic wound rings.

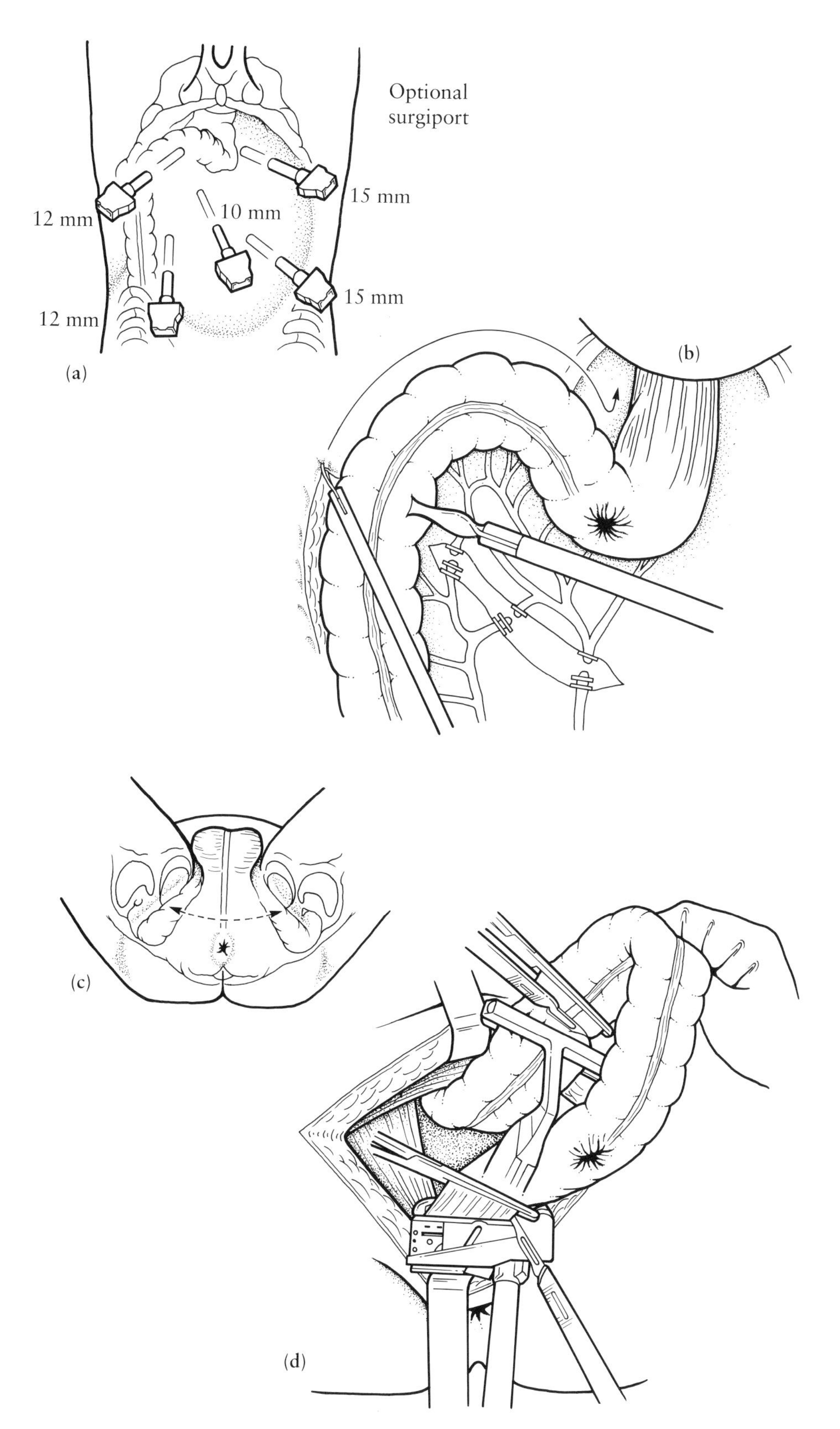

Figure 13.4: (**a**) Placement sites of laparoscope and working ports (**b**) Liberation of the sigmoid colon and rectum (**c**) Anterior perineal incision. (**d**) Exposure of rectum and preparation for resection and anastomosis.

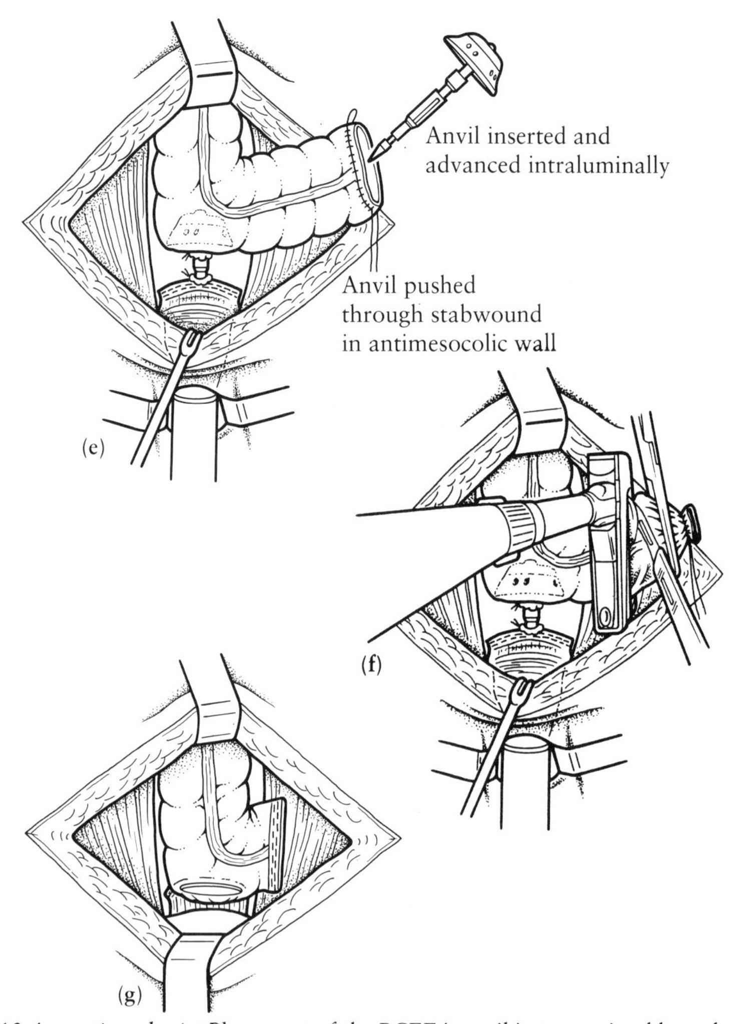

Figure 13.4: *continued* (**e**) Placement of the PCEEA anvil into proximal bowel and of the cartridge transanally. Side-to-end colo-rectostomy. (**f**) Closure and excision of blind end of proximal colon. (**g**) Final aspect of anastomosis.

At the recent second German symposium on stapling in Würzburg on 25 May 1992, F Köcherling from Erlangen and J Gastinger from Suhl presented their experimental work using functional end-to-end and triple stapling techniques similar to the ones described here[9]. They still had to resolve the proximal transportation of the anvil in the triple staple technique, but were ready to start cautious clinical trials.

On June 5th 1992, at the Congress of Eurochirurgie in Brussels, JS Azagra from the A Vesale Hospital in Montigny, Belgium, reported on his excellent experience and statistics with 95 rectosigmoid procedures and triple staple anastomosis by laparotomy between 1988 and 1992[10]. More recently he has done the same procedures on 17 patients by laparoscopy only. He removed the specimen transanally on all of them, advanced the anvil through the rectal stump into the proximal segment and then continued with the triple staple technique as shown here. In an excellent follow-up by barium enema for 80% of his 95 patients with laparotomy, Azagra noted two patients with strictures that were easily dilated from below. Two patients developed a clinically apparent anastomotic leak, and one of these patients died.

The many reports in the highly specialized literature from this country and abroad on laparoscopic colectomy and anastomosis usually performed extracorporeally (fowl or fish?) do attest to the feasibility of the dissection by laparoscopy and demonstrate that resection margins are safe; the amount of mesocolon and number of lymph-nodes are comparable or superior to those obtained by open operations for malignancy. Therefore the use of laparoscopic colectomy with a variety of anastomotic models appears justified in the hands of laparoscopically experienced surgeons, after suitable experimental preparation. The teaching of other surgeons should be encouraged on a one-to-one basis rather than through postgraduate courses.

However, in contrast to laparoscopic cholecystectomy, the headlong rush to local fame and fortune, abetted by patients and the industry, should be directed into a productive clinical study, beneficial to all concerned. While the uncontrollable enthusiasm for laparoscopic cholecystectomy was acceptable, since the event was mostly concerned with a change in technical details for the removal of benign disease, the surgical treatment of cancer imposes a different set of rules that cannot be ignored.

It is therefore important to organize study groups, similar to those that are well established for the analysis of various other cancer treatment regimens, while cases are still accruing only slowly because most surgeons are still learning the technical intricacies.

In contradistinction to cholecystectomy, where (except in rare cases of serious technical mishaps) survival from operation and disease is certain, the five- and 10-year survivals in cancer are important milestones. In a prospective randomized double blind study it would therefore not be difficult to convince our patients that, for comparable technical and prognostic risks at the present stage of knowledge, the trade-off is as follows: belly-button holes are cosmetically less unsightly, there is less pain, and there is the likelihood of earlier release from hospital and return to work, but there is also the unknown of a new course, whereas the safety of the time-proven modality carries the disadvantages of a real abdominal incision, more pain and slower recovery.

I am quite sure that, with the profession's conviction that this is the right way forward, it will be easy to explain to the public the need to accept either arm of such a study, and that laparoscopy is not a new cornerstone in the theory and practice of surgery such as wound treatment and vessel ligation, control of pain, asepsis and correction of malformations, but simply a new way to gain access to the abdominal cavity.

References

1 Flowers JL, Zucker KA, Imbembo AL *et al.* (1991) Laparoscopic cholecystectomy. *Surg Rounds*. 271–82.

2 Leahy P, Fowler D, Coller J *et al.* (1992) Laparoscopic colectomies. *Laparoscopy in Focus.* **1**:1–12.

3 Nogueras JJ and Wexner SD (1992) Laparoscopic colon resection perspective. *Colon and Rectal Surg.* 5:79–97.

4 Verdeja, JC (1992) Laparoscopic – Assisted minimal access surgery of the colon. *Laparoscopy in Focus.* **1**:7–8.

5 Leahy P (1992) Laparoscopic left hemicolectomy. *Laparoscopy in Focus.* **1**: 6.

6 Olsen DO (1991) Laparoscopic appendectomy using a linear stapling device. *Surg Rounds.* p. 873–83.

7 Steichen FM (1968) The use of staplers in anatomical side-to-side and functional end-to-end enteroanastomoses. *Surgery.* **64**:948.

8 Steichen FM (1991) Changing concepts in surgical techniques, *Current Practice of Surgical Stapling* p. 23–37, Ravitch, Steichen, Welter Ed., Lea and Febiger, Philadelphia Publ.

9 Köcherling F and Gastinger J (1992) 'Laparosckopische klammernahttechnik in der colorektalen chirurgie.' *Paper presented at the 2nd German Symposium on Stapling Würzburg, May 25.*

10 Azagra JS, Goergen M, Ceoterick M (1994). The triple-stapled technique: further progress in colorectal anastomosis. *Minimally Invasive Surgery and New Technology.* 456–63.

14

Philosophical Considerations in Laparoscopic Coloproctology

L PETER FIELDING

Introduction

Minimal access (laparoscopic) surgery is a controversial subject. It has been widely adopted without being subject to our current norms for academic development and regulatory processes, and it raises important professional, ethical and fiscal issues.

The medical profession is currently being accused of self-interest in areas of research and development where there may be conflicts of interest because of possible financial returns and/or opportunities for professional advancement. It has therefore become essential for the profession to set standards which will protect the general good while not stultifying innovation or development. This places a substantial responsibility on those who advocate the new techniques to respond to these questions and to provide reliable information upon which to base the discussion.

History

In 1878 Thomas Alva Edison began work on an electric lamp and sought a material that could be electrically heated to incandescence in a vacuum. He is credited with having produced the first electric light bulb in October 1879[1]. During the last hundred years much progress has been made to increase the strength of the light source while at the same time diminishing the heat generated by the process. Thus today we have a developed but traditional light source, with the high-intensity halogen lamps, as well as coherent light emerging from lasers[2].

To transmit light without the use of mirrors (which is very cumbersome), a coated fine-glass fibre that could be constructed into a flexible fiberoptic cable needed to be developed. This possibility was foreseen as far back as 1870 by

John Tindall, who demonstrated that light could be guided in a solid medium (light glass)[1].

The next major step in the development of laparoscopic technology was to replace the human eye with a miniature television camera at the eyepiece of the endoscope. The prototypes weighed 3600 g and produced a black-and-white image[3]. However its was the invention of the electronic chip in 1958[4] that paved the way for real miniaturization of and the ability to produce a color image.

The placement of trocars into the abdomen for investigation and some simple treatments has been widely accepted, particularly by gynecologists, over the last 20 years. However, it was the miniaturization of the color television camera which made it possible for the surgeon to lift the head away from the operative field and proceed to bimanual manipulation of instruments placed through two or more ports into the abdominal cavity.

Over the last five years, the equipment which can be placed through these different sized ports has developed at a remarkable rate. However, all these innovations have been directed towards specific mechanical problems which derive from the basic premise of television-controlled remote surgery.

Thus minimal access surgery has evolved from many different areas of science and technology (light sources, television, micro-printed circuits and surgical instruments) which have been brought together to advance the well established technique of investigative laparoscopy.

Ethical issues

The multifactorial origins of minimal access surgery raise the philosophical question of how we should view the deployment of these techniques in the clinical setting. Some would say that these developments, although quite dramatic, are a natural progression of existing ideas and technologies and need no specific thought with regard to training or credentialling of surgeons. Others view these methods as experimental and support the establishment of an institutional review board or ethics committee, which would strictly limit these technologies to the principal investigators and their research associates.

There are those who suggest that all surgeons are intrinsically reliable and always function in the patient's best interest and recommend a 'laissez faire' approach to controls. There are others who talk about academic precision and support tight restrictions. However, this approach may be motivated by an exclusive attitude which attempts to keep clinically competent non-academic surgeons out of this rapidly evolving field.

Clearly these innovations are intended to benefit the patients, and therefore we must consider what is in the public interest. We must also recognize that although the benefits and risks are describable by the physician, they are in fact borne by the individual patient undergoing the procedure. Consequently the responsibility is on the physician not only to provide proper information about efficacy and risk, but also to be accountable for the recommendations. Such accountability mandates the use of full documentation and analysis of all results.

Much of the advice that physicians provide comes from a knowledge of empirically identified conventional treatment methods, linked to and modified by additional factors such as patient age and the presence of co-morbid conditions. Even so, we can never be absolutely certain about outcome even for well characterized conditions. For example, given the diagnosis of acute appendicitis in a 25-year-old man, the likelihood of a complete and uneventful recovery is high: maybe greater than 90%. However, there are morbidity risks of 5–10%, and a finite (although small) risk of death (0.1–0.5%). In other conditions (eg adjuvant chemotherapy for breast or colon cancer), the probability of a beneficial outcome is less certain, with an increased risk of mortality and morbidity. These uncertainties make the prediction of outcome difficult.

Randomization

Since the first randomized controlled trial in medicine 45 years ago, (investigating the role of streptomycin in the management of open tuberculosis[5]), there has been an increasing reliance on the information derived from randomized controlled trials to provide the data upon which to base our clinical opinions and advice.

The main purpose of randomization is to allow for the distribution of biases so that a relatively small patient subset of the at-risk population may provide reliable information concerning the efficacy (and, to a lesser extent, the complication rates) of new treatments when compared with conventional methods. They work best when:

- the 'event rate' is high (eg the death rate from open tuberculosis in the pre-antibiotic era)
- the treatment under test is strongly efficacious when compared with conventional therapy
- the study can be double-blinded so that neither the patient nor the treating physician is aware of which treatment is being given.

All these criteria were present in the Medical Research Council's tuberculosis study; after only 100 patients had been studied, there was a clear and definitive outcome which was obviously in favor of the use of streptomycin.

There have been many useful randomized controlled trials in medicine during the last 45 years. However, as we move away from the ideal circumstances for a randomized controlled trial, the difficulty of mounting such studies increases and the usefulness of the method diminishes.

In this discussion, we must recognize that minimal access surgery is likely to replace conventional surgery in many cases, because of the benefits of shorter hospital stays, lower mortality and morbidity, and shorter postoperative recovery times. Thus the essential comparison between conventional methods and minimal access surgery is not in terms of comparative efficacy, but the possible differences in the comparative risks involved with these two methods. Because the known risks from conventional surgery are small, and the likely risks from minimal access surgery are also likely to remain numerically small (even though they may represent a several-fold difference from those in conventional therapy), it is difficult to construct studies to determine such differences. This means that there is a methodological problem to distinguish between these low event rates.

In addition to these low event rates and small risk differences, it is not possible to conduct surgical treatments on a single or double-blind basis. Both the patient and the surgeon must know from the outset the nature of the treatment being provided, thus making it impossible in this setting to distribute the associated biases inevitable with unblinded studies.

The 'coup de grâce' for the randomized controlled trial in this setting is the inevitable presence of surgeon-related variability[6], particularly in a phase of development of new operative techniques. The surgeon who is learning a new method is not, by definition, in a state of equipoise with regard to possible participation in a randomized controlled trial.

However, it is quite clear that society wants and indeed expects the medical profession to be interested in and committed to the identification of improved methods to treat disease. This is a basic mandate from which all medical development is derived. How then can we fulfill our responsibilities to both the medical profession and to society at large?

First, patients should be informed of the developmental nature of a procedure. Second, the surgeons should openly declare where they are on the learning curve of their own skill acquisition when additional skills are needed for a particular surgical intervention. Third, there should be an absolute requirement for reporting all cases in which these new methods are attempted (whether or not surgery was completed by the new methods or not). From such a registry, the early and late outcomes (both positive and negative) can be reported from the appropriate databases.

The Connecticut registry

The Connecticut state-wide cholecystectomy registry has documented the transition from mostly 'open' to mostly 'minimal access' surgical cholecystectomy[7]. The data in this preliminary report involves 4500 patients with the principal findings being for comparable mix of patients. The overall short-term (postoperative) death and complication rates were similar for the 'open' and 'laparoscopic' methods, including the rates of injury to common bile duct. However, when the data were analyzed by individual physicians, the rate of common bile duct injury was highest in the first 10 cases, and the overall complication rate gradually fell over the first 40–50 cases (from approximately 6% to 4%).

Not only has this Connecticut registry provided clinical data for professional evaluation, it also has served to provide society in general with ethically required accountability. As a phase II (observational) study, the Connecticut laparoscopic-cholecystectomy registry accomplishes a very important additional goal. The data show that there are no grounds upon which to generate hypotheses to be tested in a randomized trial format. In other words, a phase III (randomized controlled trial) is unnecessary to investigate the mortality and morbidity rates associated with laparoscopic versus open cholecystectomy.

This outcome has been achieved by a relatively straightforward process of data gathering, without the costs and complexity of a randomized controlled trial, and is an important outcome supporting the need for mandated registries for all patients undergoing minimal access surgery.

Surgeon credentialing

Having made the case for the evaluation of minimal access surgery by the development of phase II documentation studies, involving increasing numbers of surgeons in the context of a report registry, the guidelines for hospital credentialing of these new methods require discussion and agreement.

If it is accepted that the two ends of the spectrum for surgeon credentialing for minimal access surgery ('laissez faire' and 'restrictive practice') are both unacceptable, we need to define a middle ground which will serve the public interest and set a framework for the responsible acquisition of new skills.

The document generated by the Society of American Gastrointestinal Endoscopic Surgeons (SAGES) concerning the principles for credentialing physicians is well developed, and parts of it are quoted below[8–11]. (J Sackier, personal communication).

PREAMBLE

The Society of American Gastrointestinal Endoscopic Surgeons recommends the following guidelines for credentialing qualified surgeons in the performance of general surgical procedures utilizing laparoscopy (cholecystectomy, appendectomy, hernia repair and other similar procedures). The basic premise is that the surgeon must have the judgement, training and the capability of immediately proceeding to a traditional open abdominal procedure when circumstances so indicate.

DETERMINATION OF COMPETENCE IN LAPAROSCOPIC SURGERY

1. Completion of a surgical residency/fellowship program which incorporates structured experience in laparoscopic surgery. The applicant's Program Director or laparoscopic training director should confirm in writing the training, experience and actual observed level of competency as is done for other procedures in general surgery.
2. Proficiency in laparoscopic surgical procedures and clinical judgement equivalent to that obtained in a residency/fellowship program. Documentation and demonstration of competence is necessary with verification in writing from experienced colleagues.
3. For those without residency training or fellowship which included laparoscopic surgery or without documented prior experience in laparoscopic surgery, the process should be similar to a residency experience including didactics, hands-on animal experience, participation as a first assistant and performance of the operation under proctorship. The basic minimum requirements for training should be:
   a. completion of approved residency training in general surgery, with credentialing in the comparable open procedure for which laparoscopic privileges are being sought,

b. credentialing in diagnostic laparoscopy,
c. training in laparoscopic general surgery by a surgeon experienced in laparoscopic surgery or completion of a university sponsored or academic society recognized didactic course which should include instruction in handling and use of laparoscopic instrumentation, principles of safe trocar insertion and establishment of safe peritoneal access, laparoscopic tissue handling, knot tying, and equipment utilization (e.g. staplers) as well as animal experience in specific categories of procedures for which applicant desires credentialing. Attendance at short courses which do not provide supervised hands-on training and without documentation of proficiency is not an acceptable substitute,
d. experience as first assistant in patients in the category of the laparoscopic procedure for which privileges are being sought with a previously privileged individual in or outside one's community, documentation to be provided by the privileged individual,
e. proctoring by a laparoscopic surgeon experienced in the same or similar procedure(s) until proficiency has been observed and documented in writing.

MONITORING OF LAPAROSCOPIC PERFORMANCE

To assist the hospital credentialing body in the ongoing renewal of privileges there should be a mechanism of monitoring each surgical laparoscopist's procedural performance. This should be done through existing quality assurance mechanisms in the institution. This should include monitoring utilization, diagnostic and therapeutic benefits to patients, complications and tissue review in accordance with previously developed criteria.

CONTINUING EDUCATION

Continuing medical education related to laparoscopic surgery should be required as part of the periodic renewal of privileges. Attendance at appropriate local or national meetings and courses in encouraged.

RENEWAL OF PRIVILEGES

For the renewal of privileges an appropriate level of continuing clinical activity should be required, in addition to satisfactory performance as assessed by monitoring of procedural activity through existing quality assurance mechanisms as well as continuing medical education relating to laparoscopic surgery.

In summary, then, credentialing should be for surgeons already experienced in 'open' operative technique, and include provisions for:

- didactic courses
- dry laboratory experience of instrumentation
- animal laboratory experience with the procedures
- proctored clinical experience.

For the resident in training, a new segment of the general surgery residency training program should be developed to integrate these training features as a specific focus of resident activity[12].

Future developments

By the time we reach the turn of the century and the millennium, I believe that minimal access surgery will still be in a state of development. The constellation of technical developments, which have provided us with this new way of looking at and doing surgery, are as potent a source of continuing development as the introduction of anesthesia or antisepsis. I suggest that is will be some 20–30 years before its rate of exploitation and development begin to level off. If this prediction is anywhere near the mark, the future will see the introduction of:

- flexible lighted endoscopes
- high-definition television
- three-dimensional images
- advances in endoscopically controlled imaging of tissues and organs
- photochemotherapy for tumor treatments.

Furthermore, it is now possible to have multimedia medical communications for consultative purposes, links between such systems for remote robotic-assisted surgery are all possible. Such systems would, at least in theory, be able to bring a high-quality decision-making process to the patient's bedside on a worldwide basis and even be able to transmit the operative technical expertise to go along with it. These are intriguing and stimulating possibilities.

The way we train surgeons (and others) in dexterity skill development will move to the simulation laboratory, as 'virtual reality' computation systems emerge. This type of training should start in the medical schools to identify those students with particular interest and aptitude.

In addition it is to be hoped that the surgical academic colleges around the world will become active participants in these rapid changes. The importance of these technical developments will go far beyond the confines of the particular operative technique, and it will become increasingly necessary to use the complex and expensive equipment in a more time-effective and cost-efficient manner than currently occurs, to reduce reduplication of services and equipment.

None of us should forget that the rock upon which all medical transactions take place is the doctor/patient relationship. No amount of political or administrative polemic can or should change this fact; it is the basis of our mandate to treat the sick and relieve suffering.

Therefore we must remember, during these heady days of rapid technical advances, that we are doing all of this because of our primary responsibility to patient care. As we introduce these new methods, the need for open and direct discussion—including an acceptance of our limited knowledge and our ignorance—must be made clear. If we follow this approach of openness, then discussions with out patients will be ethically based and general benefit can result.

References

1 Bernstein J (1984) Three degrees above zero. In: *Bell Labs in Information Age*. Charles Scribner's Sons, New York. p. 155.

2 Maiman TH (1960) Stimulated optical radiation in ruby. *Nature*. **178**:493–4.

3 Berci G and Davids J (1962) Endoscopy and television. *Br Med J*. **xx**:1610–13.

4 Reid TR (1958) *The chip. How two Americans invented the microchip*. Simon & Shuster, New York.

5 Medical Research Council (1948) Streptomycin treatment of pulmonary tuberculosis. *Br Med J*. **ii**:769–82.

6 Fielding LP, Stewart-Brown S and Dudley HA (1978) Surgeon-related variables and the clinical trial. *Lancet*. **ii**:778–9.

7 Fritts LL and Orlando R III (1993) Laparoscopic appendectomy: A safety and cost analysis. *Am J Surg*. **128**:521–4.

8 SAGES (1991) Granting of privileges for laparoscopic general surgery. *Am J Surg*. **161**:324–5.

9 Dent TL (1991) Clinical privileges for laparoscopic general surgery. *Am J Surg*. **161**:399–403.

10 Greene FL (1991) Training, credentialling and privileging for minimally invasive surgery. *Problems in Gen Surg*. **8**:502–6.

11 New York State Department of Health Memorandum – Series 92–20, (1992) *Laparoscopic surgery*. Albany, New York.

12 Ballantyne GH, Pastena JA and Fielding LP (1993) '*Implementation of an advanced laparoscopic surgery curriculum for surgical residents.*' *Paper presented at the Association of Program Directors in Surgery meeting in Dallas, Texas, February 27.*

Index

Since the major subject of this book is laparoscopic surgery, few entries are listed under this keyword. Readers are advised to seek more specific references.